Health and Wellness

Health and Wellness

Honoring God in Body, Mind, and Spirit

by Robert T. Harper, General Editor

Triangle Publishing
Marion, Indiana

Health and Wellness: Honoring God in Body, Mind, and Spirit
by Robert Harper, General Editor

Direct correspondence and permission requests to one of the following:

Triangle Publishing
Indiana Wesleyan University
4301 South Washington Street
Marion, Indiana 46953

Web site: www.trianglepublishing.com
E-mail: info@trianglepublishing.com

Harper, Robert, General Editor

ISBN: 1-931283-04-4

Cover design: Susan Spiegel
Graphic design: Lyn Rayn

Printed in the United States of America
Evangel Press, Nappanee, Indiana

CONTRIBUTORS

Debra Drake, M.S., has been involved with nursing education for the past twenty-five years. Her nursing career has developed in a variety of settings, with obstetrics and community health as her primary areas of concentration. She has a bachelor's degree in nursing and a master's degree in nursing administration and management. She is currently serving as an assistant professor at Indiana Wesleyan University in the RN-BS program. A certified childbirth educator, Debra has completed a special education program for parish nurses and has served on several short-term mission trips.

Robert T. Harper, Ed.D., has focused on the area of personal development in the field of education. His educational background includes a master's degree in counseling and a doctorate in adult education, with a cognate in wellness management. He served for ten years as the Director of Counseling at the University of Southern Indiana. Currently, he is an associate professor for Indiana Wesleyan University, teaching graduate courses in motivation and change, as well as undergraduate courses in wellness, psychology, and career development. He is a nationally certified counselor (NCC) and a community speaker on topics of stress management, maintaining positive attitudes, and career satisfaction. Dr. Harper is the general editor of *Health and Wellness: Honoring God in Body, Mind, and Spirit.*

Lisa Larkin, M.S., has been active in the field of nursing for the past twenty-eight years as an educator, consultant, and health care provider. She currently serves as the Director of Health and Wellness Services for Marian College. Previously, she was the Director of Fitness and Wellness at DePauw University. She has a bachelor's degree in nursing and master's degrees in both nursing and health promotion. Lisa is certified through the American Nurses Credentialing Center as a college health nurse and clinical specialist, and as a family nurse practitioner.

J. Michael Manning, M.S., currently serves as the Director of Faculty Recruitment for the College of Adult and Graduate Studies at Indiana Wesleyan University. He also serves as an adjunct faculty member in the area of wellness. His master's degree is in physical education, with an emphasis in exercise science. He also has completed an internship in cardiac rehabilitation. He has coached youth and college students in track and cross-country events, and has trained adults for local road races.

Brenda K. Woods, M.D., received a bachelor of science degree in biology and psychology from Indiana Wesleyan University. She obtained a doctor of medicine degree from Indiana University School of Medicine, where she also completed her OB/Gyn internship and residency training program in family medicine. She is certified by the American Board of Family Practice and is currently in private practice in Arizona. Previously, she served five years as the Director of Primary Care Medicine at Remuda Ranch Center for Anorexia and Bulimia in Arizona.

Table of Contents

Acknowledgments

First and foremost, we would like to thank God, who directed our efforts and gave us the wisdom and the patience to complete *Health and Wellness: Honoring God in Body, Mind, and Spirit*. He knew what this textbook needed and how best to accomplish His purpose through our efforts.

A very special thanks to all of our family members without whose love, support, and encouragement this project would not have been possible. From Bob Harper, thanks to my wife Kimberly, daughter Holly, and son Todd Helfert. From Debra Drake, thanks to my husband Tom, son and daughter-in-law James and Tonya Drake, and daughter and son-in-law Cindi and Brad Lacey. From Lisa Larkin, thanks to my husband Gregory Neil and son Gregory Nicholas. From Mike Manning, thanks to my wife Tracy, son Tobey, and daughters Eleana and Rachel Mae. From Brenda Woods, thanks to my husband David and our children, Nathaniel, Amy, Jessica, and Kenneth. Your presence in our lives makes this project all the more meaningful.

To Nathan Birky, publisher of Triangle Publishing, thank you for your excellent organizational skills in bringing all of the pieces together. We especially appreciate your ready availability in answering our questions and your encouragement during challenging times.

To Bobbie Sease, editor, we cannot thank you enough for your positive guidance, suggestions, and ideas. God gave Bobbie numerous talents—the greatest of which may be patience as she worked around our busy schedules and fine-tuned our first drafts. We also would like to thank Lyn Rayn for her creative graphic design of the text, Susan Spiegel for designing the book cover, and Aimee Williams for proofreading the final manuscript.

Finally, we want to thank our patients, clients, and students over the years, who themselves have been valued teachers.

Robert T. Harper
Debra Drake
Lisa Larkin
J. Michael Manning
Brenda K. Woods

INTRODUCTION

"The health of the people is really the foundation upon which all their happiness and all their powers as a state depend."

—Benjamin Disraeli[1]

Wellness: What Is It?

Wellness. We hear this term tossed around a lot today, but what does it really mean? More specifically, what does it mean to you personally? **Wellness** as it is discussed in this textbook is a combination of *physical* well-being, *emotional* well-being, and *spiritual* well-being. The many daily choices and decisions that we make fall within the parameters of these three general areas.

We make dozens of choices every day. Each choice influences our individual well-being, resulting in benefits (positive) or consequences (negative). A primary goal of the wellness lifestyle is to help people make choices that not only will help

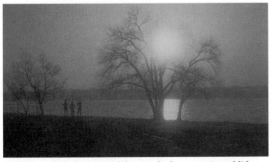

Will the quality of your life match the quantity of life you have the potential to live?

them *live longer*, but, more importantly, will allow them to *enjoy living* that longer life. In his book, *Reversing Heart Disease*, Dr. Dean Ornish reports that

what a modern medical system can provide is much less important to individual health and well-being than the lifestyle choices we make throughout each day.[2] To put it another way, the *quality* of your life and the fulfillment it provides are just as important as the *quantity* of years you live. In addition to enhancing your own well-being, positive wellness decisions also can allow you to participate more fully in the lives of those around you.

> **WELLNESS:** A combination of physical well-being, emotional well-being, and spiritual well-being.

▓ Knowing and Doing

At the college level, you will find many of the courses in which you have enrolled to be somewhat difficult. The topic of wellness can be difficult as well, but for different reasons than you might think. Many of the foundational principles of wellness are common knowledge to most of the population of the United States. Beginning as early as grade school, various courses present some of the major concepts of wellness in general ways; e.g., the need for exercise, good nutrition, and healthy social interactions.

However, many times these courses fall short in realistically explaining how to apply general principles to everyday life, making your study and practice of wellness today that much more difficult. Your personal well-being doesn't involve just knowledge about wellness. It is related directly to how well you apply this knowledge in your daily activities and choices. Personal well-being is a combination of what you know and what

> The *quality* of your life and the fulfillment it provides are just as important as the *quantity* of years you live.

you do—with the emphasis on the *doing*, the daily choices you make and the actions you take. It is not so much what you know as it is what you do with that information that really matters. How does that information direct the decisions you make?

Consider how often you or others around you know the right ("well") thing to do, but instead choose the wrong ("unwell") course of action. Knowledge directs you to make a healthy lifestyle choice, but you choose otherwise. This may be due to habit, lack of planning, and/or fear of commitment. Sometimes it is just easier to remain with long-standing, comfortable habits that fail to provide positive outcomes for your personal well-being. It is even quite common for many to hold on tightly to long-standing habits with proven negative consequences. To illustrate, consider these "unwell" choices as they relate to the three areas of well-being:

- *Physical well-being*
  Many smokers know that smoking is not good for their health, but they continue to smoke anyway.
- *Emotional well-being*
  It is commonly accepted that a positive outlook on life can help to make a day more enjoyable. However, it is easy to slip into negative thinking, focusing on failure, flaws, and worst-case scenarios.
- *Spiritual well-being*
  Many people turn to prayer in times of stress or trauma, but fewer give thanks to God for the abundance of His daily blessings.

As is readily apparent, how we act does not always match what we know—and *even take for granted*—as necessary for personal well-being. So, how do we motivate ourselves to change? One change theory states that change will occur only when the pain of remaining the same is greater than the pain of changing. The wellness perspective, however, looks at the positive, proactive side of change. It is our hope to encourage you to commit to change before you ever have to experience that level of pain in your physical, emotional, and/or spiritual dimensions.

As you read this text and participate in its assessments and learning exercises, please consider not only what you *know* about wellness, but also what you are currently *doing* to support your personal well-being. Most important, begin to target what changes you want to make. Then, consider what goals and action steps will help you to realize those changes and motivate you to better develop your personal well-being. These decisions and actions are up to you. Nobody else can "do wellness" for you. Wellness necessitates choices, decisions, and personal responsibility.

The Importance of Wellness

Why is wellness important? How will developing a proactive wellness lifestyle benefit you?

Table 1. Leading Causes of Death in the United States in 2000

Rank	Cause of Death	Number of Deaths	Percent of Total Deaths
1.	Heart Disease	710,760	29.6
2.	Cancer	553,091	23.0
3.	Stroke	167,661	7.0
4.	Chronic Lower Respiratory Disease	122,009	5.1
5.	Unintentional Accidents	97,900	4.1
6.	Diabetes mellitus	69,301	2.9
7.	Pneumonia/Influenza	65,313	2.7
8.	Alzheimer's Disease	49,588	2.1
9.	Nephritis—Kidney Disease	37,251	1.5
10.	Septicemia	31,224	1.3

Source: National Center for Health Statistics, 2000. *National Vital Statistics Report,* Vol. 50, No. 15. U.S. Department of Health and Human Services, Centers for Disease Control and Prevention.

To demonstrate how lifestyle influences health and wellness, compare the following lifestyle factors as they relate to causes of death:

1. **High Levels of Stress**
   - Heart Disease
   - Cancer
   - Unintentional Injuries
   - Suicide
   - Stroke
   - Respiratory Disease
   - Pneumonia

2. **Poor Nutrition**
   - Heart Disease
   - Cancer
   - Stroke
   - Diabetes mellitus
   - Nephritis

3. **Little Physical Activity**
   - Heart Disease
   - Cancer
   - Stroke
   - Diabetes mellitus

4. **Tobacco Usage**
   - Heart Disease
   - Cancer

5. **Alcohol Abuse**
   - Heart Disease
   - Cancer
   - Unintentional Accidents
   - Suicide
   - Nephritis

6. **Positive Emotional Outlook**
   - Can direct in positive and proactive ways the avoidance of risk factors for disease.

7. **Positive Spiritual Wellness**
   - Can direct in positive ways the outlook and attitudes necessary to address daily decisions that influence personal well-being.

It is clearly evident that lifestyle choices are relevant factors in the causes of death. This has obvious implications to those seeking a wellness lifestyle. The choices we make every day are directly related to the probability that one or more of these conditions will affect us.

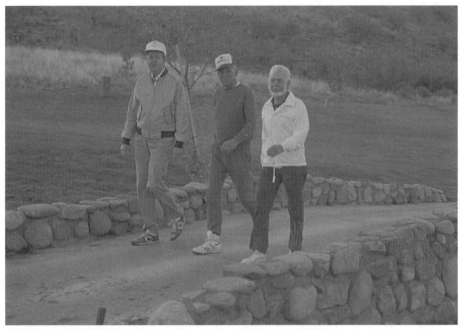

Wellness necessitates choices, decisions, and personal responsibility.

■ Disease and the Quality of Life

At the beginning of the twentieth century, infectious diseases were the primary causes of premature death. **Infectious disease** is defined as any disease or sickness that is caused by exposure to bacteria, viruses, or other microorganisms. Modern medical science has developed treatment methods essentially to eliminate infectious diseases as the primary cause of premature death. The diseases of the twenty-first century responsible for premature death include lifestyle-related chronic diseases and conditions. **Lifestyle disease** is defined as any disease or illness influenced by lifestyle habits and choices. These choices may include tobacco use, unhealthy diet, lack of physical activity, and/or drug use and abuse.

> **INFECTIOUS DISEASE:** Any disease or sickness caused by exposure to bacteria, viruses, or other microorganisms.

The seriousness of these chronic diseases and the influence they have on American quality of life is of concern to the Centers for Disease Control and Prevention, United States Department of Health and Human Services.

The following information comes from its on-line report of February 14, 2002, "Health-Related Quality of Life":[3]

- Americans report they feel unhealthy (physically or mentally) about five days per month.
- Americans say they feel "healthy and full of energy" about nineteen days per month.
- Nearly one-third of Americans say they suffer from some mental or emotional problem every month—including 9 percent who reported their mental health was not good for fourteen or more days a month.
- Americans with chronic diseases or disabilities reported higher levels of unhealthy days.

These are alarming findings. Americans today live almost twice as long as they did at the beginning of the twentieth century. However, as you evaluate your individual well-being and wellness, ask yourself this question: Will the *quality* of your life match the *quantity* of life you have the potential to live?

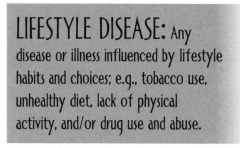

LIFESTYLE DISEASE: Any disease or illness influenced by lifestyle habits and choices; e.g., tobacco use, unhealthy diet, lack of physical activity, and/or drug use and abuse.

To repeat, the motivation for change involves choices, decisions, and personal responsibility. Information such as these statistics on quality of life and the behaviors and choices related to their prevalence can fuel the desire for change. Becoming informed is key to motivating change and establishing goals and action steps. It is also the primary reason for this book: to offer informational building blocks with which you can evaluate and adjust your personal wellness.

The Components of Wellness

At the beginning of this chapter, wellness is defined as a combination of *physical* well-being, *emotional* well-being, and *spiritual* well-being. These three general areas—body, mind, and spirit—can be further divided into six components, as illustrated in **Figure 1, The Wellness Model**:

- Physical Wellness
- Intellectual Wellness
- Emotional Wellness
- Spiritual Wellness
- Social Wellness
- Occupational Wellness

PHYSICAL WELLNESS:
Involves the activities, attitudes, and behaviors that focus on the positive development and maintenance of one's physical body.

This text is structured around the Wellness Model, with individual chapters detailing the concerns and related issues of each component. A brief overview will give you a clearer understanding of what is involved in each of these components.

■ Physical Wellness

Physical wellness involves the activities, attitudes, and behaviors that focus on the positive development and maintenance of one's physical body.

Figure 1. The Wellness Model

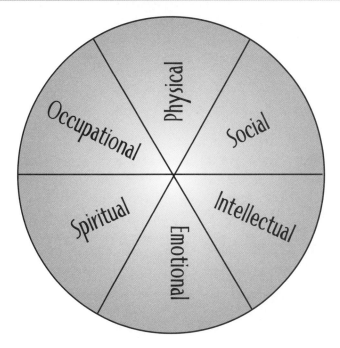

God has given you only one physical body for your time on this earth. How well do you care for your physical body? Looking through the lens of body-mind-spirit, you will see sample behaviors and attitudes that can have a positive effect on physical wellness:

Physical
- Consistently participating in physical activity
- Practicing good basic nutrition
- Getting adequate sleep
- Planning for adequate relaxation time

Emotional
- Keeping an open mind and a positive attitude regarding participation in physical activities
- Believing you are capable of achieving positive results through those activities

Spiritual
"Haven't you yet learned that your body is the home of the Holy Spirit God gave you, and that He lives within you? Your own body does not belong to you. For God has bought you with a great price. So use every part of your body to give glory back to God, because He owns it."

1 Corinthians 6:19-20

■ Intellectual Wellness

Intellectual wellness involves the activities, attitudes, and behaviors that direct the positive development and maintenance of one's mind and mental abilities.

INTELLECTUAL WELLNESS: Involves the activities, attitudes, and behaviors that direct the positive development and maintenance of one's mind and mental abilities.

The mind God has given you has tremendous potential. It is commonly reported that only a small portion of the human mind's vast potential is ever utilized. How well are you currently developing that potential? These sample behaviors can positively influence intellectual wellness:

Physical

- Developing a time management plan
- Spending more time reading
- Watching less television

Emotional

- Being open to new ideas
- Having a positive attitude about pursuing programs or classes for personal and professional growth

Spiritual

"Teach us to number our days and recognize how few they are; help us to spend them as we should."

Psalm 90:12

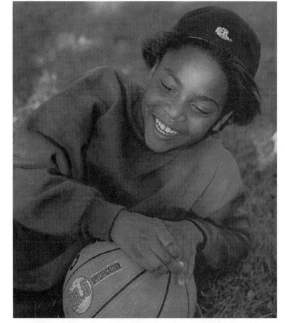

An emotionally well person strives to maintain a positive emotional outlook.

■ Emotional Wellness

Emotional wellness involves the thoughts and behaviors that help to foster awareness of personal feelings and emotions, as well as the feelings and emotions of others. An emotionally well person strives to maintain a positive emotional outlook.

> **EMOTIONAL WELLNESS:**
> Involves the thoughts and behaviors that foster awareness of personal feelings and emotions, as well as the feelings and emotions of others.

The thoughts and attitudes you choose and develop provide the guidance system for your personal behaviors. You can choose to find either positives or negatives in any person you meet or in any situation you encounter. How positive or negative is your daily outlook? These are examples of positive emotional outlooks:

Physical
- Practicing daily stress management activities
- Establishing and writing out positive personal goals

Emotional
- Developing acceptance of self and acceptance of others
- Maintaining a positive attitude

Spiritual
"Now your attitudes and thoughts must all be constantly changing for the better."

Ephesians 4:23

■ Spiritual Wellness

Spiritual wellness involves the thoughts, actions, behaviors, and values that provide a personal connectedness to God and a source of positive meaning and purpose for life.

> **SPIRITUAL WELLNESS:**
> Involves the thoughts, actions, behaviors, and values that provide a personal connectedness to God and a source of positive meaning and purpose for life.

Faith is foundational to well-being. Its presence or absence is reflected in our thoughts, words, and actions. What is the foundation that gives meaning and purpose to your life? How strong is that foundation? These sample thoughts, actions, and values can influence spiritual wellness:

Physical
- Spending time each day in prayer
- Attending a church of your choice
- Modeling personal values through your daily actions and contacts

Emotional
- Developing a personal awareness of your values
- Establishing a personal relationship with Jesus Christ

Spiritual

"Bodily exercise is all right, but spiritual exercise is much more important and is a tonic for all you do. So exercise yourself spiritually and practice being a better Christian, because that will help you not only now in this life, but in the next life too."

1 Timothy 4:8-9

Social Wellness

Social wellness involves actions, attitudes, and behaviors that facilitate the desire to communicate with others every day.

Much of your waking time each day is spent interacting and communicating with other people. Are you communicating in ways that edify people and honor God? These sample thoughts and behaviors can influence social wellness:

> **SOCIAL WELLNESS:**
> Involves actions, attitudes, and behaviors that facilitate the desire to communicate with others every day.

Physical
- Seeking out and maintaining satisfying relationships
- Modeling a spirit of kindness and support for others
- Being involved in community activities

Emotional
- Valuing time and positive communication with your family
- Being open to ways you can serve and encourage others

Spiritual
"And whatever you do, do it with kindness and love."

1 Corinthians 16:14

Occupational Wellness

Occupational wellness involves the actions, attitudes, and behaviors that support a sense of satisfaction and purpose in one's work activities and/or career goals.

How satisfied are you with your current career and your career goals for the future? These outlooks and actions can influence occupational wellness:

OCCUPATIONAL WELLNESS:

Involves the actions, attitudes, and behaviors that support a sense of satisfaction and purpose in one's work activities and/or career goals.

Physical
- Developing skills for current job enhancement and future growth
- Establishing and pursuing short- and long-term career goals

Emotional
- Building an awareness of purpose and job satisfaction, leading to the sense that you are making a difference
- Being aware of your God-given personal skills and abilities and how best to apply those gifts

Spiritual

"O Lord, I know it is not within the power of man to map his life and plan his course—so you correct me, Lord."

Jeremiah 10:23

Briefly outlined here, these six components will appear again and again in this text. They are mentioned consistently in wellness literature as foundational to personal wellness. They also are used consistently to develop various definitions of wellness. The primary focus of this text is to present information related to personal growth, awareness, and change in these and related areas of personal wellness.

Not a Vacuum

By now you are coming to the realization that wellness covers and relates to every aspect of your life. Pivotal to understanding wellness is recognizing that each of these areas of your life can and usually will influence all other areas of your personal well-being. That influence can be positive or negative, depending upon the decisions you make and the outlooks you develop.

For example, if you are experiencing stress at work, the negative consequences of this stress can influence the quality of your relationships at home. Your children may avoid you, "laying low" until you come out from under that dark cloud of pressure you've dragged home from work. Stress also can affect other relationships or contacts not related to your work or home environment. You might take out your frustrations by snapping at a store clerk. Unless you properly address these work problems or appropriately release your stress, you will find it nearly impossible to leave those problems behind at the end of your workday. They will follow you wherever you go, influencing other areas of your life.

> No component of wellness operates in a vacuum.

Problems and stress at work also may influence your physical well-being by disturbing your sleep. Lack of sleep can lead to fatigue. Fatigue may affect the quality of your work, causing you to lose your focus. This, in turn, causes more worry, which leads to even more sleeplessness, all of which reflects a downward spiral of stress and its negative impact on every area of your life. The same cycle operates if we reverse the situation. If you have problems at home, often it is very difficult to concentrate while at work.

It is important to remember that no component of wellness operates in a vacuum. All components of your life can and do influence all other areas of your life, contributing to or detracting from your overall wellness.

In evaluating your present wellness choices and decisions, ask yourself two questions before you start chapter 1:

1. What am I currently doing to influence my personal wellness, either in a positive way or a negative way?
2. What future steps can I take to influence my wellness in positive ways?

As we address these questions and related issues in this text, we will incorporate a Christian perspective of wellness and its related concepts. We encourage you to read this text with an application outlook in mind. Many chapters include self-evaluation or assessment questions and learning activities to help you move toward your goals. Look for topics or discussions in the coming chapters that are personally relevant to you at this point in your life. Then decide what concepts are applicable to your personal goals and actions toward an increased level of personal wellness.

KEY CONCEPTS

emotional wellness	infectious disease
intellectual wellness	lifestyle disease
occupational wellness	physical wellness
social wellness	spiritual wellness
wellness	

Personal Wellness Evaluation

Please rate your self-evaluated position in each of the six major wellness areas provided below. If necessary, review the discussion of that area in this chapter. Your goal in rating yourself is to develop a general personal goal in each area. As you continue your study of wellness, focus on gaining additional information regarding your goal or developing new goals in that area.

Physical:

1	2	3	4	5
Low		Average		High

Goal: _____

_____

_____

Intellectual/Educational:

1	2	3	4	5
Low		Average		High

Goal: _____

_____

_____

Emotional:

1	2	3	4	5
Low		Average		High

Goal: _____

_____

_____

Spiritual:

1	2	3	4	5
Low		Average		High

Goal: _____

_____

_____

Social:

1	2	3	4	5
Low		Average		High

Goal: _____

_____

_____

Occupational:

1	2	3	4	5
Low		Average		High

Goal: _____

_____

_____

Endnotes

1. As quoted in "American Medicine and Public Health: Key Issues," a speech given by Dr. Robert Graham at the Iowa Governors Conference on Public Health, June 2001. Archived by Center for Policy Studies in Family Practice and Primary Care; available at: www.aafppolicy.org.
2. Dr. Dean Ornish, *Reversing Heart Disease* (New York: Ballantine Books, 1990).
3. "Health-Related Quality of Life," in National Center for Chronic Disease Prevention and Health Promotion (United States Department of Health and Human Services, Centers for Disease Control and Prevention), updated 14 February 2002; available at: www.cdc.gov/hrquol/findings.

1

WELLNESS v. HEALTH

"Yesterday is gone. Tomorrow has not yet come.
We have only today. Let us begin."

—Mother Teresa[1]

The terms *health* and *wellness* often are used interchangeably. But do they really mean the same thing? If so, what do they have in common? If not, what sets them apart? What does each term mean and what are the implications for us?

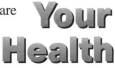

OBJECTIVES

- Recognize the differences between the concepts of *health* and *wellness*.

- Name concepts important to the implementation of personal wellness.

- Express an understanding of daily wellness activities.

The Wellness Continuum

Webster's Dictionary defines **health** as "the condition of being sound in body, mind, and spirit."[2] In the 1940s, the World Health Organization defined *health* as "the state of complete physical, mental, and social well-being, not merely the absence of disease."[3] These two definitions seem to embody the essence of the wellness model in the introduction of this text.

In common, day-to-day use, however,

HEALTH: The condition of being sound in body, mind, and spirit; not merely the absence of disease.

the term *health* most often refers to the current physical condition of one's body—especially as it exhibits either the presence or the absence of the symptoms of disease. Health can be seen as one of three elements in a wellness continuum (see Figure 1.1).

Figure 1.1, Wellness Continuum										
Illness					Health					Wellness
-5	-4	-3	-2	-1	0	+1	+2	+3	+4	+5

On the wellness continuum, health is positioned between illness and wellness. It doesn't fall into the negative side of illness, but doesn't occupy the positive side of wellness either.

■ A Matter of Chance

Health, as commonly viewed today, frequently involves a reactive mind-set. What this means is that we tend not to do anything about our physical, emotional, or spiritual well-being until something happens that negatively influences our health; e.g., an injury or the onset of an illness. Most of us take our health for granted. We blindly accept our abilities to function in our various roles and activities, or complacently resign ourselves to our limitations. If we think of our health at all, we have a vague hope of retaining a "healthy" feeling, but take little or no action to ensure that this feeling continues into the next day. We don't connect tomorrow's well-being with today's positive steps to attain and maintain optimum health. This outlook demonstrates a lack of personal responsibility, relegating health to the domain of chance.

■ A Matter of Balance

In contrast, wellness involves at least five more areas than just physical well-being (emotional, spiritual, social, intellectual, and occupational). Wellness hinges on the balance of body, mind, and spirit. This involves an ongoing awareness of how one functions in all these areas, questioning and evaluating everything as it relates to balance.

If health is reactive, then we can view wellness as proactive. Someone with a "health outlook" might say, "Have a nice day!" This reactive focus emphasizes the importance of external influences on the type of day the person experiences. Someone with a "wellness outlook" would say, "Make it a nice day!" This proactive focus emphasizes personal responsibility for the goals and outlooks the person establishes each day. Control for developing and maintaining a positive physical, mental, and spiritual foundation is in the hands of the individual. While external events and conditions can influence and even interfere with established goals for well-being, internal strengths and outlooks can help to cope with and adjust to any such events and barriers.

> Keep in mind two fundamental aspects of wellness:
> 1. Wellness involves focusing on the future, not looking back.
> 2. There is no perfect human representation of wellness.

In striving for wellness, it is important to establish growth goals for the future. Glance back briefly only to provide a foundation for positive future outlooks and actions. Looking back should never focus on unproductive guilt over past actions.

Also remember that you should strive to do your best, not to be perfect. The only perfect individual departed this earth two thousand years ago. Your purpose in striving for wellness is to learn from your efforts and proceed forward.

■ Attitudes and Actions: Well or Not Well?

Let's look at another continuum. This one includes sample attitudes and actions related to wellness or non-wellness.

Figure 1.2, Non-Wellness/Wellness Continuum

Non-Wellness	Wellness
Lack of commitment	Commitment to well-being
Activities out of balance	Balanced activities in life
No sense of fulfillment	Quality contacts in life
No goals for change	Positive goals for change
Quick-fix solutions	Positive long-term habits
No sense of life's choices	Awareness of life's choices

Where do you currently fall on the continuum? Are you closer to a proactive wellness outlook or to a reactive health outlook? If the latter, what steps can you take to move closer to the wellness position on the continuum?

Internalizing the Wellness Perspective

The introduction of this text introduces the six components of the Wellness Model. This chapter clarifies the concept of personal wellness by examining some important terms as they relate to personal wellness. Study this statement carefully:

> It is important to assume responsibility for the daily choices you make in life that influence personal well-being; to be aware of and plan for positive change in your life; to help create a physical, emotional, and spiritual balance that can add to the quality of your life and provide lifestyle habits to maintain a state of positive well-being.

The following section "diagrams" that statement into its elemental parts. As you examine these elements, evaluate how relevant these terms may be to your current understanding of wellness.

TAKE CARE

◼ Responsibility

*It is important to assume **responsibility** . . .*

To reiterate, wellness in one's life simply does not happen by chance. It takes the personal effort involved in assuming **responsibility** for personal well-being. No one can "do wellness" for anyone else. We are personally responsible for the daily decisions, attitudes, and actions that influence our well-being. This daily personal effort means breaking away from old established habits, initiating new actions and activities, and maintaining these activities and actions until they become new and more positive habits.

> **RESPONSIBILITY:** Personally making the daily decisions, attitudes, and actions that will influence well-being.

Responsibility involves more than personal care and well-being; we also are responsible for the care of those around us. Our words and actions not only influence our lives personally, but also those with whom we come in contact. We are an example to all those observing us. What we say and do has a rippling effect, influencing others directly or indirectly.

For example, a smoker may believe that smoking is a matter of personal choice affecting one's personal well-being only. But consider the smoker's influence on family members and/or friends. These individuals not only are exposed to potentially harmful secondhand or sidestream smoke themselves, but they may prematurely lose the family member or friend who smokes because of smoking's negative health consequences. It's worth repeating: Nothing you say or do occurs in a vacuum. You influence the lives of many people around you every day. You have a responsibility not only for your own well-being, but also for the well-being of those around you.

■ Choice

*It is important to assume **responsibility** for the daily **choices** you make in life that influence personal well-being . . .*

Everything in our lives involves *choice*. **Choice** means controlling how you respond to events and situations that involve your well-being. We cannot control all the events, situations, or experiences we encounter in life, but we can control how we respond to those events or situations. Often, we forget this and give control of our lives away to other people and/or to the external situations we encounter. To feel there is no choice or options in life can commonly lead to a sense of frustration and stress. We may begin to believe that life and its complex situations are out of our control.

> **CHOICE:** Controlling how you respond to events and situations that involve your well-being.

We can choose to look for the positives or the negatives in any daily encounter. While both negatives and positives usually can be found in any situation or person, for some reason the negative perspective is often the perspective of initial focus.

> We cannot control all the events, situations, or experiences we encounter in life, but we can control how we respond to those events or situations.

Which outlook is your primary initial focus: the positive opportunities that exist in a situation, or the negative problems that can also be present?

The awareness that both exist is an important step in moving toward personal wellness. By giving you free will, God has given you the ability to choose. He wants you to exercise that ability in ways that honor Him. He will open doors, direct your path, and help you take the necessary steps toward a life of wellness. However, in choosing which way to go, you also must choose which attitude will best propel you to your ultimate goals. Everything you encounter involves choice.

■ Change

*It is important to assume **responsibility** for the daily **choices** you make in life that influence personal well-being; to be aware of and plan for positive change in your life . . .*

CHANGE: Developing plans to modify and grow in the major areas of well-being and the roles and responsibilities of life.

We've often heard it said that we cannot expect our lives to change if we continue to do the very same things day in and day out. **Change** as it pertains to wellness means developing plans for positive change and growth in: (1) the major wellness areas of physical, emotional, and spiritual well-being, and (2) the important roles and responsibilities of our lives. This will involve establishing positive goals, attitudes, and action steps for the desired changes in our lives. Without clear goals, it is nearly impossible to develop a definition of success and then move in the direction of implementing that definition. Continually evaluating where we are and who we are in the *present* is foundational to helping us determine where we will be and who we will be in the *future*.

Change and a commitment to change involve personal motivation. We can define **motivation** as the intention or inner drive to accomplish something. The term "inner drive" seems appropriate as it pertains to wellness. It is important to develop personal internal motivators for the desired changes. External motivators for change or participation in a wellness activity—such as mandating participation, financially compensating participation, or providing support resources—often are not considered effective over the long-term because they do not address the core issues.

MOTIVATION: The intention or inner drive to accomplish something.

Internal motivation in pursuing wellness comes from understanding the positive results of participating in personally selected wellness activities. Focusing on internal motivation, such as the benefits you and those around you will receive, can help to overcome the barriers you may encounter as you progress in your wellness plan. An awareness that the actions and the steps you take may decrease the risk factors for premature death and disability, as well as increase the quality of your life, can provide a meaningful internal focus to help maintain your efforts. When your commitment to wellness activities falters, refocus on the reasons for your commitment and the benefits to your well-being. That focus can keep you on track toward your desired goals.

■ Balance

*It is important to assume **responsibility** for the daily **choices** you make in life that influence personal well-being; to be aware of and plan for positive **change** in your life; to help create a physical, emotional, and spiritual **balance** . . .*

Sometimes life seems like a juggling act! Each day we juggle family commitments, work responsibilities, school assignments, church activities, civic duties, time for self—the list goes on and on. Wellness involves balancing actions, attitudes, and outlooks as they relate to you physically, emotionally, and spiritually. **Balance** does not mean an extreme commitment to one of these areas to

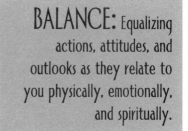

BALANCE: Equalizing actions, attitudes, and outlooks as they relate to you physically, emotionally, and spiritually.

the exclusion of the other two. Keep in mind that the ideal of perfect balance is an ideal only—there is no such thing as perfect balance. Wellness simply means striving for balance in the three major areas of wellness.

However, it is not unusual for individuals to focus on the development and maintenance of one area at the expense of the other two. We might perceive that an obviously physically fit aerobics instructor is a very "well" individual. But this presumption is not based on a clear knowledge of that instructor's emotional state or spiritual foundation. The reverse is also true. A pastor who is strong spiritually and emotionally may be weak physically.

Why is balance so important? Let's take the pastor as an example. This individual directly influences the lives of many others. Even if the pastor is spiritually strong and emotionally intact, ignoring or poorly maintaining physical health—aside from the obvious impact on the pastor's well-being—will limit abilities, restrict energy, and hinder the work God has called that pastor to perform. The pastor's witness of faith even may be compromised because of this imbalance. All three areas influence one another. It is important to establish both long-term and short-term goals that focus on developing balance in the physical, emotional, and spiritual areas of wellness.

■ Quality

*It is important to assume **responsibility** for the daily **choices** you make in life that influence personal well-being; to be aware of and plan for positive **change** in your life; to help create a physical, emotional, and spiritual **balance** that can add to the **quality** of your life . . .*

QUALITY: The kind of life one leads—positive or negative—as it relates to wellness.

One of the first benefits to come to mind when someone is interested in participating in wellness activities is the potential increase in that individual's life span; i.e., an increase in the *quantity* of years one may live. A concept just as important if not more important is people's enjoyment of their current lifestyles and their ability to participate in the meaningful activities of life. This outlook focuses more on the **quality** of one's life, the kind of life one leads—positive or negative—as it relates to wellness.

Negative habits can increase the risk of disability and decrease one's independence at an older age. Negative habits can seriously affect quality of life and can lead to the following conditions:

- Dependence on medications
- Chronic fatigue and pain
- Decreased mobility
- Inability to participate in family events or social activities

Happiness and *success* are difficult terms to define, as they mean different things to different people. To develop a life characterized by *quality*, define happiness and success as they pertain to each of your roles and responsibilities in life; e.g., parent, spouse, friend, employee, community member, etc. These meaningful, personal definitions can help you define goals for a higher quality of life. As you seek quality in your life, consider these questions:

- Are you currently happy with your lifestyle?
- What sense of accomplishment, satisfaction, and purpose do you experience from the contacts in your life?
- What future goals do you envision for your life as these goals relate to happiness and success?
- Are these goals aligned with the meaningful roles in your life?

■ Lifestyle

*It is important to assume **responsibility** for the daily **choices** you make in life that influence personal well-being; to be aware of and plan for positive **change** in your life; to help create a physical, emotional, and spiritual **balance** that can add to the **quality** of your life and provide **lifestyle** habits to maintain a state of positive well-being.*

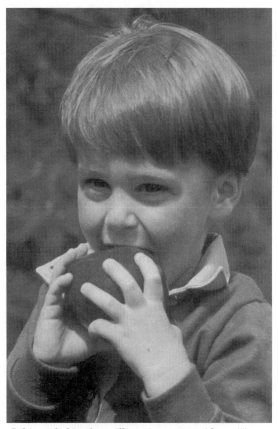

Cultivate habits that will continue to provide positive benefits for your well-being.

We often hear that we live in a society of "quick-fix" solutions. We're also told that the motivating factor for many of our actions is "instant gratification." Among today's most popular diet plans are those that advertise substantive weight loss in a minimal amount of time. How long the dieter can maintain a normal lifestyle on such a diet, however, is conveniently left out of the advertisements and promotional materials.

Exhibit 1.1, Benefits of a Wellness Lifestyle

Benefits of a Wellness Lifestyle

- A sense of humor
- Inner peace, a sense of spiritual significance
- Interest in physical activities
- Positive attitudes and outlooks
- Goals for personal and professional development
- Enjoyable and fulfilling social relationships
- A sense of positive, personal responsibility
- Clear thinking, open-mindedness
- Energy to participate in life's activities
- Positive self-esteem and self-respect

LIFESTYLE: Cultivating long-term habits that will continue to provide positive benefits for physical, emotional, and spiritual development and well-being.

Lifestyle in wellness means cultivating long-term habits that will continue to provide positive benefits for physical, emotional, and spiritual development and well-being—hopefully, for the rest of one's life. This may mean that it will take longer to experience the results of positive change. Wellness is not a "quick-fix." A short-term fix generally leads to relapse into a negative, long-term habit. Results in lifestyle wellness are achieved through a plan that can be maintained, continuing to provide positive benefits for a long time.

Taking Positive Steps

What day-to-day steps or actions are considered part of a positive wellness plan? In some of the initial research linking lifestyle factors to health and well-being, a five-year study found that well-being and even life expectancy were related to seven distinctive lifestyle habits:[4]

1. Eating three meals a day at regular intervals instead of daily snacking
2. Eating breakfast every day
3. Engaging in moderate exercise two to three times per week
4. Getting adequate sleep every night (seven to eight hours)
5. Not smoking
6. Maintaining moderate weight
7. Consuming little or no alcohol

We will discuss these and many other positive action steps in subsequent chapters of this text. Following this initial study, other perspectives have added to a menu of wellness activities from which to choose daily activities. In *Healthy Pleasures*, Drs. Robert Ornstein and David Sobel emphasize the importance of relaxation through activities such as the following:[5]

- Set aside time each day to pursue an activity you enjoy.
- Satisfy your "skin hunger" with regular hugs or a massage.

- Take saunas.
- Spend time with nature.
- Listen to soothing music.
- Take afternoon naps.

Drs. Ornstein and Sobel also discuss activities and outlooks for positive well-being. Among their suggestions are these:

- Maintain positive outlooks and expectations.
- Achieve muscular relaxation through deep breathing.
- Take a hot bath.
- Develop humor—an ability to laugh at yourself.
- Spend time with pets.
- Maintain positive communications and relations with others.
- Focus on past successes instead of past failures.
- Develop healthy altruism—caring for others.
- Pursue small moments of happiness.

The American Cancer Society also has suggested action steps for overall well-being. Among the suggestions are these:[6]

- Stay out of the sun.
- Avoid consumption of saturated fat.
- Eat lots of fresh fruits and vegetables.
- Get regular cancer screenings.

It is obvious that wellness activities are many and varied. As you examine the chapters to follow, it will be important to develop the priority activities and contacts you feel will best support your continued well-being. You will find many areas to review and evaluate as you establish goals for the future. Please remember this: You and the people you care about will be the primary beneficiaries of these goals and their related action steps.

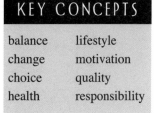

KEY CONCEPTS

balance	lifestyle
change	motivation
choice	quality
health	responsibility

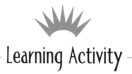

Learning Activity

1. In which areas of wellness do you need to assume a greater personal sense of responsibility?

   _____

   _____

   _____

   _____

2. What steps can you take to assume this responsibility?

   _____

   _____

   _____

   _____

3. What priorities and goals may allow you to live what you would define as a "quality" lifestyle?

   _____

   _____

   _____

   _____

4. Review the following resources to gain additional insights and information concerning personal health and wellness:

   www.yahoo.com/health

   www.mayoclinic.com

   www.healthfinder.gov

Endnotes

1. As quoted on the Stress Management and Emotional Wellness Web site: www.imt.net/~randolfi/stresspage.html.
2. Merriam-Webster, Inc., *Merriam-Webster's Collegiate Dictionary*, 10th ed. (Springfield, MA: Merriam-Webster, Inc., 2001), 534.
3. Curtis O. Byer and Louis W. Shainberg, "Introduction to Wellness," in *Living Well: Health in Your Hands* (New York: HarperCollins, 1995), 5.
4. Nedra Belloc and Lester Breslow, "Relationship of Physical Health Status and Health Practices," *Preventative Medicine* 1 (August 1972): 409-21.
5. Robert E. Ornstein and David S. Sobel, *Healthy Pleasures* (Reading, MA: Addison-Wesley, 1989).
6. For more information, visit the American Cancer Society's Web site at www.cancer.org.

2

SPIRITUAL WELLNESS

"What matters supremely, therefore, is not, in the last analysis, the fact that I know God, but the larger fact which underlies it—the fact that He knows me. I am graven on the palms of His hands."

—J. I. Packer[1]

Spirituality is a trendy topic in today's society. Magazines, newspapers, and television regularly feature stories and news items related to spirituality of all types. In local bookstores the spirituality section is growing by leaps and bounds. Society's inquisitiveness about spirituality should not surprise us—that is the way God made us. Our deep longing to know God is a basic human need.

The concept of spiritual wellness, on the other hand, is seldom mentioned. Because of this, many of us are not as comfortable discussing this aspect of wellness. However, the central theme of this book is that spirituality is the core from which all other wellness variables flow. The perspective in this text is biblical and Judeo-Christian—not to be confused with other modern worldviews.

OBJECTIVES

- Define the concepts foundational to spiritual wellness.

- Differentiate between spirituality and religion.

- Describe how spiritual wellness relates to other areas of wellness.

- Identify actions that will embody the daily living concepts of spiritual wellness.

- Assess your spiritual wellness.

Forming a Christian Worldview

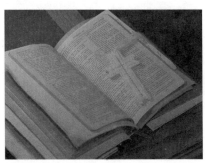

The Bible is the Word of God.

■ Foundational Components

A Christian worldview as it relates to this text includes the following foundational components:[2]

- God created everything that exists. He himself was not created. He has always existed. He created everything to have a purpose. Before sin entered the world, His creation was perfect.

- God deeply loves men and women. He handcrafted them and longs for intimate fellowship with them.

- God became human in the person of Jesus Christ. God Himself bore the penalty for humanity's sin by suffering and dying on a cross, an instrument of execution.

- God gave human beings free will in the choices they make during their earthly existence.

- The Bible is the Word of God.

> Spirituality is at the center of wellness, the core from which all other variables flow.

To repeat, spiritual wellness is the core of all other wellness actions. It is foundational, undergirding the personal values that will determine attitude, behaviors, and actions in the pursuit of total well-being. Our values about physical wellness will determine the steps we take, or do not take, to care for our physical bodies. Whether we focus on positive attitudes and outlooks or their negative counterparts is largely responsible for our mental/emotional wellness. The core values and attitudes we develop also can influence our perspective as we interact with other people, develop our careers, or pursue additional education and training.

What, then, are your core values? What are the foundational building blocks of your worldview?

- Have you formed them because they were "handed down" to you?
- Have you based them on what seems to be popular at the moment?
- Are they constant or are they changing?
- Are they based on a principle or a circumstance?

The Judeo-Christian perspective mentioned above is the pivotal core value of this text. We believe that reading the Word of God in the Bible is the key to developing the positive personal values and priorities that distinguish a Christian worldview from other worldviews. The Bible establishes core values that will guide all areas of personal well-being in positive ways. These Christian values as they relate to personal wellness are the primary subjects of discussion in this text.

■ The Wholeness Wheel

Human Care Ministries of the Lutheran Church-Missouri Synod uses a Wholeness Wheel to depict spiritual well-being as totally encompassing the other core aspects of personal well-being.[3] This clearly demonstrates how spiritual wellness relates to all other areas of wellness in our lives. At the center of this model is the statement: "I am a new creation and a member of the body of Christ."

Figure 2.1. The Wholeness Wheel

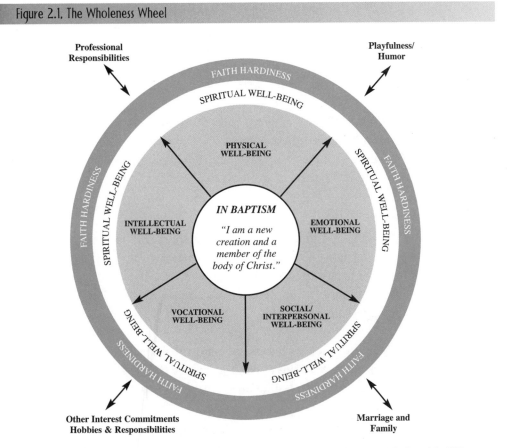

Source: The Lutheran Church-Missouri Synod (LCMS), Human Care Ministries, St. Louis, MO. Copyright 1997. Adapted from the InterLutheran Coordinating Committee on Ministerial Health and Wellness. Used by permission.

■ Foundational Attitudes

In *Christian Attitude toward Attitudes*, author Keith Hinton states that Christian attitudes are deeply rooted in the truth of God's Word and in the realization of God's power at work in our lives. "Your attitudes play an important role in directing your actions and decisions."[4] Attitudes thus naturally play an important role in the wellness decisions you make. Pointing to Jesus Christ as the beginning and end of all proper attitudes, Hinton explains that Christian attitudes develop primarily from three Christian attributes: joy, peace, and hope.

- Joy founded on the reality that our sins are forgiven; joy that is not dependent on external circumstances.

- Peace from knowing our lives have purpose and meaning; peace from the abiding presence of the Holy Spirit in our lives.

- Hope anchored in God Himself; hope from knowing that as we persevere through each tribulation, we build more hope.

Hinton concludes by stating that Christians have joy deeper than emotions, peace greater than circumstances, and hope that is anchored in more than wishful thinking.[5]

The Wholeness Wheel (Figure 2.1) illustrates spiritual wellness as completely surrounding the other components of wellness. Joy, peace, and hope can bolster positive attitudes, outlooks, and foundations for the choices and decisions we make in all areas of wellness.

■ Spirituality v. Religion

This chapter begins with the observation that spirituality is "trendy" today. It also points out that not all "spiritual" worldviews are Christian. Just what is spirituality? Is it the same as religion? If not, how do these two concepts differ?

At a recent conference on spirituality, attendees shared the following definitions of spirituality:[6]

- "Extraordinary union with a sacred energy that reaches beyond ordinary knowledge of the everyday world to embody the virtues of life in the form of hope, courage, faith, honor, love, acceptance, and a meaningful encounter with death."

- "Spirit is a non-corporeal and nonmental aspect of people that provides unity and gives meaning to life."

- "The image of God within a person; a drive for bonding with the transcendent; an intangible principle that gives life to the physical organism."

- "Equates spirit with the inner self and ties it to a greater sense of self-awareness, a higher degree of consciousness and inner strength. A power that can expand human capacity and allow people to move beyond their usual selves."

Our spiritual side or spiritual nature is the core of our being. It is the soul, the real person, the part of a person that does not die when the physical body dies. We can define **spirituality** as one's sense of relationship with the transcendent. It is that aspect of personhood concerned with incorporeal matters. E. Arnold suggests that there is both a vertical and horizontal dimension to a person's spirituality.[7] The vertical dimension has to do with a person's transcendent relationship—that person's relationship to God. The horizontal dimension demonstrates how a person lives out the vertical dimension. A person's values, lifestyle, quality of life, and interactions are captured in the horizontal dimension. (See Figure 2.2.)

> SPIRITUALITY: One's sense of relationship with the transcendent; that aspect of personhood concerned with incorporeal matters.

Figure 2.2. Vertical and Horizontal Dimensions of Spirituality.

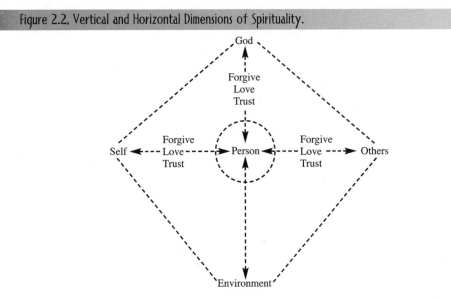

Source: Adapted from Ruth Stoll, "Spirituality and the Nursing Profession," in *Spiritual Dimensions of Nursing Practice*, ed. Verna Benner Carson (Philadelphia: Saunders, 1989), 8, with permission from Elsevier.

Another interesting definition of spirituality comes from David Moberg. He states that the definition of spirituality is not so clear and rigidly fixed that it cannot be separated from the physical, psychological, material, and other aspects of human existence. Instead, it is a component or dimension that runs through *all* of the person and that person's behavior. This provides orientation and focus, both for all the positively valued joys and experiences of life, as well as for all of the negatively framed experiences (problems, anxieties, fear of death).[8]

> **RELIGION:** Serves primarily as a vehicle to express one's spirituality; encases spirituality within a distinctive framework.

Although many equate spirituality with religion, they are two entirely different entities. **Religion** serves primarily as a vehicle to express one's spirituality. As such, we encase our spirituality within a distinctive framework, which allows us to structure our faith through doctrinal emphases and religious practices. Religion as a broad concept differs from what we commonly refer to as "religions" such as Christianity, Judaism, Buddhism, or Islam. Further subsets of these religions allow for more diversity in the "framework" of

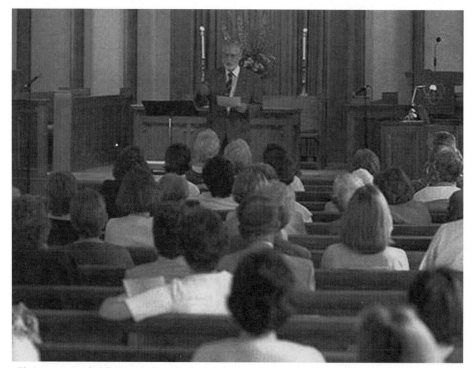

Christian attitudes develop primarily from three Christian attributes: joy, peace, and hope.

religious expression. For example, Hasidic Jews are a subset of Judaism. Mahayana Buddhists operate under the broad umbrella of Buddhism. The Wesleyan Church is a denomination of Protestant Christianity. Religions and their subsets differ in doctrine, worship style, and rituals. All Christians adhere to certain nonnegotiable articles of faith (e.g., Jesus Christ is the Son of God), but exercise diversity in how they practice Communion, baptism, special holy days, Bible study groups, prayer, and other expressions of faith.

Spiritual Wellness: A Model

While spiritual wellness may be the most difficult component to define, it is the most important component of personal well-being. John J. Pilch believes that spiritual wellness is not synonymous with religion. Instead, it involves the development of the inner self and one's soul. He sees spiritual wellness as a way of living that views and lives life as purposeful and pleasurable, seeking out life-sustaining and life-enriching options that are freely chosen at every opportunity.[9]

David Moberg states, "Spiritual well-being is evidenced when a person is free to function with a meaningful identity and purpose to relate to reality with hope."[10] This definition highlights the concepts of hope and meaning in life. Other concepts foundational to spiritual wellness are peace, love, and forgiveness. These concepts are diagrammed in Figure 2.3, A Model of Spiritual Well-Being.

Figure 2.3, A Model of Spiritual Well-Being

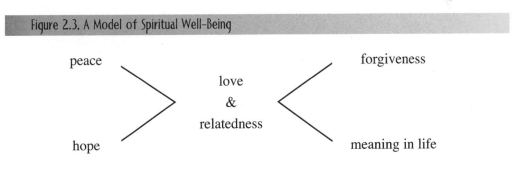

Source: Anita Robertson, from a presentation titled *"Spiritual Care: The Nurse in Life's Critical Moments"* (Greenwood, IN: October 2, 1995).

This model illustrates that love and relatedness hinge on peace, hope, forgiveness, and meaning in life. Let's look at these concepts in more detail.

◼ Meaning and Purpose

What brings meaning and purpose to our lives? What influences or shapes our life goals? The answers to these questions help to determine what "drives" us to be who we are. Our perspective on death and what happens after death also plays a part here.

> **MEANING:** The significant quality of something; e.g., how we view our place in life.

Everyone needs to feel a sense of meaning in life and purpose in daily living. We can define **meaning** as the significant quality of something or how we view our place in life. Spiritual wellness equates to life as a positive and fulfilling experience.

The Christian life—centered on a personal relationship with Jesus Christ—offers even more meaning and purpose in life. This happens when people realize two things: (1) that they are loved *so* much another Person died to save them, and (2) that same Person is preparing an eternal home for them in heaven. John 3:16 says, *"For God so loved the world that he gave his one and only Son, that whoever believes in him shall not perish but have eternal life"* (NIV). This gives us purpose and meaning. **Purpose** is the reason we exist. It is the object or end to be attained in life.

Our values are a natural extension of our spirituality, reflecting how we perceive and act out our purpose and meaning in life. Values include intangible things like honesty, autonomy, and love, as well as tangible things like wealth and family. When we have or can express what we value, we tend to be satisfied with life. When we are unable to act out our true values, we can experience feelings of inner

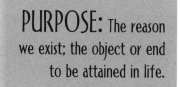

> **PURPOSE:** The reason we exist; the object or end to be attained in life.

emptiness and purposelessness. When our values are "out-of-sync" with those of our workplace or family, stress can ensue.

However, Christians give priority to a higher set of values than their own: God's values, which include forgiveness, sacrifice, and love. So, even when things around Christians are not functioning as they would like, when they feel stress because their values clash with another's values, they can still find meaning and purpose in life—based on God's higher values, love, and promises.

What values are important to you? At the end of this chapter, you will find a *Values Clarification Worksheet* to help you identify what values characterize your life. The focus of this exercise is to draw a correlation between your personal values and how they play out in specific circumstances.

■ Forgiveness

Forgiveness is a key aspect of spiritual wellness. In looking at this important concept, ask these questions:

- When you feel bitterness and resentment toward someone, how does this affect your overall attitude toward life?

- How do guilt feelings affect you?

- How do you handle guilt?

- How have you experienced forgiveness from a friend?

- How have you experienced forgiveness from God?

> **FORGIVENESS:** Pardon; ceasing to feel resentment against someone who has offended you.

■ Yours for the Asking

Those who know God's **forgiveness** can be at peace with God, with other people, and with themselves. When we forgive someone, we pardon that person. We cease to feel resentment against the one who has offended us. How do we gain forgiveness from God? 1 John 1:9 says, *"If we confess our sins [to God], he is faithful and just and will forgive us our sins and purify us from all unrighteousness"* (NIV). Jesus alone can forgive sin. We have only to ask. When we confess sin and ask for forgiveness, we acknowledge personal sin, accept responsibility for it, and then turn away from it.

Daniel Fountain, M.D. says, "When the assurance of forgiveness comes, it can remove the guilt, fear, and shame of sin, and defuse the tension and stresses caused by it."[11] Peace and hope begin to emerge and spiritual wellness begins.

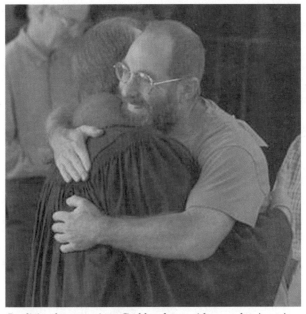

Realizing how gracious God has been with us makes it easier to forgive others.

Realizing how gracious God has been with us makes it easier to forgive others. Research continues to verify that when we do not forgive others who have wronged us, we are the ones to suffer. The inability to forgive breeds bitterness and anger, which are totally at odds with spiritual wellness. In Matthew 18, Peter asks Jesus how many times he must forgive someone who has wronged him. Jesus replies, *"I tell you, not seven times, but seventy-seven times"* (v. 22 NIV). Jesus is telling us that forgiveness of others is not an option—it is an ongoing essential in life.

■ Your Imperfect Nature

In general wellness terms, forgiveness often is overlooked or downplayed. It is easy to develop unrealistic goals and expectations of ourselves and those around us. However, forgiveness helps us remember an important truth: no one on earth is a perfect being. We will make mistakes daily. We will not achieve perfect progress toward our desired behaviors, attitudes, and goals.

The Bible captures the essence of our imperfect nature in Romans 3:23-24: *"Yes, all have sinned; all fall short of God's glorious ideal; yet now God declares us 'not guilty' of offending him if we trust in Jesus Christ, who in his kindness freely takes away our sins."* An honest realization that we are fallible human beings can provide a healthy perspective regarding setbacks or temporary lack of progress toward desired goals and changes. This is a key ingredient in a Christian worldview of wellness.

Romans 8:1 gives us another key ingredient: *"So there is now no condemnation awaiting those who belong to Christ Jesus."* No matter how terrible we perceive our failure or lack of progress to be, our earthly perspective is temporal. If our faith and foundation remain in Jesus Christ, God's eternal perspective has no room for condemnation.

■ Regroup and Refocus

We are not God. Thus, we are going to make mistakes. Sometimes we will get offtrack, drifting away from some of our daily action steps or the goals we have established. This may result in setbacks regarding our short- and long-term goals. Bear in mind that these setbacks are temporary. In fact, they are inevitable; we cannot realistically expect to make perfect progress toward our goals all the time.

When our actions or attitudes stall out, we must regroup and refocus on the positive steps we can take in the next hour, the next day, or the next opportunity to put us back in contact with our goals. We also need to celebrate the efforts and progress we have made to this point!

It can become an unhealthy habit to look back on past decisions and actions that did not focus on positive personal wellness. Doing so causes guilt. As we have seen, guilt provides no positive direction for future well-being and does not foster a beneficial outlook for positive well-being. Erase guilt through forgiveness and focus on positive goals and actions for the future.

The danger in emphasizing imperfections instead of positive progress toward spiritual wellness is that the former leads to negative thinking about ourselves and our abilities. Along with those negative thoughts comes the sense that we are not worthy of the desired change and its resulting positive benefits. Instead of forgiving ourselves for our flaws and failings (and forgiving others for theirs), we rationalize our failure as a way to pull away from positive efforts and goals.

Forgiving ourselves and others can remove many barriers to progress and can lift tremendous pressure from our shoulders. Forgiveness is not meant to replace our personal responsibility for goals and the actions necessary to achieve those goals. However, it can help us understand that we are not perfect and that we should not expect ourselves or others to achieve perfect progress every day. Positive progress toward spiritual wellness translates into this: forgive, take responsibility, and remain focused on positive goals.

■ Peace

PEACE: Inner calm; a state of tranquility or quiet.

Peace as it relates to spiritual wellness is an inner calm—a state of tranquility or quiet that can be sustained even when circumstances are chaotic. Psalm 29:11 says, *"The LORD gives strength to his people; the LORD blesses his people with peace"* (NIV). That verse underscores the source of true peace: God.

When the prophet Isaiah foretold the birth of Jesus, he said He would be the Prince of Peace (Isa. 9:6). And that He is! This kind of peace dispels fear. Health care providers often witness this kind of peace in their critically ill patients. Even as they confront death, the spiritually well patients exhibit no fear, only peace. Jesus said, *"Peace I leave with you; my peace I give you. I do not give to you as the world gives. Do not let your hearts be troubled and do not be afraid"* (John 14:27 NIV).

In *Wisdom for the Way*, Charles Swindoll says, "A peacemaker is . . . at peace with himself—internally at ease . . . not agitated, ill-tempered, in turmoil

. . . he/she works hard to settle quarrels, not start them . . . [is] accepting, tolerant, finds no pleasure in being negative . . . Few things are more godly than *peace*. When we promote it, pursue it, model it, we are linked directly with Him."[12]

Wow! What a beautiful way to live! People who are spiritually well are at peace with God, others, and themselves.

■ Hope

Hope essentially is looking forward to something that we believe is good. It is often a belief in something for which we have no tangible proof. In

> **HOPE:** Looking forward to something we believe is good, often something for which we have no proof.

Keeping Hope Alive, author Lewis Smedes suggests that hope "is a combination of wishing, imagining, and believing for things in an unknown future. Hope is the spiritual power for living successfully as creatures endowed with godlike ability to imagine the future but stuck with humanlike inability to control it."[13]

What is the source of hope? Psalm 71:5 says, *"O Lord, you alone are my hope."* The Christian echoes this, calling God our Savior and Christ Jesus our only hope (see 1 Tim. 1:1 LB). How can we have hope? Read the Bible—it offers encouragement and teaches perseverance, both necessary for fostering hope. Romans 15:13 says, *"May the God of hope fill you with all joy and peace as you trust in him, so that you may overflow with hope by the power of the Holy Spirit"* (NIV). God does not want us to live lives of despair—He wants His people to have hope. God gives us this gift of hope to keep us going, even in the face of uncertainty. To paraphrase Lewis Smedes, our spirits were made to hope, just as our hearts were made to love, our brains were made to think, and our hands were made to create things.[14]

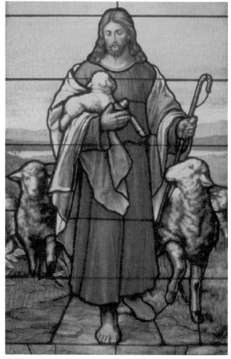

"The LORD gives strength to his people; the LORD blesses his people with peace." Psalm 29:11 NIV

■ When Hope Dims

What happens when we have no hope? Generally, losing hope means we lose the desire for good things. We lose the ability to dream and we lose our inner drive. We lose faith in God, other people, and ourselves. It is easy to fall into depression when hope is gone, keeping spiritual wellness out of reach. Charles Swindoll explains how the absence of hope can cripple someone:

> Take from us our wealth and we are hindered. Take our health and we are handicapped. Take our purpose and we are slowed, temporarily confused. But take away our hope, and we are plunged into deepest darkness . . . stopped dead in our tracks, paralyzed.[15]

False hope is worse than no hope. That is why spiritual wellness only can exist if hope is in the right place. Our hope should be in a Person—Jesus Christ. When we involve God in our hope, hope becomes *trust* in God and the promises He makes. God gives us hundreds of promises in Scripture, but they focus on three things: (1) He promises to be with us even when life tells us that He has abandoned us, (2) He promises that His children will live in heaven after they die, and (3) He promises to make our world right again.[16]

■ Nothing Helps Like Hope

Hope is basic to Christian faith. It allows us to face suffering and crisis because we never stop believing that things will get better. Charles Swindoll's words capture the essence of Christian hope:

> Hope is a wonderful gift from God, a source of strength and courage in the face of life's harshest trials. When we are trapped in a tunnel of misery, hope points to the light at the end. When we are overworked and exhausted, hope gives us fresh energy. When we are discouraged, hope lifts our spirits. When we are tempted to quit, hope keeps us going. When we struggle with a crippling disease or a lingering illness, hope helps us persevere beyond the pain. When we fear the worst, hope brings reminders that God is still in control. When we are forced to sit back and wait, hope gives us the patience to trust. Put simply, when life hurts and dreams fade, nothing helps like hope.[17]

■ Love and Relatedness

Love and relatedness issues involve our relationship to God and to other people. They involve such questions as these:

- Do you feel God loves you? Why?
- With whom do you have significant relationships?
- How do you perceive love?
- What makes you feel insecure about someone's love?

The answers to these questions help to evaluate the significance of our relationships. As a general rule, when we are in a right relationship with God, our interactions with others will be healthy, stable, and intact.

Sometimes it is hard to accept the fact that God loves us. But this is foundational to spiritual wellness. Simply put: "Jesus loves me, this I know, for the Bible tells me so." He knows us intimately—faults, fears, and frailties—and still He loves us.

In *Knowing God*, J.I. Packer says this:

What matters supremely, therefore, is not, in the last analysis, the fact that I know God, but the larger fact which underlies it—the fact that *He knows me*. I am graven on the palms of His hands. I am never out of His mind. All my knowledge of Him depends on His sustained initiative in knowing me. I know Him, because He first knew me, and continues to know me. He knows me as a friend, one who loves me; and there is no moment when His eye is off me, or His attention distracted from me, and no moment, therefore, when His care falters. This is momentous knowledge.[18]

Our goal should be to love others the way God loves us. Because we are only human and not divine, we will never be able to do this perfectly. But because His love is unconditional and sacrificial, it is the standard to which we should strive with all our strength.

■ Spiritual Distress

A person in spiritual distress lacks one or more of the positive foundational concepts of spiritual wellness (meaning and purpose, forgiveness, peace, hope, love and relatedness). Notice how the model below (Figure 2.4, A Model of Spiritual Distress) contrasts to the previous model of spiritual well-being (Figure 2.3):

Figure 2.4. A Model of Spiritual Distress

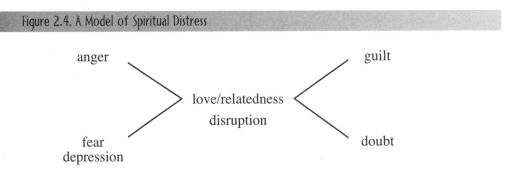

anger

guilt

love/relatedness
disruption

fear
depression

doubt

Source: Anita Robertson, from a presentation titled *"Spiritual Care: The Nurse in Life's Critical Moments"* (Greenwood, IN: October 2, 1995).

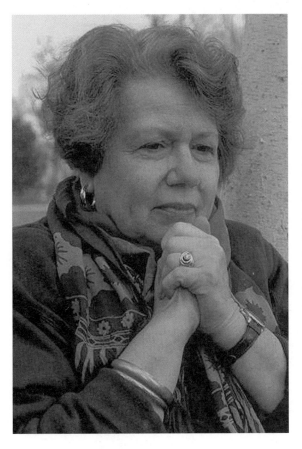

Spiritual distress is characterized by negative concepts; e.g., anger, despair, fear, depression, guilt, doubt, and disruption in love and relatedness. Spiritual distress is the result of a breakdown in a person's relationship with God. This often results in confusion and questions about one's identity and purpose in life. Donald and Nancy Tubesing echo this thought in *Seeking Your Healthy Balance*, in which they chart the intangible but very real damage of spiritual distress.[19] (See Excerpt 2.1.)

Spiritual distress is the result of a breakdown in a person's relationship with God.

Excerpt 2.1, Spiritual Health v. Spiritual Atrophy

Spiritual Health	Spiritual Atrophy
Hope	Emptiness
Positive outlook	Anxiety
Acceptance of death	Loss of meaning
Forgiveness, self-acceptance	Self-judgment, self-condemnation
Commitment	Apathy
Clear values	Conflicting values
Sense of worth	Need to prove self
Peace	Hurried and harried
In touch with God	Dead at the core
Prayer, worship	Without meaningful foundations

Source: Donald A. Tubesing and Nancy L. Tubesing, *Seeking Your Healthy Balance: A Do-it-yourself Guide to Whole Person Well-Being* (Duluth, MN: Whole Person Associates, Inc., 1992), 87. Used by permission.

Building a Spiritual Foundation

In chapter 1, we discussed several terms related to the overall concept of general wellness. Understanding spiritual wellness also involves foundational terms, especially as they relate to a Christian perspective of well-being.

> We will look at four important terms in this section:
> 1. Temptation
> 2. Faith
> 3. Patience
> 4. Obedience

■ Temptation

TEMPTATION: An attempt to persuade, induce, and/or entice, especially toward something sensually pleasurable or immoral; something that seeks to distract us from positive well-being.

Temptation is generally defined as an attempt to persuade, induce, and/or entice, especially toward something sensually pleasurable or immoral. In this respect, temptation not only is applicable to spiritual wellness, but also to general wellness. Temptation can include anything that might persuade us to think or act in a way that detracts from our positive well-being. It can lead us to procrastinate in achieving wellness goals or distract us from our wellness program. Temptation comes in a variety of forms:

- We may be tempted by foods or substances that are not good for our physical well-being.
- We may be tempted by negative thoughts and attitudes that undermine our emotional well-being.
- We may be tempted to waste time in unproductive pursuits.
- We may be tempted by thoughts or behaviors that could pull us away from our core values or our Christian faith and principles.

No one is immune to temptation. Temptations are ever present and "custom-tailored" to every person. But they have one thing in common: they are hazardous to our well-being because they may negatively impact our bodies, minds, and/or spirits.

First Corinthians 10:12-13 succinctly captures the Christian perspective regarding temptation: *"So, if you think you are standing firm, be careful that you don't fall! No temptation has seized*

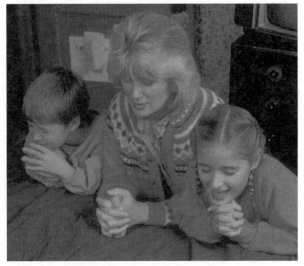

When we are tempted to veer from the path of spiritual wellness, we have only to turn to God in prayer and faith.

you except what is common to man" (NIV). In other words, even if we think we can stand up to temptation, we must be careful not to fall. We are tempted in the same way that everyone else is tempted. We are not perfect. Asserting that we can resist temptation when it strikes is a dangerous assumption, one that belittles temptation's power to catch us in a weak moment or in the guise of peer pressure. It is all too easy to fall prey to the pleasures of the moment, to relax one's commitment "just for this one time."

However, becoming informed about the temptations we will face gives the insight and the ability to develop positive methods, thoughts, and actions to counteract individual temptations. If we read further in 1 Corinthians 10:13, we will discover the source of support in responding to temptation: *"And God is faithful; he will not let you be tempted beyond what you can bear. But when you are tempted, he will also provide a way out so that you can stand up under it."*

When we are tempted to veer from the path of spiritual wellness, we have only to turn to God in prayer and in faith. Ask Him for guidance, strength, and support in making the decisions necessary for dealing effectively with temptation. God is our first line of defense. Include these coping methods in your second line of defense:

- Avoid tempting environments or situations.
- Assertively say no to self and others concerning tempting situations.
- Surround yourself with people of similar values and goals.
- Remain focused on your well-being goals and the positive thoughts and actions that support your goals.

■ Faith

> # FAITH IN SELF:
> Belief in one's ability to achieve wellness.

Faith as a foundation for spiritual wellness is twofold: faith in self and faith in God. **Faith in self** (or personal faith) in the context of this textbook does *not* mean faith as opposed to God (e.g., agnosticism or atheism). It is a belief that what you are attempting will provide positive results for your well-being. It involves confidence in your ability to perform desired actions or behaviors. Do you have enough faith in yourself and in your abilities to persist toward the goals you have established for yourself? Do you have a strong belief in the benefits your efforts will produce? Without that kind of faith, your confidence will erode and your potential for well-being will be compromised.

A Christian worldview expands the concept of personal faith to **faith in God,** the "Highest Power," who gives strength and guidance beyond our abilities. It is belief and trust that God will help us achieve what we cannot achieve on our own. In Matthew 17:20-21, Jesus illustrates the importance of faith as it relates to what

> # FAITH IN GOD:
> Belief and trust that God will help us achieve what we cannot achieve on our own.

we can accomplish. Explaining to His disciples why they were unable to perform a miracle, Jesus states: *"Because you have so little faith. I tell you the truth, if you have faith as small as a mustard seed, you can say to this mountain, 'Move from here to there' and it will move. Nothing will be impossible for you"* (NIV).

Sound amazing? It is. Faith provides a springboard for successful outcomes. Consider the fact that a placebo pill—nothing more than a pill made of sugar or some other innocuous substance—is successful in treating approximately one-third of the conditions for which it is prescribed. Why? Because the individual taking the pill has faith in the person who prescribed it and/or faith in the curing potential of the pill itself.

■ A Sure Foundation

What is the foundation of your personal faith? Is it something that is consistently available? Or is it founded on something that may be strong today but may weaken or disappear tomorrow? Faith in worldly concepts and/or individuals is important and supportive in many ways, but it also can be inconsistent in its availability and fleeting in its duration.

> Jesus Christ is always available to you. His power is constant and unchanging.

Jesus Christ is always available to you. His power is constant and unchanging. Faith in Him means that all you need to do is ask, and you will receive the strength, wisdom, peace, and courage you need to deal with daily demands, issues, and situations. This foundation of faith is solid, one that never wavers: *"The Lord your God goes with you; he will never leave you nor forsake you"* (Deuteronomy 31:6).

Your faith in yourself and in your personal abilities is important in achieving your wellness goals. However, faith in Jesus Christ is foundational to your success in staying the course toward personal well-being.

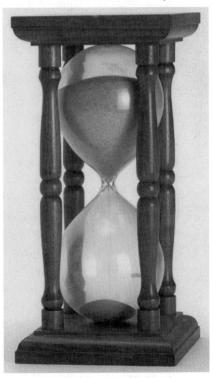

Patience is the key to establishing long-lasting, positive habits, benefits, and outcomes.

■ Patience

As a virtue, patience is often overlooked. To wait for something to occur, happen, or change almost seems contrary to today's fast-paced culture. In the area of general wellness, people often do not maintain the patience necessary to incorporate new and positive habits into their lives. Many prematurely turn away from positive growth because the desired results do not occur fast enough. They then jump into the so-called "quick fix," receiving a "quick" but not a long-lasting "fix." Common examples of these kinds of short-term solutions can include:

> **PATIENCE:** The capacity to remain steadfast despite opposition, difficulty, or adversity.

- The "quick" weight-loss program that sacrifices healthy nutrition
- The "quick" get-rich scheme that overlooks solid financial stewardship and positive career planning
- The "quick" emotional/stress relief through the use of alcohol or other substances

Too many times the short-term methods only address the signs and symptoms of what is occurring in your life, not the actual *causes* of your signs and symptoms. While some positive wellness action steps may result in immediate benefits, **patience** is key to establishing long-lasting, positive habits, benefits, and outcomes. It is the capacity to remain steadfast despite opposition, difficulty, or adversity.

Through the lens of a Christian worldview, patience means replacing your time frame with God's schedule of events and happenings. The apostle Paul reflected this emphasis in these words: *"Be glad for all God is planning for you. Be patient in trouble, and prayerful always"* (Romans 12:12).

■ God's Planning

"Be glad for all God is planning for you." Being patient is difficult. As we have seen, today's culture places great emphasis on immediate gratification. You want that promotion now. You want to be in better physical shape instantly. You want that "perfect someone" to walk into your life immediately—or tomorrow, at the latest. But Romans 12:12 tells us to be patient regarding these and other aspirations because they are part of *"all God is planning for you."* While they may not happen within the time frame you have set, if you pray and continue to work toward your goals, God will address them in His time frame. God has a definite plan for your personal and professional experience on this earth. Cultivate patience, knowing that God's timing is better than any earthly time frame you could ever establish.

■ Through Trouble

"Be patient in trouble." The second part of Romans 12:12 advises patience in troubled or stressful times. These are the times we all want to avoid, the situations we wish would disappear immediately. But Paul tell us to remain patient—*especially* in these times. Patience can help us rely on our faith and keep our focus. Knowing that troubled times are *to be expected*, we can make informed choices to cope in positive ways. Impatience often leads to frustration and a sense of helplessness, which then can lead to negative responses to the stress. Patience helps clear the air of negativity, allowing us to see the positive response options available to us and to take the steps necessary to counteract the stress.

■ Always Prayerful

". . . and prayerful always." The final portion of Romans 12:12 offers a framework for our preparation and actions during times that require patience. We should ask for God's support and direction in realizing our goals and aspirations, as they align with His will. In prayerful communication with God, we will learn the steps we should take to fulfill the purpose God has in mind for us. Second Thessalonians 3:5 explains the true source of patience: *"May the Lord bring you into an ever deeper understanding of the love of God and of the patience that comes from Christ."*

■ Obedience

In general wellness terms, **obedience** is defined as the willingness to commit to the goals we have established for personal well-being. Obedience begins when we establish positive goals for personal well-being. It continues when we follow through on the actions necessary to successfully complete our goals.

Obedience is a key component of the Christian worldview. Jesus considered it so important that He paid the ultimate price in His obedience to His Father: *"And even though Jesus was God's Son, he had to learn from experience what it was like to obey, when obeying meant suffering"* (Hebrews 5:8).

> **OBEDIENCE:** Willingness to commit to a wellness plan and complete the actions necessary to achieve personal well-being.

A wellness program, of course, will not require us to suffer in the same way that Jesus suffered. However, this passage emphasizes that obedience to personal goals for personal growth often does involve sacrifice. We learn almost immediately that the time we previously spent cultivating unhealthy habits will be in direct conflict to the time required to achieve goals for personal well-being.

■ The Danger of Apathy

Apathy is a common and dangerous barrier to obedience, both in establishing goals and then in taking the necessary steps to follow through on

> ## APATHY: Indifference; lack of interest or concern.

those goals for personal well-being. Apathy equates to indifference, a lack of interest or concern. It is a negative perspective that easily can sneak into our lives, quickly derailing positive actions and thoughts. It can surface as a belief that the changes we have planned are not worth the effort, or that our efforts will not make any real difference. It can turn our thoughts and attention away from the positive results we achieve and, instead, lead us to focus on the things that we might not be able to achieve. We may begin to believe our efforts are pointless. This results in negative thinking: "I have tried this before and didn't succeed, so why should it work now?"

Apathy also expresses itself as indifference to well-being; i.e., no interest in taking responsibility for improvements in our lives, or choosing to remain uninformed about how to achieve positive benefits for ourselves or those around us.

■ Active, Not Passive

God's plan for your life is active, not passive. It emphasizes active obedience to the goals and actions that will add quality to your life. James 2:26 accentuates this point: *"Just as the body is dead when there is no spirit in it, so faith is dead if it is not the kind that results in good deeds."*

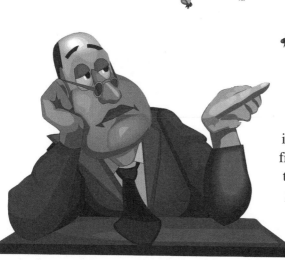

This reinforces a key wellness concept: it is not just *what you know* that is important, it is *what you do* with that knowledge that matters. Thoughts and good intentions can be a meaningful first step to positive change, but they will trip and fall flat if the follow-through and the action steps do not match the good intentions.

■ Walking the Talk

Did you know that Jesus can be seen as a role model for healthy living? His life demonstrated balance and healthy behaviors. We sometimes forget that Jesus was human. He was a child, experienced adolescence, and grew into manhood. He had feelings and lived with human limitations.

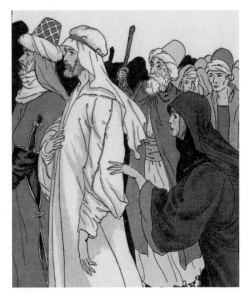

Like almost everyone else in ancient Israel, Jesus walked everywhere He went. He had been a carpenter before embarking on His three-year mission. Carpenters needed stamina and physical strength. Jesus also followed a simple diet that included fish, grains, vegetables, and little red meat. Although He must have experienced stress, especially when the crowds pressed in, He knew when to step away and rest. The Gospels mention that He often took time to be alone with His Father. He prayed regularly, not only at the prescribed times, but early in the morning before anyone else was up.

Jesus cultivated fellowship. He developed healthy relationships with people and expressed His concern and love for them. He didn't try to "do it all alone," however. Jesus often looked to others for support, allowing them to minister to Him and assist in His ministry. He carefully handpicked and mentored twelve apostles and certain disciples to be in His inner circle. These were men and women with whom He could relax, share His successes and disappointments, and prepare to carry on His work when He departed. He taught them well. That small group of believers has grown to millions of Christians around the world today. In body, mind, and spirit, Jesus embodied the principles of the wellness lifestyle.

Body, Mind, and Spirit

In the introduction of this book, we explained that wellness generally involves the body, the mind, and the spirit. All too often we judge or evaluate people by their exterior appearance—the image they project to the world. We're all prone to "size up" people by their physical appearance or clothing. We praise or criticize them for the way they handle themselves in public. We are impressed when they advocate a principle that we also value as a priority for life. However, these are surface judgments only. It takes time to learn a person's inner core values, the deeper things that motivate and direct that person. This internal value base is what lies behind the external appearance. The *Values Clarification Worksheet* located at the end of this chapter will help you determine your internal value base and, more important, whether your "visible external" is an accurate reflection of your "guiding internal." We sometimes avoid two important questions:

- How strong are our core values?
- How well does our walk match our talk (our actions match our speech)?

Spiritual wellness examines external appearances on a deeper internal level. Its focus is to establish internal values and foundations that: (1) balance the components of body, mind, and spirit, and (2) reinforce our ability to model these values in our daily contacts and actions.

God has given each of us a body, mind, and spirit. Understanding the interaction and balance of this threefold dimension of the human being is crucial to a solid foundation of spiritual wellness.

- **Body**: The physical, material aspect of the human being. As Christians, we cannot help but remember 1 Corinthians 6:19-20: *"Your own body does not belong to you. For God has bought you with a great price."* Your body is not your own. We were purchased at a costly price—the blood of Jesus Christ. That alone should motivate us to care for our bodies in order to serve God and others.

- **Mind**: One of two immaterial aspects of the human being. It also is called the "**soul**" of a person, the center of thinking, emotion, and personality. It houses the will, which is responsible for making decisions.

- **Spirit**: The second of two immaterial aspects of the human being, and the most important. The spirit is the conduit through which the Holy Spirit works, the aspect that seeks a relationship with God. In blessing the Thessalonians, Paul said: *"May your whole spirit, soul and body be kept blameless at the coming of our Lord Jesus Christ"* (1 Thessalonians 5:23 NIV).

For a deeper understanding of how basic Christian theology relates to spiritual wellness, see Addendum E at the end of this chapter. Looking at spiritual wellness through the lens of body, mind, and spirit can provide a core for our values, perspectives, and decisions. How we develop and activate our core values is up to us. God will not force us to do anything. He has given us free will to make our own decisions. We have no automatic "right" to health and wellness, but we have the right to make choices that will affect the level of wellness we incorporate into our lives.

KEY CONCEPTS

apathy	faith in God
faith in self	forgiveness
hope	meaning
obedience	patience
peace	purpose
religion	spirituality
temptation	

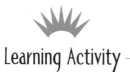

Learning Activity

1. Take a personal value assessment to help identify what values characterize your life. (See Values Clarification Worksheet, Addendum A.)

2. Take a personal spiritual assessment. (See Spiritual Assessments, Addendums B and C.)

3. Describe what difference God makes in your life. Do you have a personal relationship with Him?

   _____

   _____

   _____

   _____

4. Write your personal definition of spiritual wellness. From your definition, develop two or three action steps that will help you support a lifestyle that consistently models your definition.

   _____

   _____

   _____

   _____

   _____

   _____

   _____

5. In behavioral terms, explain how you express your spirituality.

_____

_____

_____

_____

6. In your life, what personal temptation works against your positive well-being? What can you do to overcome this temptation?

_____

_____

_____

7. List areas of your life in which you need to practice more patience. Are they related to your goals for well-being? How can you learn to be more patient in realizing these goals?

_____

_____

_____

_____

_____

_____

8. Is there anyone in your life you need to forgive? What can help you attain a sense of forgiveness?

_____

_____

_____

9. Memorize the four spiritual laws. (See Addendum D.)

Addendum A
Values Clarification Worksheet

The following worksheet is a values clarification exercise. Fifty values are listed. They come from literature, past and present, and the teachings of philosophy and religion (both Christian and non-Christian). Read through the entire list first, and then mark in column:

A: the ten values that are *most important to you*. In other words, which values most affect your personal attitudes and behavior?

B: the ten values that *you believe most commonly govern actual practice in your work setting*. This includes policy, priorities set by administration, and actual attitudes and behavior of your colleagues.

C: the values that you believe are *most needed as a corrective to problems in your work setting*. What values would you or others need to act upon to cause change?

D: Mark *all* the values that *you believe are compatible with your religious beliefs*.

	A	B	C	D		A	B	C	D
altruism	☐	☐	☐	☒	excellence	☐	☐	☐	☒
ambition	☐	☐	☐	☒	faith	☐	☐	☐	☒
assertiveness	☐	☐	☐	☐	fidelity	☐	☐	☐	☒
authority	☐	☐	☐	☒	forgiveness	☐	☐	☐	☒
autonomy	☐	☐	☐	☐	freedom	☐	☐	☐	☒
beneficence	☐	☐	☐	☒	group approval	☐	☐	☐	☐
compassion	☒	☐	☐	☒	happiness	☐	☐	☐	☒
competence	☐	☐	☐	☒	health	☐	☐	☐	☒
confidentiality	☐	☐	☐	☒	hope	☐	☐	☐	☒
cost effectiveness	☐	☐	☐	☒	human dignity	☐	☐	☐	☒
courage	☐	☐	☐	☒	humility	☐	☐	☐	☒
duty	☐	☐	☐	☒	integrity	☐	☐	☒	☐
education	☐	☒	☐	☒	interdependence	☐	☐	☐	☐
efficiency	☐	☐	☐	☒	justice	☐	☐	☐	☒
encouragement	☒	☒	☒	☒	love	☐	☐	☐	☒
equality	☐	☐	☐	☒	patience	☐	☐	☐	☒
esthetics	☐	☐	☐	☒	peace	☐	☐	☒	☒

	A	B	C	D		A	B	C	D
power	☐	☐	☐	☐	self-actualization	☐	☐	☐	☒
productivity	☐	☒	☐	☒	serving	☐	☐	☒	☒
progress	☐	☐	☐	☒	technology	☐	☐	☐	☒
prosperity	☐	☐	☐	☒	tolerance	☐	☐	☐	☒
quality of life	☐	☐	☐	☒	tradition	☐	☐	☐	☒
respect	☐	☒	☐	☒	truth	☒	☐	☐	☒
sanctity of life	☐	☐	☐	☒	vengeance	☐	☐	☐	☐
security	☐	☐	☐	☒	wisdom	☐	☐	☒	☒

■ Scoring the Values Worksheet

Count the number of values marked in **Column A** that are also marked in **B**:
_____ x 10 = _____%

Count the number of values marked in **Column A** that are also marked in **D**:
_____ x 10 = _____ 0 _____%

Count the number of values marked in **Column B** that are also marked in **D**:
_____ x 10 = _____%

Count the number of values marked in **Column C** that are also marked in **D**:
_____ x 10 = _____%

■ Interpreting Your Results

The correlation between Column A and Column B (#1) indicates how your personal values compare with the values you encounter on the job. The correlation between Column A and D (#2) shows how your personal values compare with your religious beliefs. The relationship between B and D (#3) provides a picture of how you perceive your work environment in relationship to your religious beliefs. The correlation between C and D (#4) shows how you act in difficult situations in comparison to how you think you ought to act.

Source: Adapted from *Values in Conflict* by Judith Allen Shelley and Arlene B. Miller. ©1991 Judith Allen Shelley and Arlene B. Miller. Used by permission of InterVarsity Press, P.O. Box 1400, Downers Grove, IL 60515. www.ivpress.com

Addendum B
Spiritual Assessment #1

Are you spiritually well? This is not something most people think about very often. In order to answer this question correctly, you will need to do a spiritual assessment. The purpose of a spiritual assessment is: (1) to determine the nature of a person's relationship to God and, (2) to determine the nature of a person's relationship to other people.

Many helpful spiritual assessment tools are available today. The bottom line for all of them is this: Do you have a personal relationship with God? How does this relationship affect your relationship with others? As you read through the questions of two sample spiritual assessments (Addendum B and Addendum C), examine your relationship with God in the context of your human relationships.

■ Assessment Guide

1. In one paragraph, how would you describe your childhood?
2. Describe your relationships with your parents and siblings—while growing up and now.
3. If you are or have been married, describe your relationship with your spouse or former spouse(s). If you have never been married, describe the most significant person in your life and how that relationship developed.
4. If you are a parent, describe your relationship to your child(ren). If you do not have children of your own, who are the significant children in your life? Describe your relationships with them.
5. What were the most significant *positive* events in your childhood? Adulthood? Why?
6. What were the most significant *negative* events in your childhood? Adulthood? Why?
7. How did you learn about God?
8. In what ways did you experience God while you were growing up?
9. How would you describe God?
10. What were the crisis points in your relationship with God over your lifetime? What issues were involved? How did your relationship to God change?
11. Who was the most significant person in your faith development as a child? As an adult?

12. If married or formerly married, how has your marriage influenced your faith in God? If never married, how has your closest friend influenced your faith?

13. Describe your faith community (your church and other fellowship groups). In what ways has that community nurtured your faith? How has it hindered your faith?

14. What rituals, disciplines, or other religious practices have been particularly helpful or meaningful to you? (For example, sacraments, worship experiences, devotional habits, spiritual direction, etc.)

15. Where do you find the most support in your relationship with God?

16. What kind of spiritual support do you need at this point in your life? Are you receiving it?

17. Describe a time when you were angry with God. How did you get through that period?

18. How is God at work in your life right now?

19. In what ways is your faith helpful to you in your daily life?

20. How has your faith influenced the major decisions in your life?

21. How has your relationship with God influenced your care for others?

22. What spiritual resources do you draw upon when you feel overwhelmed?

Source: Adapted from *Spiritual Care: A Guide for Caregivers* by Judith A. Shelley. ©2000 by InterVarsity Christian Fellowship/USA. Used by permission of InterVarsity Press, P.O. Box 1400, Downers Grove, IL 60515. www.ivpress.com

Addendum C
Spiritual Assessment #2

1. What gives your life purpose and meaning? What/who is the source of your strength and hope? What is your concept of God or a Supreme Being?

2. What are your thoughts about your health in relation to your spiritual beliefs?

3. How has illness affected the way you view yourself?

4. How have you coped in the past through times of difficulty or pain? What religious rituals or practices are important to you?

5. How has this situation affected your thoughts about God/Supreme Being or the practice of your faith?

6. At the end of life, are there things you want to do or people you need to speak with? What unfinished business remains? Do you want to forgive anyone or seek forgiveness?

Source: Linda Treloar, "Spiritual Care: Assessment and Intervention," *Journal of Christian Nursing* (Spring 1999): 17.

Addendum D
The Four Spiritual Laws

1. God loves you and offers a wonderful plan for your life. John 3:16; 10:9-10

2. Man is sinful and separated from God. Therefore, he cannot know and experience God's love and plan for his life. Romans 3:23; 6:23

3. Jesus Christ is God's *only* provision for man's sin. Through Him you can know and experience God's love and plan for your life. John 14:6; Romans 5:8; 1 Corinthians 15:3-6; 20-22

4. You must individually *receive* Jesus Christ as Savior and Lord. Then you can know and experience God's love and plan. John 1:12; 3:1-8; Ephesians 2:8-9; Revelation 3:20

Source: Bill Bright, *Have You Heard of the Four Spiritual Laws?* © Copyright 1965, 1994 by Bill Bright, *NewLife* Publications, Campus Crusade for Christ. All rights reserved. Used by permission.

Addendum E
Basic Christian Theology and Spiritual Wellness

Note: All scriptural references in this addendum are from the NIV.

■ The Core of Spiritual Wellness

When we consider wellness from a wholistic viewpoint, we need to address the area of spiritual wellness. You may be familiar with the term *holistic*, as related to a system of treating the complete human being: body, mind, and spirit. *Wholistic* wellness addresses the same concerns from a Christ-centered perspective. Basic Christian theology derives from the belief that a personal relationship with Jesus Christ is the only way to a right relationship with God. This is fundamental to spiritual wellness. As we consider the very core of spiritual wellness, we need to look at three important things: the character of God, the character of man, and the life of Jesus Christ.

■ The Character of God: Holiness

John 1:1-3 says, *"In the beginning was the Word, and the Word was with God, and the Word was God. He was with God in the beginning. Through him all things were made; without him nothing was made that has been made."*

God is the Creator and Originator of life. We are the creation of His hands. As we read further in the Gospel of John, we see that God sent the Word into the world. The Word in human form is Jesus.

When we characterize God as *holy*, we need to have a good understanding of the word holiness. If you were to look up "holy" in the dictionary, you would find definitions that indicate perfection, purity, sacred, or something set apart. These definitions offer an excellent glimpse of who God is—pure, perfect, sacred, and set apart. God *alone* is holy. *"Exalt the LORD our God and worship at his holy mountain, for the LORD our God is holy"* (Psalm 99:9). As we will discuss further when we examine the character of man, God is set apart from man because of His holiness. Man is not holy. *"There is no one holy like the LORD; there is no one besides you; there is no Rock like our God"* (1 Samuel 2:2).

■ The Character of Man: Sin

Mankind is separated from a holy God by sin. You may not think of that as much of a problem until you read Romans 3:10-12: *"As it is written, 'There is no one righteous, not even one; there is no one who understands, no one who seeks God. All have turned away, they have together become worthless; there is no one who does good, not even one.'"*

We go on to read in Romans 3:23 that we (all of us) not only have been unrighteous and worthless, but also have sinned: *"For all have sinned and fall short of the glory of God."* You might be thinking, "Wow! Even I have sinned? But, wait. I don't remember sinning." Psalm 51:5 says, *"Surely I was sinful at birth, sinful from the time my mother conceived me."*

Sin in mankind is inherent; it is passed down from generation to generation to *everyone*. We—all of us, all of mankind—are flawed by sin. Even worse, when we live according to our sinful nature, we are *actually dead* (spiritually speaking). *"As for you, you were dead in your transgressions and sins"* (Ephesians 2:1).

Nothing puts an end to wellness like death! Obviously, spiritual death cannot coexist with spiritual wellness. Scripture explains how spiritual death is the inevitable result of being flawed by sin *when we live according to our sinful natures*. However, God has a solution for this dangerous problem.

■ The Life of Jesus Christ: Intercession

Romans 5:7-8 tells us, *"Very rarely will anyone die for a righteous man, though for a good man someone might possibly dare to die. But God demonstrates His own love for us in this: While we were still sinners, Christ died for us."*

That's a stunning thought! Remember, according to the Scripture you read earlier (Romans 3:10-12), we are considered unrighteous, worthless, no good, and without understanding. Don't fool yourself into thinking that you could be that "good" man that someone might possibly die for. However, Christ died for us while *we were still sinners*. He not only saved us, He made us righteous. *"But now a righteousness from God, apart from law, has been made known, to which the Law and the Prophets testify. This righteousness from God comes through faith in Jesus Christ to all who believe"* (Romans 3:21-22). This righteousness is ours free for the asking, confessing, and receiving:

> *"That if you confess with your mouth, 'Jesus is Lord', and believe in your heart that God raised him from the dead, you will be saved. For it is with your heart that you believe and are justified, and it is with your mouth that you confess and are saved"* (Romans 10:9-10).

This isn't a limited offer, available only to certain people: *"Everyone who calls on the name of the Lord will be saved"* (10:13). Furthermore, when we accept Christ's righteousness, we shall not be separated from His love:

> *"Who shall separate us from the love of Christ? Shall trouble or hardship or persecution or famine or nakedness or danger or sword? As it is written: 'For your sake we face death all day long; we are considered as sheep to be slaughtered.' No, in all these things we are more than conquerors through him who loved us. For I am convinced that neither death nor life, neither angels nor demons, neither the present nor the future, nor any powers, neither height nor depth, nor anything else in all creation, will be able to separate us from the love of God that is in Christ Jesus our Lord"* (Romans 8:35-39).

God has a plan for our spiritual wellness. God's plan is to make us righteous through Christ's redemptive death for us. His plan guarantees that if we confess and believe, we will be saved. That plan is good for everyone. Finally, God's plan is sure—nothing can separate us from His love. When we look at Jesus' life, it points toward His role as our Savior. Jesus is pivotal to God's plan for our spiritual wellness.

■ Your Identity in Christ

When you accept Jesus Christ as your personal Lord and Savior, you take on a new identity as a Christian. Jesus' death and God's grace, combined with our confession of faith in Christ, are responsible for bringing about this change of identity. *"Therefore, if anyone is in Christ, he is a new creation; the old has gone, the new has come!"* (2 Corinthians 5:17). That is great news, especially when we consider that the "old" was sinful, unrighteous, and altogether worthless.

■ A New Creation

However, what is this new creation that we have become? *"Yet to all who received him, to those who believed in his name, he gave the right to become children of God—children born not of natural descent, nor of human decision or a husband's will, but born of God"* (John 1:12-13). Being a new creation means that we have become God's children—children of God! Now, that is indeed a new creation! *"How great is the love the Father has lavished on us, that we should be called children of God! And that is what we are!"* (1 John 3:1).

■ Perfect in His Sight

Galatians 2:20 outlines another miraculous aspect of our new identity: *"I have been crucified with Christ and I no longer live, but Christ lives in me. The life I live in the body, I live by faith in the Son of God, who loved me and gave himself for me."*

If Christ—Who is perfect, pure, and holy—lives in us, what does that do to us? It makes us perfect, pure, and holy. Does that mean that everything we do is perfect or that we are perfect? No, but it does make us perfect *in the sight of God*. It is vital to understand that the only way we can move from unrighteousness and sinfulness to holiness is by God's grace. *"For it is by grace you have been saved, through faith—and this not from yourselves, it is the gift of God—not by works, so that no one can boast"* (Ephesians 2:8-9).

Because we are flawed, we don't always behave or do things perfectly. If we could behave and live perfectly on our own, Christ would not have had to die. Just as the verses above explain, if we could earn our salvation by works, we would end up boasting—hardly a pure, perfect, and holy attitude. Galatians adds to this: *"I do not set aside the grace of God, for if righteousness could be gained through the law, Christ died for nothing!"* (2:21). Grace is our ticket to righteousness and holiness. It allows us to be children of God.

This is the new identity of the Christian. By accepting Christ, we become new. He changes us and sees us differently. Righteous, pure, and perfect children of God—that is spiritual wellness.

Endnotes

1. J. I. Packer, *Knowing God* (Downers Grove, IL: InterVarsity Press, 1973), 37.
2. R. Keith Iddings, *Ten Across Workbook* (Marion, IN: Indiana Wesleyan University, 1995), 10-13.
3. The Lutheran Church-Missouri Synod (LCMS), Human Care Ministries, St. Louis, MO. Copyright 1997. Adapted from the InterLutheran Coordinating Committee on Ministerial Health and Wellness. Link to the Wholeness Wheel from http://www.humancare.lcms.org/hm/wheelinfo.htm.
4. N. Keith Hinton, "A Christian Perspective on Attitude," in *A Christian Attitude toward Attitudes*, ed. Everett Leadingham (Kansas City: Beacon Hill Press, 1995), 15.
5. Ibid.
6. Cited during the Nurses Christian Fellowship Conference on Spirituality. Indiana University School of Nursing, October 5, 1998, Indianapolis.
7. E. Arnold, "Burnout as a Spiritual Issue: Rediscovering Meaning in Nursing Practice," in *Spiritual Dimensions in Nursing Practice*, ed. Verna B. Carson (Philadelphia: Saunders, 1989), 324.
8. David Moberg, *Spiritual Well-Being: Sociological Perspectives* (Washington, DC: University Press of America, 1979), 14.
9. As quoted in Gwen Robbins, Debbie Powers, and Sharon Burgess, *The Wellness Way of Life* (Dubuque, IA: Brown, 1989), 12.
10. Moberg, 14.
11. Daniel Fountain, *God, Medicine, and Miracles: The Spiritual Factor in Healing* (Wheaton, IL: Shaw, 1999), 178.
12. Charles R. Swindoll, "Promote Peace," in *Wisdom for the Way: Wise Words for Busy People* (Nashville: Thomas Nelson, 2001), 348.
13. Lewis B. Smedes, *Keeping Hope Alive: For a Tomorrow We Cannot Control* (Nashville: Thomas Nelson, 1998), 6.
14. Ibid.
15. Swindoll, "Hope Revived," in *Wisdom for the Way*, 232.
16. Smedes, *Keeping Hope Alive*, 27.
17. Swindoll, "Nothing Helps Like Hope," in *Wisdom for the Way*, 220.
18. J. I. Packer, *Knowing God*, 37.
19. Donald A. Tubesing and Nancy L. Tubesing, *Seeking Your Healthy Balance: A Do-it-yourself Guide to Whole Person Well-Being* (Duluth, MN: Whole Person Associates, Inc., 1992), 87.

3

PHYSICAL WELLNESS

"Do you not know that your body is a temple of the Holy Spirit, who is in you, whom you have received from God? You are not your own; you were bought at a price. Therefore honor God with your body."

—1 Corinthians 6:19–20 NIV

As we have explained thus far, it is important to examine many dimensions of wellness in order to develop a wholistic wellness perspective. This book considers the spiritual, emotional, physical, social, and occupational aspects of wellness. The purpose of this chapter is to provide a detailed analysis of physical wellness.

Wellness Misconceptions

▪ "But I feel okay"

Many people automatically

OBJECTIVES

- Recognize and define the five elements of physical fitness.

- Recognize the significance the five elements of physical fitness have on daily activities.

- Accurately and objectively evaluate levels of fitness in each of the five areas of physical fitness.

- Develop the capabilities to improve fitness scores in each of the five areas of physical fitness.

- Define and apply the principles of progression, overload, specificity, frequency, intensity, and duration to an individual physical wellness plan.

- Identify and avoid common injuries associated with physical activity.

associate the term "wellness" strictly in terms of physical wellness. This understanding of physical wellness is an oversimplification that often is based on misconceptions. It also can lead to some grave errors in the way we address the various aspects of wellness.

For example, it is not uncommon for people to consider themselves "physically well" simply because they "feel okay" and are not currently in a diseased state. Certainly the idea of "feeling okay" is subjective and nonspecific. We may say, "I feel okay," and then add qualifiers: "as long as I don't overdo it . . . if I pace myself . . . most days . . . with the exception of my (condition; e.g., heartburn, bad knee, etc.)." Additionally, we may be engaging in behavior that is a clearly recognized risk factor for disease. So while we may "feel okay," it is quite possible that our performance in a variety of physical wellness assessment tests would indicate a level of low fitness or poor health.

> # HYPOKINETIC DISEASE:
> A form of lifestyle disease that is directly linked to little physical exercise or activity.

Based on valid research data, many tests provide a clear and objective assessment of one's state of physical wellness. Often, people are surprised that such assessments of their physical wellness are so different from their own assessment of "feeling okay." In the earlier discussion of the World Health Organization's definition of disease, we saw that the idea of physical wellness as strictly *the lack of disease* could not be further from the truth. Many lifestyle diseases are directly associated with a lack of physical activity. This lack of physical activity causes a poor state of physical wellness, placing an individual at an increased risk of lifestyle disease. An example of a **hypokinetic disease** (a form of lifestyle disease directly linked to too little physical exercise or activity) is adult onset diabetes (Type II diabetes). Over 80 percent of Americans with Type II diabetes are considered obese.[1] Obesity, an excessive accumulation of body fat, often is directly related to a lack of physical activity.

■ "But I'm Not Athletic"

Another commonly held misconception regarding physical wellness follows this train of thought: "I surely am not physically well because I am not athletic." The very basis of this argument equates athletic skill with physical wellness. While genetics is a factor, being "athletic" or "good at sports" generally is a result of specific training to learn or master a skill, such as catching a ball or clearing a hurdle. Physical wellness is not skill focused or dependent, but rather is health focused. That is to say, when we focus on health-related outcomes, we strive to increase physical capacity and decrease our risk for disease.

The Five Components of Physical Wellness: An Overview

Physical wellness is the ability to perform daily activities in a safe, capable, and efficient manner, as well as the physical capacity to respond effectively in unusual situations. The goals of physical wellness should be to decrease the risk of disease and to increase overall function and efficiency. We can improve our physical wellness by regularly participating in activities that decrease our risk of disease or injury. Lifestyle choices also affect our risk of injury or disease and run the gamut from dietary habits to our level of physical activity. This chapter focuses on physical activity practices that address and enhance the five components of health-related fitness:[2]

> **PHYSICAL WELLNESS:**
> The ability to perform daily activities in a safe, capable, and efficient manner, as well as the physical capacity to respond effectively in unusual situations.

1. Cardiovascular fitness
2. Body composition
3. Muscular strength
4. Muscular endurance
5. Flexibility

When considering activities and programs for the purpose of enhancing health, it is critical to address all five components. It is possible to have a "high level of fitness" in one area, but a "low level of fitness" in other areas. For this reason, physical fitness programs should include activities designed to enhance each of the five areas of health-related fitness.

■ Cardiovascular Fitness

Cardiovascular disease is the leading cause of death in the United States.[3] It encompasses a wide variety of conditions that negatively impact the heart and/or the arteries and veins that carry blood to and from the heart. While many of these conditions are a direct result of lifestyle choices, regular physical activity can decrease the risk for developing cardiovascular disease. In fact, regular physical activity is one of the primary measures recommended for preventing the onset and reoccurrence of cardiovascular disease. To understand how regular physical activity can help, it is important first to understand some of the basics regarding the cardiovascular system.

■ How It Works

The function of the cardiovascular system is to circulate blood throughout the body. The blood transports oxygen to muscles and organs, which require oxygen to function. The primary components of the cardiovascular system are the heart, arteries, and veins. The heart serves as the pump, circulating blood into the lungs and throughout the body. The veins and arteries serve as the channel or pipeline to deliver blood to all parts of the body. When blood comes into the heart from the body, it is oxygen poor; that is, at the cellular level, a gaseous exchange has occurred in which oxygen is taken out of the blood and exchanged with carbon dioxide (CO_2). The heart pumps the blood into the lungs where CO_2 is discharged from the blood. The blood then picks up oxygen to be circulated through the body. Arteries carry oxygenated blood from the heart to all of the muscles and organs of the body. Veins carry oxygen-poor blood from the body back to the heart.[4]

■ How Physical Activity Helps

Regular physical activity causes a number of changes to occur that allow the cardiovascular system to function more efficiently. The heart is a muscle, and like any muscle, it becomes stronger when exercised. A stronger heart results in an increased **stroke volume,** which is the amount of blood pumped per contraction. An increased stroke volume allows the heart to become more efficient, pumping more blood with less effort. This results in a lower heart rate (HR).

STROKE VOLUME:
The amount of blood pumped by each contraction of the heart.

Another physiological change that occurs in the cardiovascular system as a result of regular physical activity is a lowered resting heart rate (HR_{rest}). A person's resting heart rate is the heart's rate of contraction per minute while the person is at rest, seated, or not performing any activity. Regular physical activity trains the heart to "work" at a higher rate for longer periods of time. While the maximal heart rate (HR_{max}) does not necessarily change with regular exercise, the heart rate reserve ($HR_{reserve}$) does increase. The heart rate reserve is the rate of contraction to which the heart can be elevated for sustained exercise bouts. The $HR_{reserve}$ is calculated based on the HR_{max} and the HR_{rest} (see "Cardiovascular Fitness: Application" later in this chapter). As a result of regular exercise, the $HR_{reserve}$ increases as the HR_{rest} decreases.

Physiological changes in the cardiovascular system are not limited to the heart. They also take place in the veins and arteries. The veins and arteries are flexible and elastic. Certain lifestyle choices (diet and smoking) can cause a decrease in elasticity. Additionally, the arterial walls are more likely to become clogged due to plaque. As the arterial walls become more rigid and thick, blood flow capacity decreases. Regular aerobic physical activity aids in the production of high-density lipoproteins (HDL) or "good cholesterol." Increased HDL levels combat the buildup of plaque. Veins and arteries free of plaque can deliver blood easily and efficiently to the organs and muscles of the body.

In general, as a result of regular cardiovascular activity, the heart is able to pump more blood for longer periods of time at a higher level of intensity. Additionally, the arteries and veins are able to deliver blood throughout the body just as God designed them to do. A strong heart and clean elastic veins and arteries decrease the risk for cardiovascular disease. For more detailed information on the cardiovascular system, refer to chapter 11, "Wellness and Disease Prevention."

> ## Heart Rate
>
> **HR_{rest}:** The rate at which the heart beats when at rest; measured in beats per minute.
>
> **HR_{max}:** The highest heart rate a person can achieve; measured in beats per minute.
>
> **$HR_{reserve}$:** The rate of contraction to which the heart can be elevated for sustained exercise bouts; the HR_{max} minus the HR_{rest}, measured in beats per minute.

■ Body Composition

In health-related fitness, body composition is the component that compares the amount of fat to lean body mass. At first glance, it appears that body composition is an area that scores of people are interested in addressing. However, many of these people mistakenly mean body weight. The difference between body weight and body composition is that body weight only considers total body weight, not the makeup of that weight. The idea behind body composition is to address the makeup of the body and to maintain a low level of body fat regardless of total body weight.

People who only consider total body weight as significant completely miss the importance of the percentage of body fat to good health and reduced risk for disease. It is quite possible to have what is considered to be an acceptable or low body weight and still have a dangerously high level of body fat. As the percentage of body fat increases, so does the risk for lifestyle disease. When the percentage of body fat becomes excessive (>30 percent), a person is considered obese.

Furthermore, as the percentage of body fat increases, the percentage of lean muscle mass decreases, which causes decreased efficiency in movement. It is very common for people with a high percentage of body fat to exercise less because of the difficulty and discomfort in movement. Without regular movement or daily physical activity, the percentage of fat can continue to increase, rising to dangerous levels. It then becomes a vicious cycle: inactivity, increased body fat, increased risk for disease. Extremely obese people often don't exercise because it is too painful. In some cases, unsupervised exercise can lead to injury.[5]

Unless we are involved in regular physical activity, we cannot address the other components of health-related fitness. Without regular physical activity, our risk for lifestyle diseases skyrockets. Proper consideration of body composition is a critical component of health-related fitness. Improved body composition allows for more efficient movement and a better quality of life, along with a reduced risk for lifestyle-related disease.

■ Muscular Strength and Muscular Endurance

Two components of health-related fitness deal specifically with muscular function: muscular strength and muscular endurance. **Muscular strength** is the ability of a muscle or muscle group to exert a maximal amount of force a single time. The classic example of muscular strength is the Olympic athlete who musters all of his energy to lift an incredible amount of weight in a single judged event.

Muscular endurance is the ability of a muscle or muscle group to repeatedly exert a given force. An example of muscular endurance is the worker who daily lifts weight many times throughout the day. The auto mechanic who routinely installs new tires on cars or the delivery woman who handles packages weighing two to fifty pounds both represent muscular endurance. The amount of weight may change drastically, but in all cases it is a sub-maximal amount that is lifted repeatedly. The majority of people can relate to the concept of muscular endurance, because it is something that most of us experience on a daily basis.

> **MUSCULAR STRENGTH:**
> The ability of a muscle or muscle group to exert a maximal amount of force a single time.

■ Learning Your Capability

When considering muscular strength in our daily lives, it is important to remember the occasional need to lift or move very heavy objects. While most people don't perform

MUSCULAR ENDURANCE:
The ability of a muscle or muscle group to repeatedly exert a given force.

"maximal exertion lifts" on a daily basis, we are sometimes required to "give it our all" to lift or move a heavy object. Poor muscular strength can place people in a dangerous situation on those occasions. If we are trying to lift or move something that is near the limits of our muscular strength, safety becomes a paramount issue. Exceeding one's muscular strength can result in torn or strained muscles or connective tissue. Other potentially serious problems include falls, dropping heavy objects on oneself or someone else, broken bones, and entrapment.

MAXIMUM EXERTION:
An effort that is one's maximum capability of work; usually can be performed only once.

A physical activity program that addresses the component of muscular strength can reduce the risk of injury. First, it helps people develop an acute awareness of what they are actually capable of doing. That knowledge is critical in helping to avoid injury. Presuming that the object someone wants to move is within that person's capability (which has been determined because of regular physical activity), this person should be more capable of handling it safely. The proper lifting techniques and practices that we also have learned through routine physical activity decrease our risk of injury when we are required to make a maximal effort. **Maximum exertion** is a person's maximum capability of work. Usually, it can be performed only once. When regular physical activity programs properly address muscular strength, our muscular strength will increase, making us capable of lifting or moving heavier objects. Finally, the training involved

"For physical training is of some value, but godliness has value for all things, holding promise for both the present life and the life to come."
1 Timothy 4:8 NIV

in increasing muscular strength aids in strengthening skeletal structure, which in turn helps to prevent osteoporosis. Increased muscular strength allows us to perform our daily activities safely, effectively, and efficiently, including the occasional maximal lift.

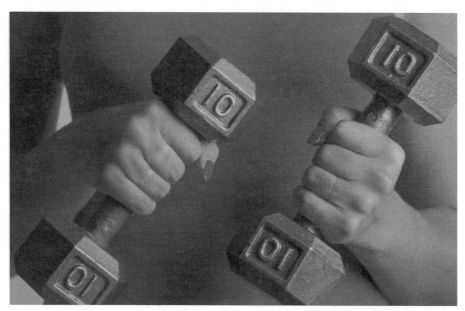

A physical activity program that regularly addresses muscular endurance can directly impact our quality of life.

■ Enhancing Your Performance

Muscular endurance is utilized on a daily basis more than muscular strength. Repeated sub-maximal exertions are far more common in daily life than single maximal exertions. Almost every job requires some type of repeated sub-maximal exertion. The exertion may be as minor as opening mail or as significant as moving furniture or appliances. Low levels of muscular endurance can lead to early fatigue, exhaustion, and lack of concentration. These conditions contribute significantly to the risk of injury or accident. Increased muscular endurance allows workers to end the workday less fatigued and less likely to have an accident due to fatigue.

A physical activity program that regularly addresses muscular endurance can have a direct impact on quality of life. Increased muscular endurance will allow us to do more, to have "energy," to "run and play with the children," and to "finish that project." Increased muscular endurance will enhance recreational pursuits by allowing us to perform better, participate longer, and be less fatigued in the process. As our muscular endurance increases, our ability to perform a given task improves. Along with improved efficiency, increased muscular endurance allows us to be more effective and reduces our risk of injury due to fatigue.

■ Flexibility

When people consider developing a plan for physical activity, they often overlook flexibility. You may think, "Big deal, so I can't touch my toes. What disease will that cause?" One very common ailment associated with poor flexibility is lower back pain. Muscles and muscle groups tend to shorten and become weak if held in one position. Many jobs and lifestyles now involve sitting for prolonged periods of time. The hamstrings, the major muscle group in the back of our legs, can shorten and become weak with prolonged sitting. The hamstrings are anchored in the pelvic region. Shortened or tight hamstrings cause the pelvis to tilt, creating pain in both the hamstring area and the lower back. The problem of lower back pain is widespread and can be very debilitating. Suddenly, touching your toes is indeed a "big deal."

The lives of people who are physically active differ substantially from those who are inactive. Flexibility is very critical in the performance of our daily physical activities in a safe, effective, and efficient manner. After all, how effective are you if you are flat on your back recovering from lower back pain? Regular flexibility exercises improve and maintain joint mobility and range of motion. Another benefit of regular flexibility activity is the correction of muscular imbalances due to tight muscles. Regular physical activity not only helps people feel better and move more efficiently, it triggers several physiological changes in the body that reduce the risk for lifestyle-related disease.

■ Summary

A person involved in a regular physical activity program that addresses cardiovascular fitness, muscular strength, muscular endurance, body composition, and flexibility increases overall capability and reduces the risk for lifestyle disease. Through muscular strength and muscular endurance activities, the regular exerciser strengthens muscles and the skeletal structure, helping to prevent osteoporosis. One muscle that is strengthened with regular exercise is the heart. As the heart is strengthened, cardiovascular function and capability increase and the risk of cardiovascular disease decreases. That translates to a better quality of life, reducing the risk that you will fall to the number-one killer in the United States: cardiovascular disease.

The Principles of Physical Activity

Upon realizing the great benefits of regular physical activity, you may be ready to make some lifestyle changes. Where do you start? How do you know

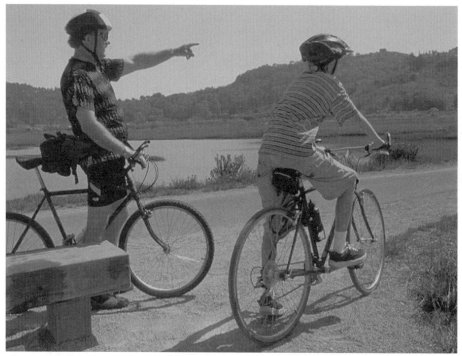

One muscle that is strengthened with regular exercise is the heart.

if you are doing the "right" thing? Just exactly what do you need to do to gain the benefits described previously? In this section, we will outline the basic principles of physical activity. These principles will help you understand the five components of health-related fitness as they relate to your life. Following this section, we will explain how to accurately determine your level of fitness and develop a plan that addresses each area.

▪ The Training Effect

When people begin to participate in regular physical activity, they will experience a condition known as the training effect. The **training effect** is the actual physiological changes that begin to occur as a result of regular physical activity. Some of these changes are a decreased resting heart rate, lower blood pressure, increased cardiac capacity and function, and changes in body composition. So, what does it take to achieve the training effect? Is it necessary to quit one's

TRAINING EFFECT:
The actual physiological changes that begin to occur as a result of regular physical activity.

job and devote oneself to six-hour exercise bouts seven days a week? No. By the same token, it is not reasonable to expect to safely achieve the training effect from one workout session per week. To safely achieve the training effect, people need to utilize multiple workout sessions or exercise bouts per week. Normally, they can begin to experience the training effect with a routine that includes aerobic activity three times per week at twenty to thirty minutes per session.

■ The F.I.T. Formula

One of the very first issues you will address when you consider a physical activity program is time.

- How long do I exercise?
- How often do I exercise?
- Are there minimums or maximums?
- Am I capable of immediately starting a program three times per week for twenty to thirty minutes per session?
- How can I objectively determine how many sessions are right for me, how hard they should be, and how long they should last?

> To answer these questions about the specifics of an individual exercise program, the F.I.T. formula is extremely useful:[6]
>
> **F** stands for **frequency** or how often you exercise.
> **I** stands for **intensity**, which is how hard you exercise.
> **T** stands for **time** or how long you exercise in each session.

Of particular importance is the direct correlation between the number of calories people expend and the number, intensity, and duration of exercise sessions in which they participate. As they increase any aspect of the F.I.T. formula, they increase the number of calories they will expend. Every carefully thought-out physical activity program addresses the F.I.T. formula. Table 3.1 shows the number of calories expended per hour for several popular activities.

A word of caution should go out regarding the F.I.T. formula. Most likely, beginning exercisers will be at a low level of fitness that requires very short exercise bouts and fewer sessions per week. As beginning exercisers continue to improve, their bodies will begin to adapt. The body changes because the effort required for the physical activity is an overload of the normal workload. Progress occurs because of this overload.

Table 3.1. Physical Activity Calorie Use Chart

The chart below shows the approximate calories spent per hour by a 100-, 150- and 200-pound person doing a particular activity.

Activity	100 lb	150 lb	200 lb
Bicycling, 6 mph	160	240	312
Bicycling, 12 mph	270	410	534
Jogging, 7 mph	610	920	1,230
Jumping rope	500	750	1,000
Running, 5.5 mph	440	660	962
Running, 10 mph	850	1,280	1,664
Swimming, 25 yds/min	185	275	358
Swimming, 50 yds/min	325	500	650
Tennis singles	265	400	535
Walking, 2 mph	160	240	312
Walking, 3 mph	210	320	416
Walking, 4.5 mph	295	440	572

Source: American Heart Association, Inc. Retrieved 5-20-2003 at www.americanheart.org.

■ The Overload Principle

The overload principle states that for physical improvement or adaptation to occur, the activity performed must be at a level that is greater (overload) than the normal level. The overload can come in the form of increased frequency, intensity, or duration, or a combination of all three. Care must be taken to avoid too much overload; otherwise, you risk physical injury, which then prevents you from further exercise and any health benefits that would result. Typically when applying the overload principle to an exercise routine, you only would overload one or two elements of the F.I.T. formula at a time.

Common injuries that can occur as a result of an overly aggressive application of the overload principle include muscle soreness, inflammation, blisters, general fatigue, and a decrease

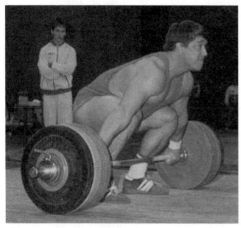

Care must be taken to avoid too much overload.

in physical capability. More serious injuries include overuse injuries such as stress fractures, tendonitis, and muscle tears or strains. It is important to remember when applying the overload principle that there is a point of diminishing returns. What this means is that if you increase frequency, intensity, and/or duration too rapidly, your risk for injury is far greater than your potential for any physical or health-related benefits. The key to safely applying the overload principle is to utilize the principle of progression.

■ Principle of Progression

When a person regularly and consistently participates in a physical activity program, physiological changes begin to take place as a result of overload and adaptability. The changes are a response to the body's adaptation to the increased physical workload of the exercise program. In practical terms what happens is that the exerciser learns how to complete the same amount of work faster, or accomplish more work at the same or lower intensity levels. As the body changes due to adaptation, what once was an overload is no longer an overload.

> "The average American takes 20 years to get out of condition and he wants to get back in condition in 20 days— and you just can't do it."
>
> **Dr. Ken Cooper**
> *Faith-Based Fitness*

Suppose a beginning exerciser develops a program in which she walks twenty minutes per session, three times per week at a moderate intensity. During the twenty-minute exercise bouts, she normally covers one mile. After a few weeks of regular and consistent exercise, she realizes that she is covering more distance than one mile without changing her intensity level or exercise duration. Her body has adapted to that particular form of exercise. The body adapts to physical activity in a gradual and normal progression. You are following the principle of progression when to achieve continued increases in capability you gradually and progressively increase the frequency, intensity, or duration of your exercise routine by utilizing the overload principle.

■ Combining the Overload and Progression Principles

The safest way to increase performance and health-related benefits is to successfully combine the overload principle and the principle of progression. The first step is to determine your physical activity goals.[7] Compare your goals to your current capabilities and consider an appropriate time frame for reaching your goals. One point to bear in mind is that when an unconditioned (out of shape) person begins a regular physical activity program, that person's gains in physical capability (progression) can sometimes be very large and occur quickly. As physical conditioning improves, the gains occur in smaller increments over longer periods of

BASELINE PERFORMANCE:
The level of performance achieved at the onset of a physical activity program; the starting point.

time. The better an individual's physical condition, the slower the rate of progression.

A clear illustration is to compare the beginning exerciser with a world-class track athlete. The new exerciser begins a walking program after years of physical neglect. At the onset of his activity program, it takes him twenty minutes or more to walk one mile. After four years of regular, consistent, and progressive aerobic training, the previously inactive person is capable of running multiple miles in ten minutes or less. During that same time period, the world-class athlete performs a very strenuous activity program, a program that is far greater in intensity, frequency, and duration than the beginning exerciser's program. Yet the world-class athlete only improves his physical performance in the mile run by a few seconds or even fractions of a second.

Be Conservative and Systematic

When developing an exercise program, determine your current level of fitness, and what you want it to be. Plan the program with reasonable progression and allow adequate time to achieve your goals. You will find several health-related physical activity assessment tests later in this chapter to help you determine baseline capabilities and reasonable health-related fitness ratings and goals. **Baseline performance** is the level of performance at the onset of a physical activity program—the starting point. When combining the overload principle and the principle of progression, the safest alternative is to be conservative (gradual) and systematic. To repeat, avoid overloading all three elements of the F.I.T. formula at once, or even overloading any single area. Journaling or logging your routine specifics is a wonderful way to safely apply the principle of progression.

Avoid increases in frequency, intensity, or duration that are greater than 10 percent of current F.I.T. levels. Allow time for your body to

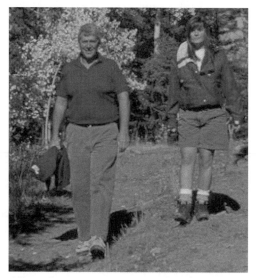

Allow adequate time to achieve your fitness goals.

recover and adapt to the overload. If you exercise three times per week and are increasing one of the elements of the F.I.T. formula by 10 percent each week, every fourth week remain at the same level without an increase. After a week without an increase, you can continue your normal rate of progression.

As your physical capability increases, allow longer amounts of time for adaptation to occur. You may not be able to increase every week—it may be reasonable to increase only once per month. Your rate of progression is highly personal and you should monitor it closely, both to stay on track for health-related fitness goals and to avoid injuries. Once you achieve your goal, realize that you may need to readjust your goals for further improvement as your body adapts. If you are satisfied when you reach your goal, maintain that level of activity to stay at the goal level. As adaptation occurs, it even may be possible to decrease your amount of activity and stay at the goal fitness level.

> "My life is a gift to me from my Creator. What I do with my life is my gift back to the Creator."
>
> **Billy Mills**
> **1964 Olympic 10,000-meter champion and former world record holder in the six-mile run.**

■ Why People Don't Exercise

Hundreds of thousands of people don't exercise on a regular basis. Hundreds of thousands of others begin an exercise program, but soon quit. Think about the people in your circle of acquaintance. How many of them regularly exercise? How many have started an activity program and then quit? In order to achieve any health-related benefits from a physical activity program, you must adhere to the program. People list many reasons for not taking part in a regular physical activity program. Among the most common excuses are these:

- Not enough time
- Don't know what to do
- Lack of equipment
- Self-conscious about appearance
- Too hard or painful

If the proper motivation is in place, you easily can address any or all of the above excuses. What motivates people to exercise? People who regularly take part in physical activity cite the following:

- Health-related fitness benefits
- Physical challenge
- Recreation
- Enjoyment
- Improved physical appearance
- Competition

Move Past the Excuses

If people can move past the excuses and focus instead on the benefits of regular physical activity, they easily will overcome these perceived barriers to greater health. The most prevalent excuse for physical inactivity is time. However, health-related fitness benefits can be achieved by exercising as little as three times per week for twenty minutes—a mere one hour per week! To ensure that you make the time for exercise, write this hour into your schedule.

Some people prefer to exercise first thing in the morning before any of their other commitments. That way, nothing in their busy day will push exercise out of their schedule. Others prefer to exercise at lunchtime or in the evening. Whatever time best fits your schedule, write it into your routine. Scheduling exercise is important, because it is easier to stick to a schedule than to "make time" later in the day.

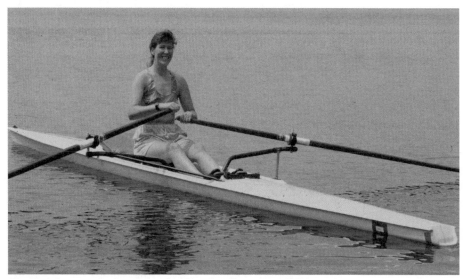

The idea that exercise has to be "hard" to be effective is invalid.

With a good understanding of the F.I.T. formula, the overload principle, and the principle of progression, the excuse of "not knowing how" becomes invalid. Also invalid is the idea that exercise has to be "hard" to be effective.

That brings us to the excuse of being "too self-conscious" about one's current physical appearance. There are several ways to address that issue. With exercise videos or home equipment, self-conscious people can begin an exercise or activity program in the privacy of their own homes. With some creativity, they don't even need special equipment to exercise at home. Other options for the self-conscious exerciser include exercising after dark, exercising in a gender-specific environment or with family members. After achieving some health-related fitness benefits and changes in body composition and shape, many people overcome self-consciousness and are able to exercise more freely in public settings. The reluctant exerciser also may see that the benefits are too valuable to lose, regardless of the excuse.

■ The Principle of Specificity

With the groundwork completed on how long, how often, and how hard to progress, the next question to ask is: "What do I do?" Proper activity selection is critical for achieving desired health-related fitness goals. The principle of specificity states that in order to improve performance or fitness in a particular health-related fitness area, the training must be specifically for that area of health-related fitness. For example, to improve cardiovascular fitness, we need to perform a cardiovascular activity. To improve muscular strength or endurance, we must perform muscular strength or endurance activities.

While some activities provide "crossover" improvements, the greatest gains come when activity specifically matches fitness goals. An example of crossover improvement would be the modest cardiovascular gains achieved from a circuit-training routine geared toward development of muscular endurance. Muscular endurance gains will occur at modest levels from aerobic training, but the greatest gains for muscular endurance come from a routine of resistance training.

To apply the principle of specificity to the five components of health-related fitness, select activities that provide the greatest gain for the particular area you are trying to develop. To carry the principle of specificity even further, activity selection should be specific to the activity you want to improve. While swimming, walking, and cycling all improve cardiovascular fitness, the best way to improve cardiovascular fitness *and* running performance is to run. When applying the principle of specificity to muscular strength and muscular endurance, the training must be specific for both the muscle/muscle group *and* the movement.

■ The Categories of Physical Activity

Exercises are often grouped into broad terms that are developed based on the physiology of the activity. It is important to be familiar with these terms when planning an activity program.

Aerobic v. Anaerobic

Aerobic exercise is a widely used term and can include any number of specific types of exercise from dance to stair climbing. **Aerobic activities** require the use of large muscle groups, are performed at a sub-maximal intensity, and can be maintained for sustained periods of time. The cardiovascular system is able to provide the body with enough oxygen to continue the activity for extended time periods. Other examples of aerobic activity include walking, jogging, running, swimming, cycling, cross-country skiing, continuous calisthenics, and skating.

AEROBIC ACTIVITY:
Any activity that utilizes the large muscle groups, is performed at a submaximal intensity, and can be maintained for a sustained period of time.

We do not hear the term anaerobic exercise as much as we hear aerobic exercise. **Anaerobic activities** require the use of large muscle groups, are high intensity (maximal or near-maximal efforts), and are performed for short periods of time. Anaerobic activity may be intermittent, but not continuous. During anaerobic activity, the body is not able to provide sufficient oxygen to continue the activity for sustained efforts. Examples of anaerobic activities include sprinting, football, baseball, some forms of weight training, and interval training.

ANAEROBIC ACTIVITY:
Any activity that utilizes the large muscle groups and is performed at maximal or near-maximal intensity for short periods of time.

Some activities can be considered aerobic or anaerobic, depending on the skill level of the participant. Tennis, racquetball, handball, and volleyball are good examples of such activities. Someone with a high skill level, who is able to play continuously for more than twenty minutes, would consider these activities aerobic. However, someone with a low skill level, who is unable to play for a long period of time, would consider these activities anaerobic.

Resistance Training

Resistance training involves contracting muscles or muscle groups against some type of resistance. The resistance can be a movable object or an immovable object. It even can involve contracting against the force of another muscle or muscle group. Resistance training falls into one of three groups based on what type of muscular contraction is involved.

1. **Isotonic contractions** are contractions in which the resistance is a movable object, and the muscle or muscle group changes length. Equipment used for isotonic contractions is readily available and familiar to most people. It includes free weights, resistance bands, weight machines, and even the weight of one's own body.

2. **Isokinetic contractions** are contractions in which the resistance also comes from a movable object and the muscle/muscle group changes length. However, in an isokinetic contraction, the rate of contraction, intensity of resistance, and angle of contraction are controlled by a piece of exercise equipment. The equipment used for an isokinetic contraction is specialized and substantially more expensive than other types of resistance equipment.[8]

3. **Isometric contractions** are contractions against an immovable object; consequently, the contracted muscle or muscle group does not change length. Isometric contractions require little or no equipment and can be performed virtually anywhere. For example, stand in a door frame and press your hands against either side of the door frame. You have just completed an isometric exercise. However, muscular strength and endurance are improved only for the specific movement you practice, and only for the specific angle of the joint. Generally speaking, isometric contractions are not the most practical for improving overall muscular strength and endurance.

> **Resistance Training**
>
> **isotonic:** A contraction in which the resistance is a movable object and the muscle/muscle group changes length.
>
> **isokinetic:** A contraction in which the intensity, angle of contraction, and rate of contraction are constant.
>
> **isometric:** A contraction in which the muscle/muscle group does not change length and the object of resistance is immovable.

■ Goal Setting for Health-Related Fitness

Aerobic, anaerobic, isometric, isotonic, and isokinetic are all categories of physical activity with positive and negative attributes. How do you determine what type of exercise to include in your activity program? Which exercise is best for you? Which activity is most available? You should ask all these questions before designing a personal physical activity program.

However, one question needs to precede all others: "What are my health-related physical wellness goals?" The more specific your goals are, the easier it will be to develop a safe and effective physical activity program. It is not enough to simply say, "I want to get in better shape." Your goals must be measurable; otherwise, you won't be able to determine your progress toward your goals. "Better shape" is too vague and not accurately measurable.

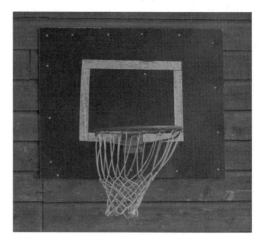

Select an activity that you enjoy.

The key in setting measurable goals is to be specific. To be able to jog two miles in twenty minutes is a very specific and measurable goal. So is the goal to lose ten pounds. Progress towards measurable goals can be monitored and adjustments made as necessary. Sometimes progress will be so swift that the difficulty of the goal will have to be increased. At other times it may become apparent that the goal is not realistic. You then adjust and continue.

When thinking of your physical activity goals, think in specific terms for each of the five components of health-related fitness: cardiovascular fitness, muscular strength, muscular endurance, body composition, and flexibility. A great way to determine health-related fitness goals is to perform a number of different health-related assessment tests and set goals for improvement over your (initial) performance. Think through your goals and then record them for future planning, monitoring, and adjustment.

■ Activity Selection

After you have determined your health-related fitness goals, you need to consider the specificity principle. What activities will actually help you to reach your goal? Make a list of all the activities you can think of that would aid you in reaching your goals. Be creative, specific, and exhaustive when developing your list of activities. Start by itemizing your goals into categories: cardiovascular fitness, muscular strength, muscular endurance, body composition, and flexibility. Under each category, brainstorm and list as many activities as you can that might help you in that category. Be bold and inclusive; this is still the selection process. Just because you list an activity, doesn't mean that activity will be included in your personal program. Although you might think you really would enjoy a particular activity, your current fitness or skill levels may not allow you to participate in that activity. List it anyway! Fitness and skill can be developed; maybe later down the road, you actually will be able to participate in those activities.

What Would You Like to Do?

After you have developed an exhaustive list of activities that will help you to reach your health-related fitness goals, ask yourself, "What do I like to do?" What activities on the list do you actually enjoy or think you would enjoy? Go a step further and consider whether you like to exercise in a group or alone. If you like to exercise with others, be cautious when selecting an exercise partner. Make sure that person's goals and objectives match and do not contradict your goals and objectives. If your cardiovascular goals are to exercise for health-related benefits three times per week at a moderate intensity, don't select an activity partner who is

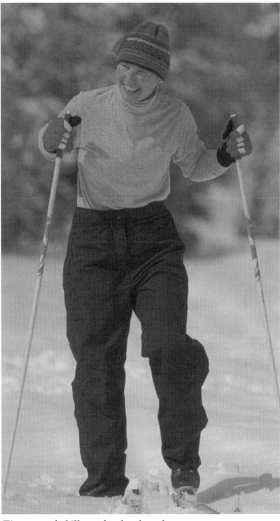

Fitness and skill can be developed.

preparing for a fifty-mile ultra-marathon. Both sets of goals are too different for either one of you to achieve your objectives.

If you prefer to exercise alone, don't join a basketball league or aerobic dance class. Selecting an activity you enjoy may sound basic, but all too often people begin an exercise program that centers on an activity they really don't enjoy. The outcome of that choice is very predictable—they don't adhere to the exercise program and eventually quit. After you have decided what activities you like or think you would enjoy, highlight them on your list.

What Is Available?

The next question to ask is: "What is available?" It is important to select activities that are readily available to you. Cross-country skiing is an excellent cardiovascular activity that many people enjoy. However, if you live in Florida, it is not practical to develop your activity plan around cross-country skiing—unless you plan to use a cross-country ski machine. More common examples might be, "I enjoy lifting weights, but live forty-five minutes from a gym" or "I love to swim, but there's no indoor pool available to me." If you enjoy seasonal activities or those that are available only when you take a vacation, include those as supplemental activities. Don't plan to build your exercise routine around those activities. Look at your list of highlighted activities and circle the items that are readily available to you.

What Will You Stick With?

Next ask yourself: "What will I stick with?" Examine your list and think about activities that you will continue for the long term. What activities can become part of your lifestyle? It is important to include a few options in this area. Your first and second options should be activities that are readily available, are enjoyable, will provide some variety to your routine, and will help you meet your goals.

Be sure to have a third option. Maybe it is something that is seasonal or not always available on a daily basis. Maybe it is a weekend activity. For example, perhaps you are developing your cardiovascular fitness level by walking daily, but also enjoy long mountain-bike rides on the weekend. Allow enjoyable activities to serve as additional motivation to continue consistently in your primary routine. For your primary activity option, choose something you will stick with. You won't receive any health-related fitness benefits if you quit because you either don't like the activity or you can't always perform the activity due to unforeseen

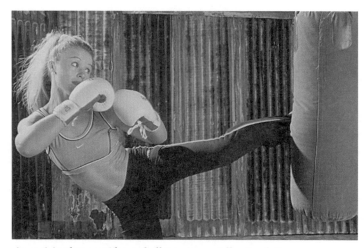

An activity that provides a challenge is mentally stimulating.

circumstances. Circle the items on your list that you believe will be your three best options for reaching your goals.

What Will Challenge You?

Finally, ask yourself: "What will challenge me?" An activity that provides a challenge is mentally stimulating. If the activity of choice provides a challenge, there is room to raise your goals as your fitness and skills improve. Place an asterisk beside the items on the list that provide an element of challenge.

If you were exhaustive and specific, you should have listed several activities in each area that will help you reach your goals. If you asked yourself the aforementioned questions, you likely have selected what best will help you attain your goals. Once you have selected your activities, it becomes clear that you don't necessarily have to think in terms of aerobic v. anaerobic, or isometric, isokinetic, or isotonic. There are times when the type of exercise you select is critical for specific performance goals. However, when you select activities meant to help achieve health-related fitness goals, adherence is a far more important issue. Exercise adherence is best achieved when you are involved in an activity that meets the four criteria above (enjoyment, availability, variety, and goal/objective completion). When you adhere to your exercise plan, the health-related fitness benefits will follow. The activities on your list that you have highlighted, underlined, and marked with an asterisk should be the basis for your physical activity plan.

Measuring the Components of Wellness

In the first section of this chapter, we briefly outlined the five components of physical wellness: cardiovascular fitness, muscular strength, muscular endurance, body composition, and flexibility. In this section, we will look at these components in more detail, with an emphasis on applying them to your personal wellness program.

■ Cardiovascular Fitness: Application

To reiterate, cardiovascular fitness has to do with the body's ability to perform aerobic activity. Improved cardiovascular fitness increases functional capacity for daily activities, helps in maintaining body composition, and lowers the risk of developing lifestyle-related diseases.

Cardiovascular fitness can be determined or measured in a variety of ways. The most accurate method involves measuring maximum oxygen uptake ($\dot{V}O_2max$); i.e., the maximum amount of oxygen the body can utilize during a maximal intensity physical assessment test.[9] A maximal intensity physical assessment test involves exercising at increasing intensities to the point of exhaustion. The test can be conducted by way of a few different modalities, including the most common types: stationary cycling and treadmill running. However, there are some hindrances to widespread $\dot{V}O_2$max testing. The equipment is expensive and not readily available, the tests are complex and must be administered by trained professionals, and most people are not interested in exercising to the point of exhaustion.

Other laboratory tests that calculate $\dot{V}O_2$max are sub-maximal in nature and rely on mathematical equations to extrapolate a $\dot{V}O_2$max score. Sub-maximal tests are accurate and can be performed in a variety of protocols. Other cardiovascular fitness tests that are available don't necessarily provide a $\dot{V}O_2$max score, but rather provide a rating of fitness level. One such test is the Rockport Walking Test.[10]

■ The Rockport Walking Test

To conduct this cardiovascular fitness test, you need a measured mile course, and a stopwatch. You should warm up sufficiently and then walk one mile as fast as possible without running. After walking one mile, record your time and check your pulse rate. It is best to take a fifteen-second heart rate (HR) and multiply that figure by four to determine your per-minute heart rate. To perform a fifteen-second HR, locate either your carotid or radial pulse and count the number of contractions that occur during a fifteen-second time span. Longer or shorter HR counts can skew accuracy of the actual per-minute HR. After you have your mile time and your ending HR, determine your fitness rating from the tables below:

Table 3.2, One-Mile Fitness Zones

Male

Mile Time			
	18:00-22:00	with a HR of 220-140	Low Fitness Zone
	15:00-22:00	with a HR of 220-120	Marginal Fitness Zone
	12:00-20:00	with a HR of 220-120	Good Fitness Zone
	8:00-17:00	with a HR of 220-120	High Performance Zone

Female

Mile Time			
	16:00-20:30	with a HR of 220-138	Low Fitness Zone
	14:00-20:30	with a HR of 220-120	Marginal Fitness Zone
	12:00-19:00	with a HR of 220-120	Good Fitness Zone
	10:00-17:00	with a HR of 220-120	High Performance Zone

Once you have determined your level of cardiovascular fitness, you can begin to plan your activity program to improve or maintain your level of fitness.

According to the principle of specificity, the best way to improve cardiovascular fitness is to be physically active in cardiovascular (aerobic) activities. If regularly performed, the following aerobic activities will in time lead to improved cardiovascular fitness:

Exhibit 3.1, Aerobic Activities to Improve Cardiovascular Fitness			
Walking	Rowing	Stationary Cycling	Hiking
Jogging	Cross-Country Skiing	Aerobic Dance	Continuous Calisthenics
Running	Skating	Stair Climbing	Skipping Rope
Cycling	Swimming		

Also: Use of Aerobic Exercise Equipment (Elliptical Trainers, Recumbent Cycles, Ski Machines, and Arm Ergometers)

Compare this list to the list of activities you compiled earlier. Select the activities that you plan to include in your personal activity plan.

■ Calculating Heart Rate

While preparing an aerobic activity plan, it is a good idea to set intensity based on HR calculations.

1. First determine your maximum heart rate (HR_{max}) HR_{max} = 220 - Age (years)

2. Next determine your resting heart rate (HR_{rest}) by checking your pulse first thing in the morning, or when you are completely at rest. Count for one full minute or take a fifteen-second HR count and multiply by four.

3. After you have determined your HR_{max} and HR_{rest}, calculate a value known as heart rate reserve ($HR_{reserve}$) using the Karvonian Method:

$$HR_{reserve} = HR_{max} - HR_{rest}$$

4. Finally, for best health-related benefits, aerobic activity should be performed at an intensity of 60-80 percent of $HR_{reserve}$. The beginning exerciser should start at 60 percent $HR_{reserve}$ and increase as fitness improves.

Lower Limit for Aerobic Training = $HR_{reserve}$ x 60 percent
Upper Limit for Aerobic Training = $HR_{reserve}$ x 80 percent

Once you have calculated your lower and upper heart rate limits, you have a range of heart rates in which you should try to stay for best progress towards cardiovascular fitness goals. Inexpensive heart rate monitors that can aid the exerciser in training are readily available at most sporting goods stores. Some heart rate monitors have alarms that allow you to program your lower and upper limits; if your intensity changes in such a way that you are no longer in the 60-80 percent zone, the alarm will sound. You then check your current rate and adjust your intensity level as needed to stay within the appropriate zone.

If you don't have a heart rate monitor, you can check your pulse rate periodically throughout your exercise routine. You should have a good idea of your intensity level by taking a reading midway through your routine and again at the end of your routine. The more you participate in the activity, the better you will become at accurately gauging your level of intensity.

■ A Good Place to Begin

When considering the F.I.T. formula for cardiovascular fitness training, a frequency of three times per week is a good place to begin. This allows the body adequate time to recover between sessions. It is also easier for beginning exercisers to fit three times per week into their schedules. Regarding intensity, it is important to remember that beginning exercisers should start at an intensity level of approximately 60 percent of their $HR_{reserve}$. As the body adapts, there is room to increase intensity, which is not to exceed 80 percent of $HR_{reserve}$. While activity duration should start within a conservative time frame, it should still be an overload. As adaptation occurs, exercisers can progressively increase any of the elements of the F.I.T. formula to provide continued improvement for cardiovascular fitness.

Remember not to do too much too soon or you will risk injury. After several weeks or a few months of regular and consistent cardiovascular training, you may want to take the Rockport Walking Test again to see how your fitness rating has improved. Make sure not to "test" yourself too often—it takes time to improve fitness. The higher the level of fitness, the longer improvement will take. A good recommendation for cardiovascular fitness testing is once every six to twelve months. This can provide valuable information for adjusting your activity plan as needed.

■ Body Composition: Application

The area of body composition is very important for health-related fitness. As the percentage of body fat increases, the risk for lifestyle-related diseases also increases.

Additionally, as body fat increases, functional capacity decreases. Body composition is measured by the percentage of the body that is made up of fatty tissue. A wide variety of testing procedures can determine the percentage of body fat, but hydrostatic weighing is recognized as the most accurate method.[11] Hydrostatic weighing means weighing the body while under water to determine the percentage of body fat. Although accurate, hydrostatic weighing involves a great deal of expensive and specialized equipment, must be conducted by trained professionals, and can be a scary and time-consuming process for the individual being tested.

A more common method to determine body fat composition is known as a skin fold test. When determining body composition by a skin fold test, measurements are taken with skin fold calipers at several specific points on the body. The scores are mathematically compiled to arrive at a percentage of body fat. For best health-related fitness,

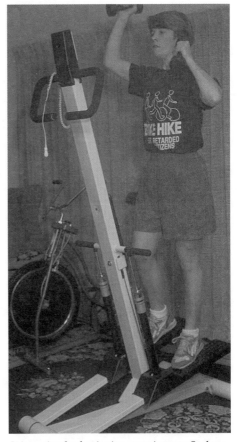

It is easier for beginning exercisers to fit three times per week of exercise into their schedules.

men should be between 10-20 percent body fat and women should be between 18-25 percent body fat. Scores in excess of 25 percent for men and 30 percent for women carry the rating of obese. Some deterrents to skin fold testing include skewed accuracy if more than one test administrator is used, the reliability of test administrators, and the availability of accurate equipment (which is quite expensive; however, inexpensive and modestly accurate equipment is widely available). In addition, modest people are often uncomfortable with the sites that require measurement.

■ Calculating BMI and WHR

Other testing protocols for body composition provide a fitness rating, require a minimum of equipment, and can be self-administered. The Body Mass Index (BMI) is one such testing protocol. The Waist-to-Hip Ratio Test (WHR) is also easy to conduct and provides a general fitness score as opposed to a percentage of body fat.

The Body Mass Index is calculated by dividing body weight by height squared.

$$\text{BMI Score} = \frac{\text{body weight (kg)}}{(\text{height in meters})^2}$$

Calculate your weight in kilograms by dividing your weight in pounds by 2.2. To determine your height in meters, multiply your height in inches by the constant of .0254. The following is an interpretation of BMI Scores:

Exhibit 3.2, BMI Risk Zones

	Male	Female
High Risk Zone	$\geq$27.8	$\geq$27.3
Marginal Risk Zone	25.0-27.7	24.5-27.2
Good Fitness Zone	19.0-24.9	18.0-24.4
Low Fitness Zone	17.9-18.9	15.0-17.9

A low score does not equate to lower risk. On the contrary, a low BMI score or too little percentage of body fat is associated with a myriad of health problems and increased risk for lifestyle-related disease. The ideal is to score in the Good Fitness Zone.

The Waist to Hip ratio is easily calculated by dividing the hip measurement into the waist measurement.[12] The waist circumference is measured 2-3 inches above the belly button. Measure the largest circumference around the buttocks for the hip measurement. Ideally, the waist circumference should be smaller than the hip circumference.

Exhibit 3.3, WHR Risk Zones

Classification	Male	Female
High Risk	>1.0	>.85
Moderately High Risk	.90-1.0	.80-.85
Lower Risk	<.90	<.80

Average Waist/Hip Ratio Scores

Men 17-39 years old	.80
Women 17-39 years old	.90
Men over 39 years old	.90
Women over 39 years old	.98

After determining a body composition classification by either a BMI test or WHR test (or both), the beginning exerciser can make specific body composition goals. Be sure to remember when developing goals that body composition is more critical to health-related fitness than body weight. Furthermore, muscle weighs more than fat, so it is possible that a beginning exerciser may initially increase weight because of changes taking place in body composition. That should not be a concern, because if the beginning exerciser continues regular activity, weight loss should follow. In order to lose weight, the best activities should be aerobic in nature, and the frequency should be at least five times per week. If weight loss is not a concern, frequency can begin at three times per week. The exerciser also should address intensity and duration as noted in the cardiovascular fitness section of this chapter.

■ Muscular Strength and Endurance: Application

While muscular strength and muscular endurance are different components of health-related fitness, they have some similarities during testing. The most significant similarity is that both components can be tested only on a specific muscle/muscle group and movement. In other words, there is no single test to determine total body strength or muscular endurance. It is entirely possible to have a very high level of strength or endurance in one muscle or muscle group and a low strength or endurance score in a different muscle or muscle group. To accurately measure muscular strength or endurance, you must measure each muscle/muscle group individually. The beginning exerciser can adequately determine muscular strength and muscular endurance by a combination of a few specific exercise tests.

■ Determining 1-RM Strength

The standard type of measurement for muscular strength is the one-repetition maximum (1-RM). A one-repetition maximum is the amount of weight you can lift (through a specific motion) one time; it is a maximal effort. It can be difficult to determine accurately and safely where to start when trying to do a 1-RM lift. If you start with too little resistance, you will require continual increases in resistance until you work up to 1-RM. These increases can cause fatigue, which can hinder an accurate maximal score. If you start with too much resistance, you run a substantial risk of injury. Muscle tears or strains become a real possibility, along with the risk of dropping the weight or becoming pinned beneath the weight.

For safety measures it is of vital importance to utilize at least one "spotter" during a maximal strength test. A **spotter** serves as a safety precaution in weight lifting, helping to make sure you don't lose control of the weight you are lifting. In the event of an emergency, the spotter can prevent you from dropping the weight or becoming pinned beneath the weight.

SPOTTER: Someone who serves as a safety precaution in weight lifting; prevents the exerciser from dropping the weight or becoming pinned beneath the weight.

The safest way to determine 1-RM is to perform a sub-maximal lift and extrapolate the 1-RM score. You can do this by performing a sub-maximal lift and calculating a 1-RM based on your performance of the sub-maximal lift. The type of sub-maximal lift to be used in calculating a 1-RM is known as a ten-repetition maximum (10-RM). You perform a 10-RM in the same manner as a 1-RM, except you determine the amount of weight you can lift ten times to the point of fatigue. The 10-RM is safer because you are not dealing with as great an amount of weight as a 1-RM. It also should be easier to handle than the weight of a 1-RM. Research indicates a direct relationship between 10-RM and 1-RM. As the 10-RM increases, so does the 1-RM. In general, a 10-RM is equivalent to 75 percent of the 1-RM. Determine your 10-RM weight, and you can quickly calculate your 1-RM using the following formula:

$$1\text{-RM} \ = \ \frac{10\text{-RM}}{.75}$$

While this type of calculation is an estimate and not 100 percent accurate for determining 1-RM, it is much safer than performing an actual 1-RM lift. For the beginning exerciser, the 10-RM is a great place to start when determining 1-RM strength.[13]

Establishing a Baseline

The beginning exerciser can establish a baseline of muscular strength by determining a 1-RM weight for a few different major muscle groups. The bench press and leg press 1-RM are often utilized to provide the muscular strength 1-RM baseline. However, any muscle/muscle group and motion can be tested. Remember that muscular strength is specific to each motion or muscle group tested. If you do not need to test specific movements or muscle groups to meet your personal goals, then go with the bench press and leg press. The movements can be completed in almost any weight-lifting facility, and each of these lifts requires the use of large muscle groups. You can determine a muscular fitness rating for each lift by calculating your strength per pound of body weight. Use the following formula to determine your strength per pound:[14]

$$\text{Strength Per Pound} = \frac{\text{1-RM lbs.}}{\text{Body Weight lbs.}}$$

After you have calculated your strength per pound, you can use Table 3.3 and Table 3.4 to determine your muscular fitness rating. These tables include figures for both bench press and leg press tests, categorized for males and females. While there is no single test to determine total body strength, the bench press and leg press tests are good indicators of upper and lower body strength respectively.

Table 3.3, Upper Body Strength*†

		Age				
	Percentile	20–29	30–39	40–49	50–59	60+
Men	90	1.48	1.24	1.10	.97	.89
	80	1.32	1.12	1.00	.90	.82
	70	1.22	1.04	.93	.84	.77
	60	1.14	.98	.88	.79	.72
	50	1.06	.93	.84	.75	.68
	40	.99	.88	.80	.71	.66
	30	.93	.83	.76	.68	.63
	20	.88	.78	.72	.63	.57
	10	.80	.71	.65	.57	.53
Women	90	.90	.76	.71	.61	.64
	80	.80	.70	.62	.55	.54
	70	.74	.63	.57	.52	.51
	60	.70	.60	.54	.48	.47
	50	.65	.57	.52	.46	.45
	40	.59	.53	.50	.44	.43
	30	.56	.51	.47	.42	.40
	20	.51	.47	.43	.39	.38
	10	.48	.42	.38	.37	.33

*One repetition maximum bench press, with bench press weight ratio = weight pushed/body weight.

Source: American College of Sports Medicine, *ACSM's Guidelines for Exercise Testing and Prescription,* 6th ed. (Baltimore: Lippincott Williams & Wilkins, 2000), 82. † Data provided by the Institute for Aerobics Research, Dallas, TX (1994). Study population for the data set was predominately white and college educated. A Universal dynamic variable resistance (DVR) machine was used to measure the 1-RM. The following may be used as descriptors for the percentile rankings: well above average (90), above average (70), average (50), below average (30), and well below average (10).

Table 3.4, Leg Strength*†

	Percentile	Age 20–29	30–39	40–49	50–59	60+
Men	90	2.27	2.07	1.92	1.80	1.73
	80	2.13	1.93	1.82	1.71	1.62
	70	2.05	1.85	1.74	1.64	1.56
	60	1.97	1.77	1.68	1.58	1.49
	50	1.91	1.71	1.62	1.52	1.43
	40	1.83	1.65	1.57	1.46	1.38
	30	1.74	1.59	1.51	1.39	1.30
	20	1.63	1.52	1.44	1.32	1.25
	10	1.51	1.43	1.35	1.22	1.16
Women	90	1.82	1.61	1.48	1.37	1.32
	80	1.68	1.47	1.37	1.25	1.18
	70	1.58	1.39	1.29	1.17	1.13
	60	1.50	1.33	1.23	1.10	1.04
	50	1.44	1.27	1.18	1.05	.99
	40	1.37	1.21	1.13	.99	.93
	30	1.27	1.15	1.08	.95	.88
	20	1.22	1.09	1.02	.88	.85
	10	1.14	1.00	.94	.78	.72

*One repetition maximum leg press, with leg press weight ratio = weight pushed/body weight.

Source: American College of Sports Medicine, *ACSM's Guidelines for Exercise Testing and Prescription,* 6th ed. (Baltimore: Lippincott Williams & Wilkins, 2000), 82. † Data provided by the Institute for Aerobics Research, Dallas, TX (1994). Study population for the data set was predominately white and college educated. A Universal dynamic variable resistance (DVR) machine was used to measure the 1-RM. The following may be used as descriptors for the percentile rankings: well above average (90), above average (70), average (50), below average (30), and well below average (10).

■ Determining Muscular Endurance

To test muscular endurance, determine the maximum number of repetitions (muscular contractions) you can complete. Examples include the push-up, the chin-up, and the partial curl-up (crunch) test. Tables 3.5 and 3.6 below convert raw scores into percentile by age groups and gender. Measuring muscular endurance is the same as muscular strength in that it is specific to muscle/muscle groups and motion.

To perform the push-up muscular endurance test, simply do as many push-ups as possible. If you are a male, ask a partner to position his fist under your chest, so that each time you go to the "down" position, you must touch his fist. The subject must extend arms to the "locked" elbow position. If you are a female, you may perform a modified or bent-knee push-up. Both males and females should keep their backs straight at all times during the test. After you have determined the maximum number of push-ups you can do, compare your test score to the table below for a percentile rating.

To correctly perform the partial curl-up (crunch) test, lie flat on the ground with your legs bent in a 90-degree angle and your feet flat on the floor, approximately eighteen inches apart. Your hands should be at your side touching

Table 3.5. Percentiles by Age Groups and Gender for Push-ups*

| Percentile | Age | | | | | | | | | |
| | 20–29 | | 30–39 | | 40–49 | | 50–59 | | 60–69 | |
Gender	M	F	M	F	M	F	M	F	M	F
90	41	32	32	31	25	28	24	23	24	25
80	34	26	27	24	21	22	17	17	16	15
70	30	22	24	21	19	18	14	13	11	12
60	27	20	21	17	16	14	11	10	10	10
50	24	16	19	14	13	12	10	9	9	6
40	21	14	16	12	12	10	9	5	7	4
30	18	11	14	10	10	7	7	3	6	2
20	16	9	11	7	8	4	5	1	4	—
10	11	5	8	4	5	2	4	—	2	—

Source: American College of Sports Medicine, *ACSM's Guidelines for Exercise Testing and Prescription,* 6th ed. (Baltimore: Lippincott Williams & Wilkins, 2000), 85. *Based on data from the Canada Fitness Survey, 1981. (Reprinted from Canadian Standardized Test of Fitness (CSTF) Operations Manual. 3rd ed. With permission of Fitness Canada, Fitness and Amateur Sport Canada, Ottawa, 1986.) The following may be used as description for the percentile rankings: well above average (90), above average (70), average (50), below average (30), and well below average (10).

a piece of masking tape. Place a second piece of masking tape beyond the first piece (8 cm beyond for those 45 years of age or older, or 12 cm beyond for those less than 45 years of age). The participant should slowly curl up lifting the shoulder blades off the floor. The hands should remain on the floor and slide to the tape beyond the starting position. It is important to flatten the lower back before each curl-up. At the rate of 20 curl-ups per minute (a metronome is helpful in maintaining pace; set it at 50 beats per minute), complete as many as possible (up to 75). The total number completed is your raw score. Compare it to the table below for a muscular endurance sit-up percentile rating.

Table 3.6. Percentiles by Age Groups and Gender for Partial Curl-up*

| Percentile | Age | | | | | | | | | |
| | 20–29 | | 30–39 | | 40–49 | | 50–59 | | 60–69 | |
Gender	M	F	M	F	M	F	M	F	M	F
90	75	70	75	55	75	50	74	48	53	50
80	56	45	69	43	75	42	60	30	33	30
70	41	37	46	34	67	33	45	23	26	24
60	31	32	36	28	51	28	35	16	19	19
50	27	27	31	21	39	25	27	9	16	13
40	24	21	26	15	31	20	23	2	9	9
30	20	17	19	12	26	14	19	0	6	3
20	13	12	13	0	21	5	13	0	0	0
10	4	5	0	0	13	0	0	0	0	0

Source: American College of Sports Medicine, *ACSM's Guidelines for Exercise Testing and Prescription,* 6th ed. (Baltimore: Lippincott Williams & Wilkins, 2000), 86. *Based on data from the Canadian Standardized Test of Fitness Operations Manual. 3rd ed. Ottawa: Canadian Society for Exercise Physiology in cooperation with Fitness Canada, Government of Canada, 1986. The following may be used as descriptors for the percentile rankings: well above average (90), above average (70), average (50), below average (30), and well below average (10).

■ Use Your Imagination

A common misconception regarding muscular endurance and strength training is that it requires bulky and expensive equipment or membership in a health club. On the contrary, methods of strength training are limited only by the imagination of the exerciser. For example, calisthenics utilize body weight as resistance. Other creative forms of resistance include household items. Milk jugs, juice containers, and canned goods are great sources for variable resistance training. You can adjust the resistance by how much you fill the jugs. The jugs can be filled with liquid, sand, or gravel for even greater variation in the resistance. When searching for household items to use for muscular endurance and strength training, use not only imagination, but also common sense regarding safety issues. Avoid items that are difficult to grip or that are unstable.

More traditional modalities for muscular endurance and strength training include free weights, universal style machines, resistance bands, and plyometric training equipment. In selecting the "best" exercise modality, reference your previously developed list of activities and select an activity that best fits your needs. The principle of specificity is very important in resistance training. Be sure to include motions and muscles/muscle groups that are specific to your health-related fitness goals and objectives. Remember the F.I.T. formula: the basic guideline for strength training is fewer repetitions at greater resistance (intensity). For muscular endurance training, the focus is on lower resistance (intensity) and greater repetitions. For the beginning exerciser, two days per week of resistance training is usually enough to reach health-related physical wellness goals for muscular strength and endurance.

■ Flexibility: Application

Flexibility testing is specific to joints and motions in much the same way that muscular strength and endurance training are specific to muscles and motions. Testing for flexibility is no different from other physical performance tests in that there are a myriad of testing protocols and procedures. Because flexibility is specific to the joints to be tested, no single test can determine total body flexibility. For the beginning exerciser, it would not be practical or desirable to test flexibility for all of the joints of the body. Two easily administered tests for flexibility are the Modified Sit and Reach Test and the Trunk Rotation Test. Before you conduct the Trunk Rotation Test, gather the following equipment: two yardsticks, one roll of masking tape, and one partner. You may wish to do some warm-up exercises before these tests. To perform the Trunk Rotation Test, follow the directions below:

1. Tape two yardsticks to the wall at shoulder level.
2. When facing the wall, the yardstick on the left should be placed right side up and the yardstick on the right upside down.
3. Mark a line on the floor perpendicular to the wall. The line should be at the 15-inch mark on the yardstick.
4. With your toes on the edge of the line marked on the floor, stand one arm's length (left arm, fist closed) from the wall.
5. Drop your left arm to your side and raise your right arm to shoulder height parallel to the ground.
6. Rotate at the trunk (waist) to your right —do not move your feet or bend at the trunk.
7. Rotate as far as possible and hold for two seconds.
8. Have a partner record the spot reached on the yardstick to the nearest half-inch.
9. Perform the rotation twice, average your score, and record.
10. Face the opposite direction and repeat the test for the left side, rotating to the left with your left arm raised at shoulder height, parallel to the ground.
11. Compare your scores to the Trunk Rotation Fitness Ratings in Table 3.7 below to determine a fitness level.

Table 3.7, Trunk Rotation Fitness Ratings		
Classification	**Male**	**Female**
High Performance Fitness Zone	$\geq$20"	$\geq$20.5"
Good Fitness Zone	16-19.5"	17-20"
Marginal Fitness Zone	13.5-15.5"	14.5-16.5"
Low Fitness Zone	$\leq$13"	$\leq$14"

To complete the Modified Sit and Reach test, you need a rigid box approximately 15 inches long, one yardstick, one roll of masking tape, and a partner. To perform the Modified Sit and Reach Test, follow the directions below:

1. Sit on the floor with your hips and back against the wall. Do not wear shoes.

2. Place a rigid box or bench (approximately 15 inches long) at your feet.

3. Without bending your right leg at the knee, place the sole of your right foot flat against the box/bench (you may bend your left leg at the knee).

4. While keeping your back and hips against the wall, extend your arms toward the box as far as possible.

5. Have a partner hold a yardstick on top of the box.

6. After you have extended as far as possible without moving your hips or back from the wall, have your partner slide the yardstick to your fingertips, then affix the yardstick in the new position with tape.

7. Now bend at the waist, reaching as far forward as possible without bending your right leg at the knee. Relax and repeat. Relax and repeat a third time. On your third try, when you are extended as far as possible, hold for two seconds and have your partner record the score to the nearest inch. Repeat the procedure and record the score again. Average the two scores to arrive at a right hamstring flexibility score.

8. Repeat the entire procedure with the sole of the left foot against the box/bench. Remember not to bend the left leg at the knee (you may bend the right leg at the knee).

9. Transfer your scores to the table below for a fitness rating score for each leg.

Table 3.8, Hamstring Flexibility Fitness Ratings

Classification	Male	Female
High Performance Fitness Zone	$\geq 16"$	$\geq 17"$
Good Fitness Zone	13-15"	14-16"
Marginal Fitness Zone	10-12"	11-13"
Low Fitness Zone	$\leq 9"$	$\leq 10"$

When training for improved flexibility, it is important to know that several variables directly impact flexibility. Among these are age, gender, muscle temperature, and ambient temperature. Flexibility peaks at adolescence, unless regular stretching exercises are performed to improve flexibility. Decreases in physical activity lead to decreases in flexibility. Consequently, many people have a decrease in flexibility as they age because they become less active. Females tend to be more flexible than males. The cooler the ambient and muscle temperatures, the poorer the flexibility. It is best to perform stretching exercises after the muscles have been sufficiently warmed up. Muscles generally can be warmed by five to ten minutes of light activity.

■ Stretching Exercises

Stretching exercises fall into two broad categories: static and dynamic. When you move into a stretched position and hold that position for a period of time, you are performing a static stretch. Static stretches are characterized by a lack of movement or motion. On the other hand, dynamic stretching exercises involve a great deal of movement or motion.

To perform a static hamstring stretch, stand with your feet shoulder-width apart and bend forward at the waist, reaching toward the floor. Once you have gone as far as possible, hold the position for five to thirty seconds. The dynamic hamstring stretch is performed the same way, except that once you extend as far as possible, you straighten up and then repeat the movement several times.

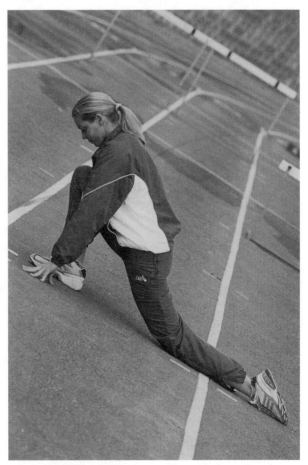

Proper flexibility training is an important component of overall physical wellness.

Static stretching is widely considered to be much safer than dynamic stretching, especially for the beginning exerciser. Brief stretches are recommended at the beginning of an exercise session to prepare the muscles and connective tissue for the ensuing activity. After exercise, stretching for longer periods of time is indicated for gains in flexibility. In flexibility stretching exercises, just as with any other of the health-related components of fitness, overload determines the amount of improvement. Overload in flexibility occurs when muscles are stretched beyond their normal capacity. The body learns to adapt, and the principle of progression can be applied for continued improvement.

> "Next to a leisurely walk, I enjoy a spin on my tandem bicycle. It is splendid to feel the wind blowing in my face and the springy motion of my iron steed. The rapid rush through air gives me a delicious sense of strength and buoyancy, and the exercise makes my pulse dance and heart sing."
>
> **Helen Keller**
> *The Story of My Life*

When applying the F.I.T. formula to a flexibility routine, be sure to coordinate it with other physical activities. Stretching easily can be worked in before and after these physical activities. Effective stretching before and after these activities will help to prevent injury and will speed recovery. Frequency for stretching exercises can be daily; a minimum frequency should be every time you perform any other exercise. Include a brief session before exercise and a slightly longer session following your exercise bout.

While intensity for stretching should be an overload, it should be a very moderate overload for the beginning exerciser. Stretch only to the point of slight discomfort. As your body adapts, you will be able to stretch further before you experience discomfort. Avoid stretching that causes high levels of discomfort or pain. The time component of flexibility training will vary greatly from individual to individual. Usually, five to ten minutes before exercise and ten to twenty minutes after exercise is enough. Some people combine stretching with deep breathing to aid in stress relief. Stretching is also incorporated into many types of martial arts. As with all physical activity, the F.I.T. formula is specific to you and your goals.

Flexibility is often overlooked when people consider an activity program. However, proper flexibility training is key to preventing injury, maximizing potential, and maintaining free movement. It is an important component of overall physical wellness.

Take Action!

Just as wholistic wellness is a whole divided into several smaller components, so is physical wellness. If we think strictly in terms of physical wellness as a whole, it can become an overwhelming and confusing notion to improve our current state of fitness. Physical wellness involves so many areas that we must break it down into manageable components. These components are cardiovascular fitness, body composition, muscular strength, muscular endurance, and flexibility.

By following the guidelines in this chapter, you can safely, accurately, and objectively determine your current level of fitness. From these assessments, you can begin to plan your physical wellness activity program. With the knowledge of some basic exercise principles, you can implement a safe and effective exercise routine. Finally, with guidelines on how to choose activities and get started, you have all the tools you need to improve your life.

Regular physical activity not only can greatly enhance the length of your life, but also the quality of your life. Many of the other components of wholistic wellness are directly related to and impacted by physical wellness. Improved

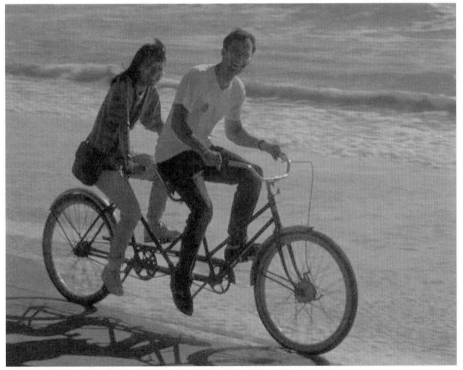

Regular physical activity can enhance the quality of your life.

KEY CONCEPTS

aerobic activity
anaerobic activity
baseline performance
hypokinetic disease
isokinetic contraction
isometric contraction
isotonic contraction
maximum exertion
muscular endurance
muscular strength
physical wellness
spotter
stroke volume
training effect

physical wellness through regular physical activity can augment every other area of wholistic wellness.

This chapter has provided the basic information you need to determine and improve your current level of fitness. Physical wellness is such a critical component of general wellness that you should be motivated to action. Take the assessment test, formulate a plan, and change your life. James 1:22 NIV says, *"Do not merely listen to the word, and so deceive yourselves. Do what it says."* What a fitting admonishment regarding physical wellness. Don't deceive yourself—do what you know needs to be done!

Learning Activity

1. According to the assessment tests available in this chapter, what were your health ratings for the five components of physical wellness?

_____

_____

_____

_____

_____

2. As a result of reading this chapter, what three physical wellness goals would you like to establish for yourself?

_____

_____

_____

3. What three exercise activities did you identify as appropriate for your goals?

_____

_____

_____

4. What two activities that you enjoy would be more enjoyable if you were at a higher level of physical wellness?

_____

_____

5. List three individuals or groups that can aid you in reaching your physical wellness goals.

_____

_____

_____

6. What are some anticipated barriers to reaching your physical wellness goals? How will you overcome these barriers?

_____

_____

_____

_____

7. Review the following resources to gain additional insights and information concerning physical wellness:

http://www.acsm.org/

http://www.americanhiking.org

http://www.bicycling.com

http://www.caloriesperhour.com/

http://www.cooperaerobics.com/

http://www.exercise.about.com/

http://www.nof.org

http://www.runnersworld.com

http://www.swiminfo.com

Endnotes

1. Robert Hockey, *Physical Fitness: The Pathway to Healthful Living*, 8th ed. (Boston: McGraw-Hill, 1996), 11.

2. Charles B. Corbin, Ruth Lindsey, Gregory J. Welk, and William R. Corbin, *Concepts of Fitness and Wellness: A Comprehensive Lifestyle Approach*, 4th ed. (Boston: McGraw-Hill, 2002), 11, 46, 149, 84.

3. Gordon Edlin, Eric Golanty, and Kelli McCormack Brown, *Health and Wellness*, 6th ed. (Sadbury, MA: Jones and Bartlett Publishers, 1999), 10.

4. Henry Gray, *Gray's Anatomy—The Anatomical Basis of Medicine and Surgery,* eds. P. L. Williams, R. Warwick, et al., 37th ed. (Edinburgh: Churchill Livingstone, 1989).

5. American College of Sports Medicine, *Guidelines for Exercise Testing and Prescription*, 5th ed. (Baltimore: Williams & Wilkens, 1995), 216, 53, 58, 59.

6. Corbin, Lindsey, Welk, Corbin, *Concepts of Fitness and Wellness*, 46.

7. American College of Sports Medicine, *Resource Manual for Guidelines for Exercise Testing and Prescription*, 2nd ed. (Philadelphia: Lea and Febiger, 1993), 337.

8. Ted Baumgartner and Andrew Jackson, *Measurement for Evaluation in Physical Education and Exercise Science,* 5th ed. (Madison, WI: Brown and Benchmark, 1982), 208.

9. G. M. Kline, J. P. Porcari, R. Hintermeister, et al., "Estimation of $\dot{V}O_2$max from One-Mile Track Walk, Gender, Age and Body Weight," *Medical Science Sport Exercise*, vol. 19, no. 3 (1987): 253-59.

10. Ibid., 206-07.

11. American College of Sports Medicine, *Resource Manual for Guidelines for Exercise Testing and Prescription*, 236.

12. Ibid., 235.

13. Matt Brzycki, "Assessing Strength: You Can Assess Muscular Strength in a Safe, Efficient Manner by Using Formulas That Do Not Require Clients to Attempt Maximum Lifts," *Fitness Management Magazine* (June 2000) [Online] http://www.fitnessmanagement.com/cgi-bin/layout.pl?htmlfile=/info/info.

14. Cedric X. Bryant and James A. Peterson, "Measuring Strength: Assessing Client's Muscular Fitness Need Not Be a Costly Process," *Fitness Management Magazine,* vol. 11, no. 7 (June 1995): 32-34, 37. Available online at http://www.fitnessworld.com/info/info_pages/library/strength/measure695.html.

Additional References

Textbox quotations in this chapter were taken from:

Kenneth Cooper, *Faith-Based Fitness* (Nashville: Thomas Nelson, 1995).

Mark Will-Weber, ed., *The Quotable Runner: Great Moments of Wisdom, Inspiration, Wrongheadedness, and Humor* (New York: Breakaway Books, 1995), 277, quoting Billy Mills.

Bill Strickland, *The Quotable Cyclist: Great Moments of Bicycling Wisdom, Inspiration, and Humor* (New York: Breakaway Books, 1997), 82, quoting Helen Keller.

4

EMOTIONAL WELLNESS
AND STRESS

"You will break the bow if you keep it always bent."

—Greek proverb[1]

Emotional wellness is a broad category that can mean many different things. In the context of this book, emotional wellness refers to one's personal foundational outlook and attitude, particularly as these relate to the people and situations encountered each day. Human emotion is a complicated subject and can involve numerous aspects that interact and influence human behavior. Among these aspects are:

- **Emotion**—a feeling that results in both physical and psychological reactions

- **Feeling**—an emotional state or reaction; an emotion or sensitivity

EMOTION: The interactions of your feelings, attitudes, and thoughts, along with a personal awareness that these factors can influence the choices and decisions you make.

- **Attitude**—a manner of feeling and an indicator of a mental or emotional state
- **Thought**—ideas and outlooks prevalent at a given time

Emotion in this text focuses on the interactions of feelings, attitudes, and thoughts, along with a personal awareness that these factors can influence the choices and decisions we make. The goal of emotional wellness is to direct these influences in a positive way so that the choices and decisions we make will have a positive impact on our lives.

Developing Awareness and Control

Personal awareness and personal control are important for developing positive emotional wellness. By personal awareness and personal control we mean:

- Awareness of personal emotions (self and others)
- Developing positive coping styles in dealing with emotions
- Developing a positive way of expressing emotional states

■ Primary Points of Awareness

Daniel Goleman emphasizes this sense of awareness and control in his book, *Emotional Intelligence*.[2] He states that emotional intelligence is a personal awareness of the choices available in responding to a given situation. Primary points of awareness in making a choice of response include these:

- Self–awareness (recognizing personal feelings)
- Recognizing the links between thoughts, feelings, and reactions
- Awareness that thoughts and feelings can direct a decision
- Seeing the consequences of a decision
- Applying those insights to a decision-making process
- Taking personal responsibility for decisions

- Following through on commitments
- Respecting differences in how individuals feel about things
- Distinguishing between what someone says or does and your reactions

■ Two Sides of the Picture

As with many topics, the topic of emotion has both a positive and negative side. Positive emotions can include feelings of hope, gratitude, peace, joy, optimism, and happiness. Negative emotions can include feelings of anxiety and/or fear, hostility, depression, pessimism, and guilt.

Medical research confirms that consistently negative emotional states can have adverse effects on individual health and longevity, not to mention the quality of one's life. Conversely, consistently positive emotional states have been shown to strengthen the immune system and positively affect personal health and well-being.[3] The appropriate expression of negative emotions, combined with the presence of positive emotions, seems to strengthen human immune system function.[4]

Before we turn our attention to cultivating positive emotional well-being, let's first look at some negative emotional states and how they can affect our

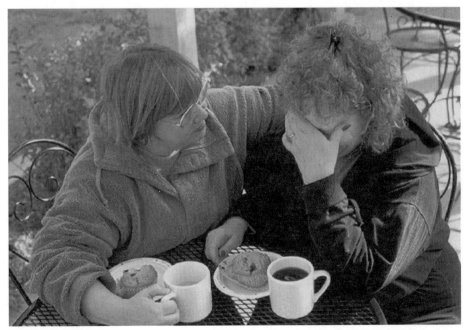

Negative emotions can include feelings of anxiety, fear, hostility, depression, pessimism, or guilt.

well-being. Being aware of these negative states, their symptoms, and their potential consequences should provide positive motivation for change.

A Look at Negative Emotional States

■ Depression: More Than Just Sad

It is normal to experience periods of sadness. However, depression is more severe than merely a state of sadness. **Depression** often is described as a loss of pleasure in life, a sense of hopelessness, and a perception that days are filled with disappointment. Along with this sense of hopelessness is a belief that one's life is meaningless and has no real purpose.[5] These feelings and perceptions can be accompanied by a sense of low self-esteem. As this vicious cycle continues, the feelings of hopelessness and lack of purpose can pull self-esteem to even lower levels.

The common symptoms of depression may include these:[6]

- Feeling sad, down in the dumps
- Not finding much to make one happy
- Feeling tired and weak
- Inability to make decisions
- Not eating or sleeping much

If these symptoms continue for an extended period of time, it can be helpful to evaluate any situations or conditions that may be causing these symptoms. Depression can significantly influence one's physical and psychological health, actually suppressing the function of the human immune system. Goleman reports that in a study involving patients diagnosed with kidney disease, depression was a stronger predictor of death than were any other related medical conditions.[7]

DEPRESSION: A loss of pleasure in life, a sense of hopelessness and/or meaninglessness.

Depression commonly takes two forms. *Mild* forms of depression are temporary and usually disappear with the passage of time. *Clinical* or severe forms of depression usually are longer in duration and can require treatment through the use of antidepressant drugs.

Physical and psychological well-being seem to have a positive correlation. Due to this relationship, exercise and various forms of physical activity can help to counter feelings of depression. However, individuals suffering from depression often do not have the internal motivation to participate in these activities. It may take the support or encouragement of another individual to overcome this barrier, helping the victim of depression to develop and maintain a positive commitment.

■ Guilt: Living "Down"

Feelings of **guilt** commonly arise from a sense either that we have done something we believe we *should not* have done or we have failed to do something we believe we *should* have done.[8] Along with the feeling of guilt can come a sense of self-blame, a feeling of culpability for an imagined offense or from a sense of inadequacy. Self-blame means we believe we are bad and that our worth as individuals will be judged in a negative way—because we did or did not do whatever our "*should* or *should not* statement" implies. Guilt feelings can degrade our sense of personal worth. In our minds, without any factual documentation, we can create a negative label for ourselves and then begin to *live down* to that label.

> **GUILT:** A feeling of culpability for an imagined offense or from a sense of inadequacy.

Another negative often associated with guilt is a lack of action. Planning appropriate action steps and committing to follow through on our action steps can help to lessen our sense of guilt (e.g., planning time to be with family members). The previous section on depression explains that support and assistance from others can help in planning and completing the necessary action steps.

■ Anxiety: A Toxic Emotion

Everyone at one time or another will experience anxiety, which is a form of fear. **Anxiety** can be defined as a sense of crisis at a particular moment, possibly involving a perceived threat, fear, tension, and/or apprehension. Anxiety is commonly associated with chronically overactive stress responses, negative thoughts that usually run wild, and a state of constant worry that focuses on a worst-case scenario. When anxiety becomes dominant in one's life, it can interfere with

> **ANXIETY:** A sense of crisis at a particular moment, possibly involving a perceived threat, fear, tension, and/or apprehension.

daily functioning.[9] Unlike people with depression, individuals who experience anxiety often are attempting some coping responses.[10]

Healthy fear is realistic and normal. Its purpose is positive since it can provide a sense of protection. Healthy anxiety also can include personal awareness of and response to our environment and what is going on around us. Healthy anxiety is beneficial because it can prepare us to deal with various situations in our lives and help us to address any challenges our environment may present.[11]

Neurotic anxiety is not realistic, but is made up of distorted thoughts. It is considered to be a toxic emotion and often creates a barrier toward positive steps for change and development.[12]

■ Two Classifications

> Anxiety is commonly classified into two types:
>
> 1. **Trait anxiety,** which means the anxiety/fear can appear in various kinds of situations, or is considered to be more of a consistent personal trait.
>
> 2. **State anxiety** is dependent upon a situation and may appear only in certain specific situations; e.g., having to present a speech or take a math exam.

The level of anxiety also can make a difference as to how it influences an individual. A high level of anxiety often can decrease one's ability to perform or to respond to a stimulus. On the other hand, a moderate amount of anxiety can increase one's ability to perform or respond. Low levels of anxiety correlate with fewer physical symptoms, while higher levels of anxiety seem to weaken the immune system, adversely affect the cardiovascular system, and become a factor in chronic pain.[13]

TRAIT ANXIETY: Appears in various kinds of situations; a consistent personal trait.

Personal well-being depends on an awareness of the danger of crossing the line between healthy fear and neurotic anxiety. There is a similar line between good stress and bad stress. Taking corrective action means knowing *when* to take corrective action.

STATE ANXIETY: Appears only in specific situations.

Excerpt 4.1, The Effects of Hostility

Young adults who scored high on a test of their hostility levels were 2.5 times more likely to have signs of heart disease 10 years later than those who were rated average or below, a study found. The study was published in the May 2000 issue of the *Journal of American Medical Association.*

Researchers studied 374 people – a nearly equal mix of women and men, blacks and whites – who were 18 to 30 in 1985. They were given a 50-question test that asked them to respond to true/false statements such as: "I have at times had to be rough with people who were rude to me" and "No one cares much what happens to you."

Ten years later, they underwent a heart scan to measure calcium deposits in their arteries, an indicator of heart disease. Seventeen percent of those who scored above average on the hostility test showed calcification, compared with 9 percent in the below-average group. Researchers put the risk at 2.5 times higher for the high-hostility group after adjusting for other factors.

The study was led by Dr. Carlos Iribarren of the Kaiser Permanente Medical Care Program of Oakland, California. He said one reason for the difference could be that hostile people release more stress hormones that raise blood pressure and can lead to heart disease.

Source: Based on Carlos Iribarren, et al., "Association of Hostility with Coronary Artery Calcification in Young Adults: The CARDIA Study," *Journal of the American Medical Association* 283 (17 May 2000): 2546-51.

■ Hostility: Injurious Anger

Hostility is a form of anger. We all experience moments of anger; however, hostility takes anger to a higher level. We generally think of the term hostility as a negative approach to other people. This usually occurs through internal, abusive thoughts or external, abusive statements to or about the individual involved. In its worst form, hostility appears as a predisposition to injure others either physically or verbally.[14]

Hostility does not foster interpersonal relationships. Generally, a hostile person is

- dominant and forceful
- easily excited
- easily frustrated
- aggressive when challenged
- usually not helpful to others

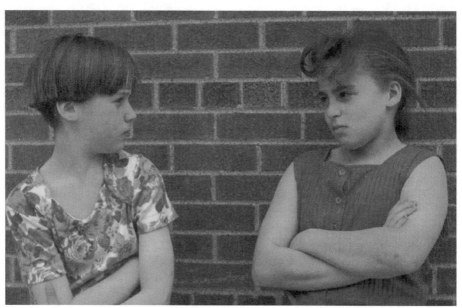

Hostility does not foster interpersonal relationships.

- unforgiving
- untrusting

HOSTILITY: A negative approach to other people; can include abusive thoughts, statements, and actions.

In addition to damaging relationships with others, hostility can damage personal health. It is classified as a significant factor in cardiovascular disease. Hostility can contribute to high blood pressure, coronary artery disease, and death. One potentially dangerous consequence of hostility is that it can decrease the pumping efficiency of the heart. This factor has not been derived from other negative emotional states—only hostility, indicating the grave consequences of this dangerous emotion.[15]

"Be gentle and ready to forgive; never hold grudges. Remember, the Lord forgave you, so you must forgive others."

Colossians 3:13

Expressions of hostility usually decrease from adolescence to mid-life. Occasional expressions of hostility may not result in dangerous physical consequences. However, chronic expressions of hostility will influence the occurrence of the negative signs and symptoms just mentioned.[16]

■ Pessimism: Progression of Defeat

We commonly define **pessimism** as a belief that negative thoughts and outlooks outweigh the positive, along with an expectation of the worst in a given situation. Our thoughts and outlooks can provide a personal foundation for how we explain daily situations and events. A pessimist believes a situation will never change and accepts the majority of the blame for negative outcomes. There's a progression of defeat as a pessimist strings together negative generalizations: (1) I did poorly on this math test, (2) I will do poorly on all math tests, (3) I will always do poorly in math, (4) I am not capable of learning math. Outlooks and generalizations such as these underscore the pessimist's reputation for being hopeless and incapable of change.[17] Considering options for change, developing a plan for change, or even simply asking for assistance seem out of the pessimist's reach.

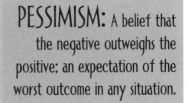

PESSIMISM: A belief that the negative outweighs the positive; an expectation of the worst outcome in any situation.

It is easy to see why pessimism can lead to depression. A sense of hopeless inevitability—that no matter what actions or changes one makes, the outcomes will be negative—can lead to carelessness about personal health habits; e.g., smoking, drinking, and lack of exercise.

Stress and Your Emotional State

Stress and negative emotional states seem to share a close relationship. Stress may be the single most significant negative factor influencing personal well-being. Stress can rob us of peace and can fuel a generally negative emotional state. This negative emotional state is mirrored in negative outlooks and attitudes, which create major barriers to positive physical, emotional, and spiritual well-being. When stress gets a foothold, we can become trapped in a cycle of negativity—unaware of options that might help us cope with stressful events or, worse still, unwilling to believe that those options can help us in any way. Further, the negative emotional states brought on by stress can lead to an increased perception that stress will always have the upper hand, leading to a belief that one's life is "out of control."

In order to cope in positive ways with negative emotional states and with stressful events, it is important to better understand how stress influences an individual's life and the negative physical, emotional, and spiritual consequences that can develop from stress.

Stress: What Is It?

What is stress?

- Is it the cause of your response to demands on your life?
- Is it your response to stressful demands?
- Is it the name given to your emotional state as the result of stressful demands, the signs and symptoms of being "under stress"?

STRESS: A combination of the demands people experience and the negative outcomes these demands create in their lives.

Ask ten people for a definition of **stress,** and you will receive ten different responses. Stress is an individualized concept and a difficult term to define. F. Roberts expresses that difficulty in his definition of stress: "Stress, in addition to being itself and the result of itself, is also the cause of itself."[18]

Stress is a negative and vicious cycle that can influence every area of personal well-being. As the above questions indicate, stress can be the actual cause of a stress response, the outcome of a stressful situation, and/or the signs and symptoms that a stressful experience can create. For the purpose of discussion in this textbook, stress is defined as a combination of the demands people experience and the negative outcomes these demands create in their lives.

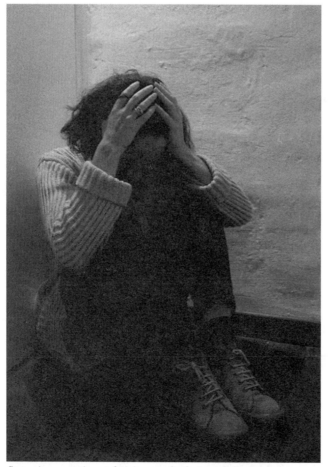

Stress is a negative and vicious cycle that can influence every area of well-being.

Excerpt 4.2, The Aspirin Age — A Formula for Success

Whoever dubbed our times "The Aspirin Age" didn't miss it by very far. It is correct to assume there has never been a more stress-ridden society than ours today. For many, gone are the days of enjoying bubbling brooks along winding pathways or taking long strolls near the beach. The relaxed bike ride through the local park has been replaced with the roar of a motorcycle whipping its way through traffic. And the easy-come, easy-go lifestyle of the farm has been preempted by a hectic urban family going in six different directions . . . existing on instant dinners, shouting matches, strained relationships, too little sleep, and too much television.

Add financial setbacks, failure at school, unanswered letters, obesity, loneliness, a ringing telephone, unplanned pregnancies, fear of cancer, misunderstanding, materialism, alcoholism, drugs, and an occasional death; then subtract the support of the family unit, divide by dozens of opinions, multiply by 365 days a year, and you have the *makings of madness*! Stress has become a way of life; it is the rule rather than the exception.

Source: Charles R. Swindoll, *Man to Man* (Grand Rapids: Zondervan, 1996), 325. Used by permission.

■ A Two-Sided Coin

Charles Swindoll sees stress as a primary reason our culture today is called the "Aspirin Age" (see Excerpt 4.2). Stress also has been referred to as the modern epidemic of the industrialized world. Hans Selye, one of the first to research stress and its influence on the human body, stated that stress is a nonspecific response of the body to any demand placed upon it. He explained that stress is not necessarily a bad thing and that stress cannot and should not be avoided.[19]

Stress in life is inevitable. We are all going to experience it, probably on a daily basis. Stress is like a coin—it is two-sided. On the positive side, stress can motivate us to think, help us to expand our awareness, and assist us in being more creative. On the reverse side, the negative side, stress can weaken the immune system, place us at a greater risk for lifestyle diseases, or spur us to develop a negative outlook toward life.

Eustress: Positive Stress

Positive stress often can motivate in a helpful, practical way. Realizing that you have a work project or a school paper due in four weeks can motivate you to begin planning an outline for the project and to take some initial action steps during the first few days. Positive stress that motivates and provides positive outcomes and actions is called **eustress.** Eustress is usually observed in the form of a cycle involving positive actions, behaviors, and/or attitudes toward the demand that has initiated your response.

EUSTRESS: Positive stress that motivates and leads to positive outcomes and actions.

Distress: Negative Stress

As opposed to eustress, if you wait until the middle of the final week or, worse yet, the night before to begin work on your project or paper, you can create a negative cycle with resulting negative outcomes. This negative cycle is called **distress.** Distress is commonly observed in the form of negative thoughts, negative behavioral patterns, negative physical symptoms, and/or negative emotions. These negatives can break your focus on positive responses to the demand you have experienced. Distress allows you to cross the line from positive benefits and results to negative consequences and outcomes. You still may complete the project, and you even may complete it on time. However, it is important to remember that how you complete a goal—with much stress or with little stress—is just as important or possibly more important than the fact that you complete the goal.

DISTRESS: Negative stress that leads to negative patterns of thought and action and that directs one's focus away from positive thoughts and actions.

■ Negative Stress: What Causes It?

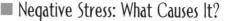

What can cause or create a stress response? For one thing, stress appears to be individualized. What may create negative consequences for one person may have no negative influence on another person.

The thought of a dental appointment may send the blood pressure of one individual soaring into the "red" zone, while another may view that same appointment as a welcome break in the day, a chance to get away from school or the work site. Two people view the same event and respond in completely different ways. To one it is traumatic; to the other, relaxing. One person may be totally indifferent to what can create negative stress for someone else.

Although the specific causes of stress can be many and varied, three general factors seem to be common in the development of stressful responses:

- Personal perceptions and appraisals
- Life events
- Change

■ Negative Stress: Perceptions and Appraisals

Factors that influence the negative outcomes of stress seem to vary greatly from person to person, adding to the difficulty of defining stress in specific terms or by specific causes. In examining the general causes of stress, Robert Sapolsky points to four major factors involved in personal perception:[20]

- Loss of control
- Loss of outlets for frustration
- Loss of sources of support
- A sense that life is getting worse

How a person perceives an encounter, event, or contact largely determines that person's level of stress. This focus on personal appraisal and perception is a familiar topic today. We often hear statements like these on the talk show circuit:

> "Stress is self-induced—induced through your personal thoughts and appraisals."
> "Events in life are neutral until you assign meaning to them."
> "Your perceptions become your reality."

Such statements may have some validity concerning personal appraisals and the relationship they have to the development of stress responses. Your thoughts and perceptions *can* create your reality. A stressful appraisal believes no choices or options—essentially no element of control—are available to you in dealing with whatever demand you encounter. This belief or appraisal seems to be a common denominator in the development of negative consequences and a negative cycle of stress. Consequences and symptoms of stress can appear in the form of negative physical, emotional, behavioral, and/or cognitive responses when someone is faced with a demand that is perceived to be out of that individual's personal control.

Primary appraisal

The perception of an event itself or an individual appraisal of the demand an event places upon someone is an important factor in the development of stress. Our appraisal process seems to involve two separate steps, report Richard S. Lazarus and Susan Folkman.[21] They explain that the initial appraisal of the demands an event will place on someone is the primary appraisal. This appraisal involves three possible response options. A person believes an event is:

1. Irrelevant—it carries no implication for personal well-being.

2. Benign or positive—the outcome of the demand is viewed as positive, something that preserves or enhances well-being.

3. Stressful—the outcome of the demand is viewed as negative, including threat, harm, and/or loss of well-being.

Secondary appraisal

If the primary appraisal of the demand someone experiences is stressful, Lazarus and Folkman report that the person has a secondary appraisal to consider. The secondary appraisal involves two response options: control through challenge or helplessness. Let's examine each of these secondary appraisal responses.

1. **Control through challenge.** The perception of personal control significantly influences one's secondary appraisal. A belief that there are choices and control options related to the demand experienced can create thoughts and outlooks of *challenge*. A sense of challenge can generate positive thoughts and actions toward the demand.

   Challenge and control can take many courses. Lazarus and Folkman compare the concept of control through challenge to a life-threatening, incapacitating illness or to a severe personal loss. In this situation, a person may face the challenge of maintaining a positive outlook or tolerating pain and distress—without falling apart. The issue of control is not so much about the demand itself, as to how the person responds to the demand. A sense of control regarding response options and/or actions complements challenge even during the most difficult of demands.

2. *Helplessness.* The second possible option in a secondary appraisal is a feeling of helplessness. A sense of helplessness indicates an outlook that sees little opportunity for positive choices or options. This outlook results in negative feelings and emotions. The negative cycle of helplessness may feed on itself and produce even more stress. Negative thoughts and outlooks can generate negative action steps—or even worse—a belief that nothing (no action) can help the situation. The negative cycle of stress continues its downward spiral, taking its victim with it.

The development of stressful responses through the appraisal process usually involves three significant steps:

1. A demand on personal resources

2. A primary appraisal of that demand

3. A secondary appraisal of possible responses to that demand

Assigning a perception or appraisal to a demand will vary from person to person. You may look forward to writing a report, seeing it as a challenge to apply the concepts and ideas you have learned and an opportunity to receive feedback about your proposed ideas. Someone else working on a similar report may view it as a threat to a job or grade point average, or even as just a waste of time. This person may feel a sense of helplessness and frustration. An identical event can create different appraisals and perceptions. The different perceptions can lead to varied reactions and responses to that demand.

When negative stress begins to build, it may be helpful to evaluate thoughts and appraisals of the events being encountered. An awareness of these personal appraisals can help in assessing and possibly reevaluating thoughts related to the stressful event, leading to a focus on other available outlooks and choices.

■ Negative Stress and Life Events

A second cause of negative stress is found in life events themselves. The factors that lead to stressful responses can derive from both the major traumatic events that occur infrequently in life and the day-to-day hassles encountered on a regular basis.

Of these two types of events, which seems to generate the most negative stress responses? You might be surprised to learn that most serious negative responses come from the day-to-day hassles!

When a person experiences a major, traumatic event that results in negative signs, symptoms, and outcomes, the cause of these negative consequences is usually very evident. Immediately after the traumatic event, many sources of support often are available (family, church, support groups, etc.) to help in dealing with the trauma and the demands the person has experienced. So while the negative stress may quickly rise to a very high level, with the passing of time and adequate support, the stress eventually will drop to a more normal level.

Hassled and Harried

The danger of daily "hassles" is that we can't always identify the cause of our negative signs, symptoms, and consequences. When a factor influencing our stress level is not evident, we begin to accept that factor as a typical part of our day. This acceptance can become a major barrier, preventing us from taking positive coping actions or seeking assistance in coping positively with the demands. This stress factor simply becomes a part of "normal" day-to-day life. This also means accepting the negative signs and symptoms associated with the negative stress factor. You accept that you will come home from work with a headache or in an angry mood. You will automatically express anger every time you come into contact with a certain individual. These negative emotional and physical responses then become a common and accepted part of your daily existence.

In looking at how a single traumatic event affects stress responses, we saw that the stress level can rise rapidly and that over time it will fall back into a more normal range. However, the stress level from daily hassles usually rises at a very slow rate, building on the person's acceptance of the stress. This dangerous acceptance means the level of stress and its negative consequences *may not fall back to a normal range* but may continue to slowly increase in intensity. The common negative consequences of these daily hassles can be:

- Emotional (anger, frustration and/or hopelessness)
- Physical (increased blood pressure, increased cholesterol levels, and/or physical pain)
- Spiritual (loss of faith, less time in prayer, decreasing church attendance)

Consequently, the residual effects of day-to-day hassles can impact the body more negatively than a major trauma. Remaining unaware of the stress buildup means one probably will not pursue methods of coping with the causes of stress.

As with appraisals and perceptions, the daily hassles that create negative consequences will vary from person to person. It is important to be aware of the daily hassles that may be creating negative stress. Certain signs and symptoms should be red flags, warning that something in the day-to-day routine is having a negative effect. When you notice negative signs and symptoms, make time to evaluate the contacts and events that may be influencing you, even in subtle ways. Life events, both traumatic and day-to-day hassles, have a direct bearing on personal well-being.

■ Negative Stress and Change

A third cause of negative stress is change. Veering from the "familiar and comfortable" can create a state of anxiety and stress. We often associate stress with change that involves a negative experience or outcome. Some examples of change that result in negative stress are a death in the family, job termination, or failing health.

However, even positive change can be stressful. A job promotion, birth, or marriage can be viewed as a very positive change in life. Although they are

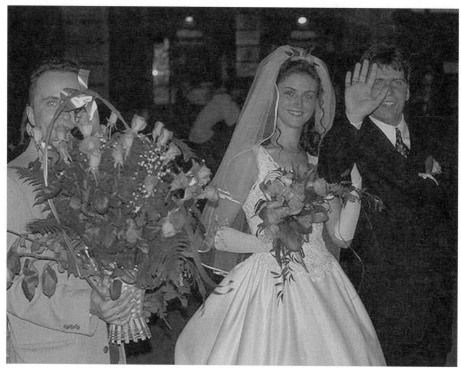

Even positive change can be stressful.

positive, they are still major lifestyle changes that can lead to stress. Let's say you leave a job that provides too little job satisfaction and too much work-related stress, and begin a new job with great career opportunities. Because you are entering an unfamiliar work environment and taking on new responsibilities, you may still experience stress. If you leave a negative relationship, you may experience stress. Even though the relationship is toxic, it is familiar. You know what to expect, but you may not know what to expect "out there" on your own. Trying something new or changing a familiar pattern of behavior can create stress. Thus, both negative and positive changes in life can result in stressful responses.

The Recent Life Changes Questionnaire (Table 4.1) lists various types of life changes common to an American lifestyle. A total of 300 life change units or more over a six-month period, or 500 life change units or more over a one-year period indicate a high degree of stress. Are your current life changes placing you at or near a high level of risk for stress?

Table 4.1. The Recent Life Changes Questionnaire

Life event	Life change units		Life event	Life change units	
	Men	Women		Men	Women
Death of son or daughter	135	103	Moderate illness	47	39
Death of spouse	122	113	Loss or damage of personal property	47	35
Death of brother or sister	111	87	Sexual difficulties	44	44
Death of parent	105	90	Getting demoted at work	44	39
Divorce	102	85	Major change in living conditions	44	37
Death of family member	96	78	Increase in income	43	30
Fired from work	85	69	Relationship problems	42	34
Separation from spouse due to marital problems	79	70	Trouble with in-laws	41	33
Major injury or illness	79	64	Beginning or ending school or college	40	35
Being held in jail	78	71	Making a major purchase	40	33
Pregnancy	74	55	New, close personal relationship	39	34
Miscarriage or abortion	74	51	Outstanding personal achievement	38	33
Death of a close friend	73	64	Troubles with co-workers at work	37	32
Laid off from work	73	59	Change in school or college	37	31
Birth of a child	71	56	Change in your work hours or conditions	36	32
Adopting a child	71	54	Troubles with workers whom you supervise	35	34
Major business adjustment	67	47	Getting a transfer at work	33	31
Decrease in income	66	49	Getting a promotion at work	33	29
Parents' divorce	63	52	Change in religious beliefs	31	27
Relative moving in with you	62	53	Christmas	30	25
Foreclosure on a mortgage or a loan	62	51	Having more responsibilities at work	29	29
Investment and/or credit difficulties	62	46	Troubles with your boss at work	29	29
Marital reconciliation	61	48	Major change in usual type or amount of recreation	29	27
Major change in health or behavior of family member	58	50	General work troubles	29	27
Change in arguments with spouse	55	41	Change in social activities	29	24
Retirement	54	48	Major change in eating habits	29	23
Major decision regarding your immediate future	54	46	Major change in sleeping habits	28	23
Separation from spouse due to work	53	54	Change in family get-togethers	28	20
An accident	53	38	Change in personal habits	27	24
Parental remarriage	52	45	Major dental work	27	23
Change in residence to a different town, city, or state	52	39	Change of residence in same town or city	27	21
Change to a new type of work	51	50	Change in political beliefs	26	21
"Falling out" of a close, personal relationship	50	41	Vacation	26	20
Marriage	50	50	Having fewer responsibilities at work	22	21
Spouse changes work	50	38	Making a moderate purchase	22	18
Child leaving home	48	38	Change in church activities	21	20
Birth of grandchild	48	34	Minor violation of the law	20	19
Engagement to marry	47	42	Correspondence course to help you in your work	19	16

Source: M. A. Miller and R. H. Rahe, "Life Changes Scale for the 1990's," *Journal of Psychosomatic Research* 43 (1997): 279-92, with permission from Elsevier.

Personal appraisals and perspectives, life events, and change are three causes of stress in life. Within these broad categories, we can find numerous common factors that influence how stress develops and damages. Awareness of these personal factors is pivotal to developing positive coping methods. Before we explore these positive ways of managing stress, let's take a closer look at the negative consequences of stress.

■ Stress and the Mind-Body Connection

The mind-body connection is a key to the consequences stress can have on the human body. Stressful attitudes and perceptions can negatively influence the physical functioning of the human body and can be a factor in the presence of physical signs and symptoms of stress.

> Stress has been called the greatest single contributor to illness in the industrialized world.

Stress has been called the greatest single contributor to illness in the industrialized world. To repeat, each person reacts differently to the demands of stress. The negative consequences of stress can be exhibited in many ways:

- Physical consequences—frequent illness or physical exhaustion
- Behavioral consequences—new or increased substance usage; avoiding a person or situation
- Cognitive consequences—persistently pessimistic outlook and/or negative thinking
- Emotional consequences—apathy, anxiety, and/or irritability

■ "Fight or Flight"

Walter Cannon discusses a "fight or flight" reaction of the body when it is exposed to a stress demand.[22] Cannon states that this reaction is the body's way of preparing and dealing with physical, life-threatening demands. It is meant to prepare the body physically to flee the perceived threat. However, most of the stress we encounter today is stimulated by psychological appraisals of events that create perceived threats to personal well-being. These appraisals can be situations such as work conflicts, exams, or public speaking. The demands we experience often do not come from life-threatening activities, nor do they typically lend themselves to physical "fight or flight" responses. Without such a response to stressful demands, the body's preparedness to do something physical can become unhealthy and lead to negative consequences.

How does this happen? The physical response to a perceived demand indicates what goes on in the body as it prepares itself to cope with the demands it has encountered—real or perceived. One's physical body prepares itself to endure what it still perceives to be a physical attack against it. The body responds by releasing adrenaline, which then causes a series of physical changes. These changes can include the following:

- The heart beats faster and stronger.
- Blood pressure rises abruptly.
- Blood flow increases to the muscles and decreases to the stomach and skin.
- Chemicals are released to make the blood clot more rapidly in case of injury.
- High-energy fats are released into the bloodstream for energy.
- Breathing quickens.
- Pupils dilate.

The body's alarm system has prepared it to physically "fight" for survival or to physically take "flight" in order to survive. Both options indicate a physical release for the stressful demand encountered. To reiterate, the problem is that in today's modern world the stress we commonly experience comes from *mental appraisals of a demand* rather than from *a physical threat to survival*. These perceived sources of stress usually do not allow for a physical kind of fight or flight response. Without the fight or flight physical release, there is no way for the body to respond to this alarm. The body has no outlet for the adrenaline-created responses it is now producing. The absence of this outlet means that negative signs and symptoms will begin to build in the body.

■ The Toll on the Body

The human body can withstand high levels of abuse for long periods of time, but eventually the abuse will take its toll. A person may begin to experience various physical negative signs and symptoms of stress. Physically, stress can decrease the number of white blood cells, which in turn can weaken the body's immune system and defenses against disease. This weakening can make the individual more susceptible to chronic conditions such as heart disease, cancer, and allergies. Along with physical signs and symptoms, there can be behavioral, emotional, and cognitive signs and symptoms of stress as well.

Some of the common negative signs and symptoms that can be experienced from demands perceived as stressful include the following:

1. Physical signs and symptoms:
   - high blood pressure
   - elevated cholesterol levels
   - headaches
   - indigestion
   - sleep disorders
   - chest pains
   - weakening of the immune system

> "A relaxed attitude lengthens a man's life; jealousy rots it away."
>
> **Proverbs 14:30**

2. Behavioral signs and symptoms:
   - critical attitude
   - increased irritability
   - lack of focus
   - overeating/drinking
   - use of drugs

3. Emotional signs and symptoms:
   - feeling of powerlessness
   - crying
   - anger
   - unhappiness
   - edginess

4. Cognitive signs and symptoms:
   - inability to make decisions
   - patterns of negative thinking
   - loss of humor
   - forgetfulness
   - easily upset

Throughout this chapter, we have recommended developing awareness as the primary tool in combating stress-related symptoms. Those who do not develop the ability to recognize these signs and symptoms, or those who recognize them and decide to do nothing about them allow them to become a part of their day-to-day existence. They accept them rather than reject them. Unless they develop a

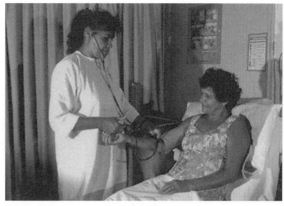

Eventually, stress will take a toll on the human body.

KEY CONCEPTS

anxiety	hostility
depression	pessimism
distress	state anxiety
emotion	stress
eustress	trait anxiety
guilt	

method of release or positive coping skills, they will allow these signs and symptoms to build to levels of chronic illness.

This does not mean that you experience stress with every headache or every incidence of forgetfulness. But if these symptoms appear consistently, view them as red flags. Use them to evaluate what is going on in your life at that time. Then determine what actions to take or decisions to make regarding the factors influencing these signs and symptoms. Responding to the demands of stress in a positive way is called stress management, the topic of the next chapter.

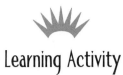

Learning Activity

1. Considering the different types of signs and symptoms an individual may experience, what are some common signs and symptoms you experience that may indicate the presence of negative stress in your life?

Physical symptoms:

_____

_____

_____

_____

Emotional symptoms:

_____

_____

_____

_____

Behavioral symptoms:

_____

_____

_____

_____

Cognitive symptoms:

_____

_____

_____

_____

2. Considering the general causes of stress discussed in this chapter, what factors could be causing negative stress in your life and influencing the negative signs and symptoms listed above? (These factors may be happening in your life at the present time or they may be events from the past that influence stress when you remember them.)

Negative appraisals or perceptions of situations or other people in your life:

_____

_____

_____

_____

Specific events or contacts in your life:

_____

_____

_____

_____

Changes in your life:

_____

_____

_____

_____

Remember: An awareness of stress factors in your life will be important as you develop stress management options and positive methods of coping.

Additional Activities and References

1. What in your life (contacts, actions, beliefs, etc.) supports a sense of personal optimism?

    _____

    _____

    _____

    _____

2. What in your life (contacts, actions, beliefs, etc.) supports a sense of pessimism?

    _____

    _____

    _____

    _____

3. What changes in your life are necessary to better support a sense of optimism and reduce a sense of pessimism?

    _____

    _____

    _____

    _____

4. What are some positive stresses in your life?

    _____

    _____

    _____

    _____

5. How do you benefit from this positive stress?

_____

_____

_____

_____

Endnotes

1. As quoted in Charles R. Swindoll, *Man to Man* (Grand Rapids: Zondervan, 1996), 325.
2. Daniel Goleman, *Emotional Intelligence: Why It Can Matter More than IQ* (New York: Bantam Books, 1995), 268.
3. Robert E. Ornstein and David S. Sobel, *Healthy Pleasures* (Reading, MA: Addison-Wesley, 1989).
4. Jane E. Myers, Thomas J. Sweeney, and J. Melvin Witmer, "The Wheel of Wellness," *Journal of Counseling and Development* 78 (Summer 2000): 254, citing K. M. Dillon, B. Minchoff, and K. H. Baker, "Positive Emotional States and the Enhancement of the Immune System," *International Journal of Psychiatry in Medicine* 15 (1985): 13-17.
5. Robert M. Sapolsky, *Why Zebras Don't Get Ulcers: An Updated Guide to Stress, Stress Related Diseases, and Coping* (New York: W. H. Freeman and Co., 1998), 258.
6. Howard Friedman, *The Self-Healing Personality: Why Some People Achieve Health and Others Succumb to Illness* (New York: Penguin Group, 1992), 52.
7. Goleman, *Emotional Intelligence*, 176.
8. Herbert Benson and Eileen M. Stuart, *The Wellness Book* (Secaucus, NJ: Carol Publishing Group, 1992), 211.
9. Friedman, *The Self-Healing Personality*.
10. Sapolsky, *Why Zebras Don't Get Ulcers*, 273.
11. Friedman, *The Self-Healing Personality*, and Benson and Stuart, *The Wellness Book*.
12. Benson and Stuart, 216.
13. Donald H. Kausler and Barry C. Kausler, *The Graying of America: An Encyclopedia of Aging, Health, Mind, and Behavior* (Urbana: University of Illinois Press, 1996).
14. Friedman, *The Self-Healing Personality*.
15. Kausler and Kausler, *The Graying of America*; Friedman, *The Self-Healing Personality*; Ornstein and Sobel, *Healthy Pleasures*.
16. Goleman, *Emotional Intelligence*.
17. Benson and Stuart, *The Wellness Book*.
18. Claudia Sowa, "Understanding Clients' Perception of Stress," *Journal of Counseling and Development* 71 (Nov/Dec 1992): 179, citing F. Roberts, "The General Adaptation Syndrome," *The British Medical Journal* 2 (1950): 104.
19. As discussed in Benson and Stuart, *The Wellness Book*, 177.
20. Sapolsky, *Why Zebras Don't Get Ulcers*, 252.
21. Richard S. Lazarus and Susan Folkman, *Stress, Appraisal, and Coping* (New York: Springer, 1984), 31.
22. As explained in Benson and Stuart, *The Wellness Book*, 33.

5

EMOTIONAL WELLNESS AND STRESS MANAGEMENT

"Nothing can keep you down if you let God lift you up."

—Norman Vincent Peale[1]

Chapter 4 emphasizes that stress may be the greatest single obstacle to spiritual, physical, and emotional wellness. Stress can rob us of a positive mind-set, which is essential for positive thoughts and actions. A positive mind-set determines the course to personal well-being, leading us to establish positive methods of coping with stress. Our general emotional outlook on life can direct the actions we take toward the specific situations we encounter each day. The spiritual faith we develop and maintain can provide the foundation for our personal attitudes and outlook. Critical to personal well-being is the concept of individual choice. It is important to be aware of the many choices and options available for dealing with stress, and to take personal responsibility for implementing those choices.

OBJECTIVES

- Discuss the purpose of positive stress management.
- Identify personal choices involved in coping with stress.
- Recognize the importance of attitude in coping with stress.
- Describe optional methods of seeking relief from stress.
- Discuss hardiness and its relationship to stress management.

Stress Management: Coping in Positive Ways

How can you deal with stress in positive ways? Chapter 4 points out that stress is present consistently in day-to-day living. Since stress can negatively affect the body, thoughts, and actions, it is important to develop positive methods of coping with the stressful demands we encounter. This is commonly referred to as developing techniques for **stress management.** The focus of a positive stress management method is to develop

> **STRESS MANAGEMENT:**
> The ability to develop positive methods of coping with stress; a technique or method that helps to "create calmness."

some type of action or thought that will help to "*create calmness*," since calmness is exactly what stress and its consequences seek to destroy. To effectively control stress, everyone should practice some form of stress management daily, several times a day if possible. This involves varying the methods of stress management, selecting from three or four different methods to create calmness.

As the causes of stress will vary from person to person, stress management methods also will vary from person to person. It is important to try a variety of methods and to determine which ones give the best results. Remember that it takes time to develop new habits. Change is often difficult. In attempting a new method or technique for stress management, allow time to feel comfortable. If a method does not create a total sense of calmness on the first attempt, be persistent. Keep trying for a reasonable length of time. A general rule is to allow three to four weeks of daily practice—not only to develop the new habit, but to reach the necessary comfort level in applying this new habit.

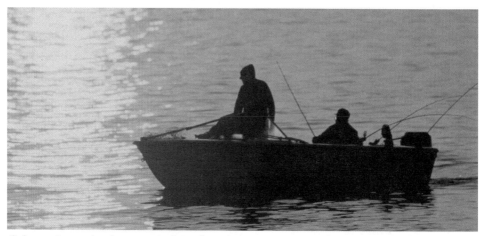

Calmness is exactly what stress seeks to destroy.

■ Personal Decisions: Change, Accept, or Leave?

To create calmness in times of stress, decide which type of coping action to take toward the stressful demand. This decision or choice involves three options: to change, to accept, or to leave. Not to choose one of these options and follow the recommendations related to that option actually may increase the severity of stressful demands.

■ Change: Focus on the Event

Change as a choice has a focus toward the particular stressful situation. Change means either taking action to change the event/person that is creating stress and resulting in negative signs and symptoms, or changing the outlook toward the event/person creating the stress. This option involves directing actions toward the *event* itself that is creating stress. This choice has three possible outcomes:

- You decide that trying to change the event/person is not worth the risk of confrontation (stress continues).

- You try to change the event, person, or personal outlook but no change occurs (stress continues).

- The event, person, or outlook does change (stress ends).

If choosing to focus on the event fails and the stressful demand continues, a second option is available.

■ Accept: Focus on Self

To accept is to realize that the stressful situation probably is not going to change in the immediate future. It has become a fixed part of one's life and will continue in this capacity for some time. In this case, accept that nothing is going to change and focus on taking care of *self* in a positive way. This is important in helping to develop the physical, emotional, and spiritual strength needed to deal with the unchanging events/people one may encounter.

The choice to accept most closely aligns itself with the specific methods of stress management detailed later in this chapter. These various methods will help strengthen the body, mind, and spirit in coping with the unchanging demands that may be encountered.

To accept is often an overlooked choice. It is common to keep hoping or thinking that something will change, even though we may not be making an active effort in that direction. Not choosing to accept can lead to feelings of frustration. This then can become a cycle of negativity—resentment, bitterness, anger—all of which feed a sense of hopelessness about the continuing stressful demand.

If the situation does not change, and the person cannot accept it, there is a third option.

■ Leave: Focus on the Positive

Often called the choice of last resort, the final option is simply to leave or get away from the stress demand. Perhaps someone has been unable to bring about acceptable change. Perhaps the stress demand contradicts that individual's personal value system, making it impossible to accept the situation. In these cases, the person needs to evaluate the merit of leaving the situation or environment that is creating the stressful demand.

> Ruts are hard to climb out of, even when they result in negative signs, symptoms, and outcomes.

Leaving something familiar is difficult, despite the fact that remaining causes great discomfort. Ruts are hard to climb out of, even when they result in negative signs, symptoms, and outcomes. The sense of security these ruts give, coupled with anxiety about change, can keep one trapped in negative contacts and environments.

Making these choices and taking any necessary steps in dealing with stress demands is a personal responsibility. Remember that not all stress demands will respond to the same option. A person may need to change one stress demand, accept another, and leave a third. Determine where you are in making these decisions (change, accept, or leave) in relationship to the stress factors in your life. The option you select will direct the appropriate actions toward your stress factor. Ask yourself two questions:

- Have you made a choice to deal with stress factors in your life?
- Are you following through on decisions and actions related to that choice?

Exhibit 5.1. Biblical Stress Management

You say: "It's impossible."
> God says: *All things are possible.* Luke 18:27

You say: "I'm too tired."
> God says: *I will give you rest.* Matthew 11:28-30

You say: "Nobody really loves me."
> God says: *I love you.* John 3:16; 13:34

You say: "I can't go on."
> God says: *My grace is sufficient.* 2 Corinthians 12:9; Psalm 91:15

You say: "I cannot do it."
> God says: *You can do all things.* Philippians 4:13

You say: "I'm not able."
> God says: *I am able.* 2 Corinthians 9:8

You say: "It's not worth it."
> God says. *It will be worth it.* Romans 8:28

You say: "I can't forgive myself."
> God says: *I forgive you.* 1 John 1:9; Romans 8:1

You say: "I can't manage."
> God says: *I will supply all your needs.* Philippians 4:19

You say: "I'm afraid."
> God says: *I have not given you a spirit of fear.* 2 Timothy 1:7

You say: "I'm always worried and frustrated."
> God says: *Cast all your cares on Me.* 1 Peter 5:7

You say: "I don't have enough faith."
> God says: *I have given everyone a measure of faith.* Romans 12:3

You say: "I'm not smart enough."
> God says: *I give you wisdom.* 1 Corinthians 1:30

You say: "I feel all alone."
> God says: *I will never leave you or forsake you.* Hebrews 13:5

You say: "I can't figure things out."
> God says: *I will direct your steps.* Proverbs 3:5-6

Stress Management: Caring for Self (Body, Mind, Spirit)

If the stress demands do not change and, at least for the present, a person chooses to accept them, the individual must pursue positive ways to create calmness in encountering these demands. Increasing and maintaining personal stamina will help in coping with stress factors. Positive stress management methods can give the physical, emotional, and spiritual strength needed to handle the stressful demands.

The next section examines some proven methods of positive stress management that incorporate the Christian worldview. Among them are these methods:

- Prayer
- Physical Activity
- Nutrition
- Time Organization
- Support Networks
- Assertion Skills
- Relaxation
- Positive Attitude (Optimism)

■ Prayer

"Don't worry about anything; instead, pray about everything; tell God your needs and don't forget to thank him for his answers." Philippians 4:6

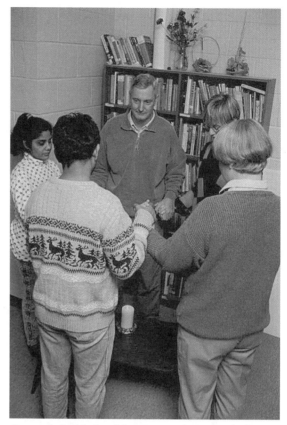

Prayer is foundational for peace and serenity during stressful times.

"Always keep on praying. No matter what happens, always be thankful, for this is God's will for you who belong to Christ Jesus."
1 Thessalonians 5:17-18

Prayer is foundational for peace and serenity during stressful times. People often compound their stress levels by thinking they *themselves* must find the "perfect" solution to the stress demands they encounter. When the problems seem beyond their abilities to "solve" them, they succumb to frustration, defeat, and hopelessness. This worldly belief can increase the level of pressure.

The Christian worldview looks beyond self to the source of strength—a source that can provide direction, timing, and wisdom in dealing with stress demands. This strength is accessible through prayer to God. In this chapter we refer to prayer as a method for dealing with stress. However, it is important to emphasize that prayer is a constant, ongoing communication with a loving God.

As we pray for strength and direction in dealing with stress, we also must pray with grateful hearts for all of the blessings and gifts that God has provided—the greatest of which is the gift of salvation. It is sometimes too easy to turn to God in difficult times, but then forget Him in times of prosperity.

Consistency is important in developing one's prayer life. Emotional wellness and stress management can include these prayer options:

- Developing specific daily prayer times
- Praying thankfully at the beginning of each day
- Praying for guidance at the beginning of each day
- Praying before an important or stressful event or contact
- Praying thankfully at the end of each day

You may be wondering how you can pray thankfully when your life seems to be under siege by stressful demands. When you begin to view prayer as two-way communication, you will understand that prayer is not simply a "formal request," in which you ask God to solve some problem in your life. It is also acknowledging all He is and all He has done. Prayer then begins to reflect a positive mind-set, the ability to look beyond the difficulties in life to the opportunities they present. It allows you to comprehend and express gratitude.

Consider starting a prayer journal in which to record your requests and the answers to those requests. You will gain insight and confidence as you see God working in your life, helping you overcome your fear and inadequacy. His past acts on your behalf will serve to remind you of how He will continue to work in the future. Pray for the wisdom, strength, and guidance to deal with any stress you encounter. Let go and let God provide.

■ Physical Activity

"Bodily exercise is all right, but spiritual exercise is much more important and is a tonic for all you do. So exercise yourself spiritually and practice being a better Christian, because that will help you not only now in this life, but in the next life too. This is the truth and everyone should accept it." 1 Timothy 4:8-9

Chapter 3 explains the significance of healthy physical activity as a means of coping with stress. Physical exercise not only provides release for the "fight

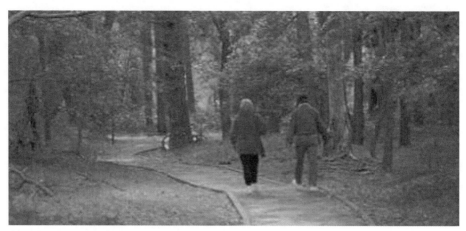

Healthy physical activity is a means of coping with stress.

or flight" responses triggered by the body, but it also builds and maintains physical strength as a safeguard against stress. When the body is fatigued or weak, we are at greater risk for the negative consequences of stress. Stress management and emotional wellness will include these physical activity options:

- Getting adequate sleep (seven to eight hours a day)
- Scheduling regular exercise times
- Having routine medical checkups
- Scheduling specific times each day for relaxation
- Maintaining a healthy body weight

■ Nutrition

"Fire goes out for lack of fuel . . ." Proverbs 26:20

Poor nourishment can put the body at a higher risk level during times of stress. An automobile will not function without fuel. Without fuel, the body can still function for a period of time—but not at its optimal level, which is what is needed when handling stress demands. Simply *taking the time to eat* in itself will provide a break from the stressful contacts we encounter. Becoming personally aware of how we respond to stress through nutrition is also important. Does stress cause you to eat more, eat less, or not to eat at all? In the area of nutrition, stress management and emotional wellness will include the following suggestions:

- Eating regular meals, including breakfast
- Taking a lunch break away from your work site
- Eliminating or restricting the caffeine and sugar in your diet
- Avoiding crash diets
- Eliminating or restricting alcohol consumption
- Including adequate amounts of vitamins and minerals
- Drinking enough water every day

■ Time Organization

"God is not one who likes things to be disorderly and upset."
1 Corinthians 14:33

Books on time management are more popular than ever before! Today's hectic pace makes fitting everything we want to do in twenty-four hours nearly impossible. This is a blueprint for stress. Stress can lead to the belief that our schedules are overcommitted and out of control. Ironically, when we are under stress, time dedicated to positive stress management activities is usually the first thing we cut from our personal schedules.

However, it is vitally important to manage time during high stress demands. Make time for yourself *during* times of stress (reacting time) and *before* times of stressful encounters (proactive time). Leave enough time in your schedule for positive forms of release and relaxation. Organizing your time can relieve stress; a lack of planning can create stress. Emotional wellness and stress management in the area of organizing time will involve these recommendations:

- Establishing and prioritizing long- and short-term goals
- Avoiding procrastination; taking initial steps toward a goal
- Making daily "to do" lists
- Minimizing schedule interruptions
- Scheduling priorities—doing things in the order of importance
- Scheduling "relaxation" times throughout the day

■ Support Networks

"Share each other's troubles and problems, and so obey our Lord's command." Galatians 6:2

It's not always easy to seek support or assistance from others. We often view this as a sign of weakness. Our independent mind-set may tell us that we *should* be able to handle our problems by ourselves—that we need to present a "Superman" or "Wonder Woman" image. However, it is not humanly possible or realistic to expect perfection in how we handle all of our life issues and stress demands.

The section above on prayer explains that the ability to reach beyond oneself to God is a sign of positive well-being. Consider support networks in the same way. Look at the need for assistance from others as a sign of strength, a positive awareness of and desire to better handle a situation. The feedback, help, and suggestions from others can provide guidance for the actions and

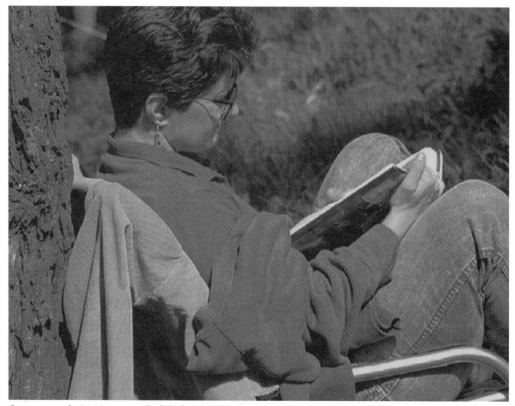

Leave enough time in your schedule for positive forms of release and relaxation.

decisions needed in handling stress demands. A support network can be a source of personal affirmation and nurturing. As you seek to bolster your support network, remember that God is always available to listen and care. Emotional wellness and stress management in the area of support networks will include these suggestions:

- Not being afraid to ask for assistance with personal problems
- Being receptive when support is offered
- Delegating responsibilities to others
- Seeking optimistic people for support
- Developing and cultivating good communication channels with family, friends, and professional networks
- Participating in community and/or volunteer activities

■ Assertion Skills

"What can we ever say to such wonderful things as these? If God is on our side, who can ever be against us?" Romans 8:31

Assertiveness often is unused as a personal stress management method. Assertiveness can be defined as openly and honestly expressing to others one's personal needs, values, and thoughts. It is important to express assertiveness in a respectful manner. Assertively expressing *our* personal values and making decisions based on those personal values are two important foundations for a true sense of personal peace. If we stray from our values and priorities in life and begin to make decisions based on what we think *others* want us to do or say, or if we base our decisions on other people's values, we are developing a foundation for negative stress and its consequences. Many people also stifle their personal values, afraid to express them for fear of "sticking out" in the crowd. A repressed value system invites stress. Expressing personal values—in a healthy, courteous way that does not overtly offend—is an important part of emotional wellness and a meaningful component of stress management

ASSERTIVENESS:
Openly and honestly expressing to others one's personal needs, values, and thoughts.

behavior. Assertion skills include the following:

- Realizing you have a choice to say "no" to the demands of others
- Understanding that it is human to make mistakes
- Developing a clear understanding of your personal values
- Assuming personal responsibility for disclosing your values, needs, and thoughts to others
- Expressing yourself clearly to prevent misunderstandings about your values, needs, and thoughts

▩ Humor

In their book *Healthy Pleasures,* authors Robert E. Ornstein and David S. Sobel explain the importance of humor in relieving stress:

> Laughter is an invigorating tonic that heightens and brightens mood, releasing us from tensions, pretensions and constraints. Humor offers a healthful perspective on ourselves and the world. Psychologist Gordon Allport suggested, "I venture to say that no person is in good health unless he/she can laugh at him/herself. During a hearty laugh your brain orchestrates a melody of hormonal rushes that rouse you to high-level alertness and that may numb pain."
>
> People who like humor, who use humor in their lives, and who themselves are funny are less likely to suffer when confronted with negative life events. By seeing humor in a stressful situation, we may be able to diffuse the threat and divert psychological arousal into merriment. When we laugh, we cannot be thinking about what is troubling us. There is some experimental research to support this. Levels of the stress hormones epinephrine and cortisol predictably fell when experimental subjects watched for an hour as a comic pummeled a watermelon with a mallet and performed other ridiculous antics.
>
> Suggestions to help indulge yourself in laughter include these options:

- Watch funny movies.
- Read joke books.

- Take in acts of comedians.
- Laugh at others' jokes.
- Collect cartoons and jokes from books.
- Use humorous exaggeration to keep things in perspective.
- Find a humorous motto and repeat it to yourself.
- Can't laugh? Smile.
- Can't smile? Fake it.[2]

■ Relaxation

"Come to me and I will give you rest—all of you who work so hard beneath a heavy yoke." Matthew 11:28

"Be still, and know that I am God." Psalm 46:10 NIV

The word relaxation has appeared in several lists above. Scheduling relaxation time in the daily schedule is common in many cultures around the world. In some countries, businesses close and people rest for a period of time in the middle of the day. Unfortunately, our country is not one of those societies. You are not alone in feeling "guilty" for making time for yourself. Guilt seems to be built into our "hurry-up" Western culture. Even if we cannot

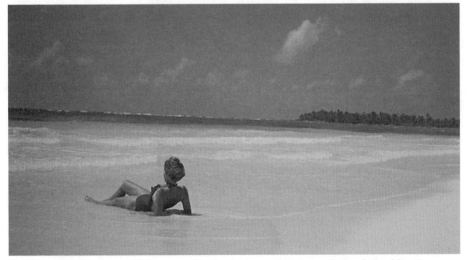

If you are refreshed, you will be more effective in the performance of your daily obligations.

"close up shop" for a couple of hours in the middle of the day, we can still carve out some time each day. Whether scheduling a real lunch period away from our work site (instead of gobbling a sandwich at the desk), taking a brief walk, using part of the lunch period to exercise, reading something inspirational, listening to a motivational tape on the drive to or from work, or relaxing in a number of other ways, we will find this time well spent in its ability to refresh us. If we are refreshed, we will be more effective in our work and better able to respond to the other contacts we have that day.

> God placed us on this earth to serve others, but to best accomplish that purpose, we first must care for ourselves.

If your daily work schedule does not allow time for relaxation, remember that taking time to relax before or after work or on your days off will provide a positive method of stress release. Looking forward to future times of relaxation is in itself a method of release.

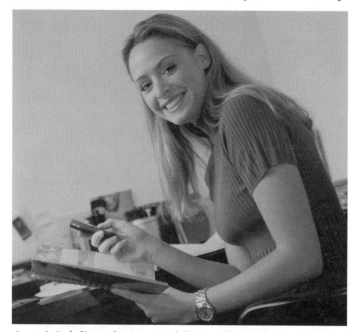

An optimist believes that in general things will turn out okay in life.

God placed us on this earth to serve others, but to best accomplish that purpose, we first must care for ourselves. Emotional wellness and stress management in the area of relaxation will include the following:

- Praying and meditating
- Breathing deeply and slowly
- Listening to music
- Writing in a journal to express personal thoughts and feelings
- Maintaining and nurturing a sense of humor
- Committing to a time of relaxation each day

■ Positive Attitude (Optimism)

"Now your attitudes and thoughts must all be constantly changing for the better." Ephesians 4:23

"A relaxed attitude lengthens a man's life; jealousy rots it away." Proverbs 14:30

Chapter 4 identifies the negative attitudes that contribute to and compound stress. One of these is pessimism, which was defined as a belief that the negative outweighs the positive—an expectation of the worst outcome in any situation.

From a wellness perspective, it is important to consider what can be done to cope with or change negative emotional states like pessimism. A foundation for a positive emotional outlook and for taking positive actions can come from the opposite of pessimism—an attitude of **optimism.** We define optimism as a strong appreciation that in general things will turn out okay in life, in spite of the possible setbacks and barriers we may encounter. An optimistic outlook believes that resources are available to help us respond to and deal with any situation we encounter.

> **OPTIMISM:** A strong appreciation that in general things will turn out okay in life, in spite of the possible setbacks and barriers we may encounter; an outlook that asserts that we can deal effectively with any situation we encounter.

■ Develop Realistic Optimism

A negative and inaccurate view of optimism sometimes is described as viewing life through "rose-colored glasses." This view translates optimism as an unrealistic, idealistic way of dealing with the difficulties of life. However, optimism as wellness refers to a *realistic* optimism. Realistic optimism is a way of explaining success and failure. A realistic optimist sees failure as something temporary, something that can be changed. Optimism involves confidence, a sense of control, and a choice. It is a belief that while we cannot control everything that occurs in our lives, we can control how we respond and the decisions we make related to that occurrence. An important thing to remember about optimism is that if it is not currently present in one's life, *it can be learned.*[3]

Optimism can keep a person from falling into the pessimistic states of hopelessness and depression. An optimistic attitude can lead to positive actions that address and help overcome negative emotions. We have already discussed some of the methods below in other areas of stress management, but they are particularly relevant to developing optimism:

- Participating in exercise or activity outlets
- Discussing and sharing personal concerns with a close confidant
- Seeking contacts for professional assistance
- Taking time to relax
- Taking time for prayer
- Developing a more trusting outlook and attitude

■ Cultivate Affirmations

Affirmations are positive thoughts that provide a direction and a focus for a specific area of life. Stress researcher Hans Selye states that "nothing can erase unpleasant thoughts more effectively than concentrating on pleasant ones."[4] What the mind hears becomes its reality. Through affirmations, we provide positives for the mind's foundation of reality. To develop affirmations, consider these guidelines:

- Select an aspect of your life that is causing you stress.
- Decide what you want to change about this situation, or how you would rather feel in this situation.
- Articulate this goal as a first-person statement:

   "I can have a relaxed body and a focused mind," or

   "I am confident in my work."

- Always state affirmations in the present tense.
- Repeat the affirmation to yourself and notice how you feel when you say it.
- Repeat your affirmation throughout the day, perhaps as part of a relaxation process.[5]

With all that happens during a day, it is easy to forget these affirmations unless we keep them visible. Write down your affirmations and post them where you can see them throughout the day. Keep them in conspicuous places, such as on a mirror, at your work desk, or on a computer screen saver. Some sample affirmations are:[6]

- "I can handle it."
- "I accept myself as I am."
- "I am peaceful."
- "I am becoming healthy and strong."
- "Let it be."
- "I am doing the best I can."

What you think is what you get—it is your reality. You and only you have the power to allow an external event or another person to upset you or create stress in your life. What you think about an event can either provide an appraisal of opportunity or an appraisal of fear or loss. You can find either positives or negatives in every situation you encounter. Evaluate each stress demand. Are you commonly seeing the negative side of a contact or experience? Or are you able to see the positive side and the learning that can come from that contact or experience?

Emotional wellness and stress management go hand in hand with a positive (optimistic) attitude. You can build realistic optimism and affirm your life by practicing the following:

- Identifying and eliminating negative thought patterns
- Identifying and reinforcing positive thought patterns
- Recognizing and developing your personal strengths
- Developing positive personal affirmations
- Developing reasonable goals and expectations for yourself and others

■ Commitment

"I am still not all I should be but I am bringing all my energies to bear on this one thing: Forgetting the past and looking forward to what lies ahead, I strain to reach the end of the race and receive the prize for which God is calling us . . ." Philippians 3:13-14

It takes almost no effort to let stress into our lives. It does take commitment and personal responsibility to cope with stress in positive ways. Taking action through any combination of the methods mentioned above—or applying one not mentioned, a method that creates calmness for an individual—is important

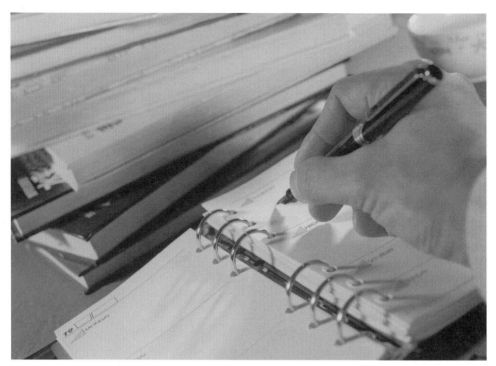

Make time for stress management a priority in your day.

in helping to release the negative buildup from stressful demands. Make a personal commitment to apply at least one method of stress management each day. This is only a partial list of the many possible methods available. The most important methods are the ones that will work best for the individual. The most important goal is to find three or four positive methods of stress release that provide a sense of calmness when daily demands seem to take over. Consider what other methods can be added to the list of stress management options.

God did not place us on this earth to be unhappy or frustrated. Stress not only can sabotage happiness, but it can seriously limit our potential. Coping positively with the stress we encounter can help us overcome the barriers that stress creates. To repeat, be particularly aware of stress's subtle ploy to lead you to believe that your schedule is too full for stress management activities. When your time seems to be limited, your responsibilities overwhelming, and your life out of control—that is exactly when you need stress management the most! Your personal commitment to emotional wellness through stress management principles will positively impact the quality of your life.

■ Hardiness

"For I can do everything God asks me to with the help of Christ who gives me the strength and power." Philippians 4:13

In addition to commitment in battling stress, we need what some stress theorists call hardiness.[7] **Hardiness** as it relates to stress management can be defined as a positive and proactive outlook about ourselves and our choices as we encounter stressful demands. Chapter 4 explains that personal appraisals of various stress demands largely determine one's course of action. Negative appraisals include feelings of helplessness and lack of control. Positive appraisals see the possibilities and potential inherent in stress demands. If we have a positive focus, we will look for positive methods of coping with the demands we experience in life.

> **HARDINESS:** A positive and proactive outlook about ourselves and our choices as we encounter stressful demands.

To briefly summarize some key points from chapter 4, we may have more control choices in our lives than we imagine. While we may not be able to control all situations or circumstances, we always can control how we respond to a demand, as well as our outlook regarding that demand. We cannot control what others may say or do, but we can control our response to what is said and done. How we act and react are important aspects of the choices we make to manage stress. Those choices are totally under our control.

Hardiness is part of a personality-based theory that can provide ways to develop personal outlook options in dealing with the stressful demands of life. Hardiness involves three appraisals toward the stressful demands we experience:

1. Commitment
2. Control
3. Challenge

We have looked at these same three terms as they relate to other concepts, but let's focus now on their relationship to the concept of hardiness. These three appraisals interconnect and influence one another, just as they influence our personal perceptions of stressful demands.

■ Commitment and Hardiness

How committed are you to being totally involved in positive living? Positive living means taking positive actions for total well-being—body, mind, and spirit. The opposite perspective, negative living, means to live in a disinterested manner, unwilling to develop your potential.

Are you committed to taking the necessary time and effort to implement wellness actions in your life? Are you assuming personal responsibility for the actions you take (or the actions you do not take) to make positive changes in your life? Focusing on positive steps and maintaining an optimistic outlook can build a strong foundation of personal responsibility. When you accept responsibility for the choices you make in dealing with stress demands, you demonstrate commitment.

■ Control and Hardiness

How strongly do you believe you can positively influence the course of your life? Do you feel that you have control over your personal choices and actions? Or do you feel powerless over the circumstances of your life?

A personal sense of control is pivotal to building wellness. It is worth repeating: you cannot control all that happens to you, but you can control how you respond. Negative emotions and outlooks can cloud your ability to see clearly the choices and opportunities that each demand can present. Do you feel and believe that a stress demand is beyond your control, or do you examine each situation, factually evaluate your choices, and take the first step to a positive coping method? Focusing on the solutions instead of the problems demonstrates a sense of personal control.

■ Challenge and Hardiness

Do you accept change and view it as an opportunity for development? Or do you see change as a threat to your security and well-being?

You have a choice to view every situation in your life through a positive lens or a negative lens. The positive lens sees a stress situation as a challenge. The negative lens sees the same stress situation as a barrier. What is your general focus? Do you expend your energy asserting that something *can't* be overcome and then listing all the reasons why? Do you throw your hands up and complain, "Why me?" Or do you focus on the possibilities and learning potential in every situation, accepting the challenge to do something constructive with the stress demands in your life?

What can you do to develop hardiness? Ask yourself this question when you appraise a stress situation. Then focus on a proactive approach that will help you meet life's challenges with optimism, defeating the negative consequences that stress demands can create.

Contentment

Applying the principles of commitment, control, and challenge to stress demands will result in another "C" term—contentment. In *Bible Power for Successful Living*, Norman Vincent Peale says this about contentment:[8]

A sense of contentment often directs actions that can help to eliminate stress in our life. The German philosopher Goethe said there are nine keys to contentment:

- Health enough to make work a pleasure
- Money enough to support your needs
- Strength enough to battle your difficulties and overcome them
- Grace enough to confess your sins and forsake them
- Patience enough to work until something good is accomplished
- Charity enough to see some good in your neighbors
- Love enough to move you to be useful and helpful to others
- Faith enough to make real the things of God
- Hope enough to remove all anxious fears concerning the future

Emotional wellness hinges on the ability to manage stress. Stress management is not something that can be pulled out of the file drawer every once in a while to deal with a "crisis." Stress management is a life principle built into a wellness lifestyle. It works best when it is practiced regularly and becomes a seamless part of daily life. It reflects respect of self as God's creation and the desire to live a life—body, mind, and spirit—that pays tribute to Him.

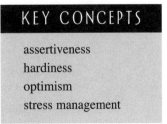

KEY CONCEPTS

assertiveness
hardiness
optimism
stress management

Learning Activity

1. Stressful situations or contacts require you to make three choices: to change, to accept, or to leave the stress demand. After reading this chapter, what choices do you need to make for each of your stress issues?

   Which conditions do you desire to change?

   _____

   _____

   _____

   Which conditions at this time do you need to accept?

   _____

   _____

   _____

   Which conditions do you need to leave?

   _____

   _____

   _____

2. If at the present time certain stress conditions in your life will not change and you cannot leave them, you must accept them. In accepting and dealing with these stress conditions, what options of release and methods of building personal strength do you wish to pursue?

Physical Stress Management Activities:

_____

_____

_____

_____

Emotional Stress Management Activities:

_____

_____

_____

_____

Spiritual Stress Management Activities:

_____

_____

_____

_____

Additional Activities and References

1. What changes/decisions do you need to make to ensure that you commit twenty to thirty minutes each day to relaxation and the pursuit of calmness?

   _____

   _____

   _____

   _____

2. Which contacts give you a sense of relaxation and peace?

   _____

   _____

   _____

   _____

3. Review the following resource for additional information regarding stress management:

   www.stressrelease.com

Endnotes

1. Norman Vincent Peale and Donald T. Kauffman, *Bible Power for Successful Living: Helping You Solve Everyday Problems* (Grand Rapids, MI: Fleming H. Revell, 1993), 49.
2. Robert E. Ornstein and David S. Sobel, *Healthy Pleasures* (Reading, MA: Addison-Wesley, 1989), 219-20, paraphrased.
3. Daniel Goleman, *Emotional Intelligence: Why It Can Matter More than IQ* (New York: Bantam Books, 1995), 89.
4. Herbert Benson and Eileen M. Stuart, *The Wellness Book* (Secaucus, NJ: Carol Publishing Group, 1992), 235, quoting Hans Selye.
5. Ibid.
6. Ibid.
7. Ibid., 178, referencing Suzanne Kobassa.
8. Peale and Kauffman, *Bible Power*, 67.

6

SOCIAL AND FAMILY WELLNESS

"Effective family life does not just happen; it's the result of deliberate
intention, determination, and practice."

—Charles Swindoll[1]

Why do you participate in wellness activities? One primary benefit is that in doing positive things *for* yourself, you gain a more positive outlook *about* yourself—an increased sense of confidence and an improved perspective about life in general. This improved outlook is foundational to more positive interactions with people, both personally and professionally.

Participating in wellness activities decreases risk factors for many of the leading causes of premature death in this country. By decreasing risk factors, we take steps to ensure as much quality time as possible with our family and others important to us. Only God knows how many days we have in this life. However, positive wellness steps may enable us to follow the paths God has set before us, as well as increase the quality of the days God has given us. Family can be both the

OBJECTIVES

- Identify the three main components of caring communication.

- Describe personal goals that will help create positive communication with others.

- Explain how communicating with God is important to overall communication.

- Discuss a personal definition of family wellness.

- Recognize actions that promote positive family wellness.

greatest gift and the greatest responsibility God offers. It is important to provide family members with positive lifestyle examples and role models in the areas of physical, emotional, and spiritual well-being. Others always learn more from what we *do* than from what we *say*.

Persons Are Gifts

Persons are gifts the Creator God sends to us . . . wrapped.

Some come wrapped very beautifully,
Some come in ordinary wrapping paper.
Some persons are very loosely wrapped,
Others very tightly.
Sometimes the gift has been mishandled in the mail.
Once in a while there is a special delivery.

But the wrapping is not the gift.

I AM A PERSON. THEREFORE, I AM A GIFT, TOO.

A gift to myself, first of all.
God my Creator gave myself to me.
Have I ever really looked inside my wrapping?
Am I afraid to?
Perhaps I have never accepted the gift that I am.
Could it be that there is something else inside the wrappings
other than what I think is there?
Maybe I have never seen the wonderful gift that I am.
Could God's gift be anything but beautiful?
I love the gifts which those who love me give to me.
Why not the gift of me?

AND I AM A GIFT TO OTHER PERSONS.

Am I willing to be given to others?
To be a person for others?
Do others have to be content with the wrapping,
Never permitted to enjoy the gift?

EVERY MEETING OF PERSONS IS AN EXCHANGE OF GIFTS.

Love is a relationship between persons who
see themselves as they really are.
Gifts are given by God
to be given to others.

—Author Unknown

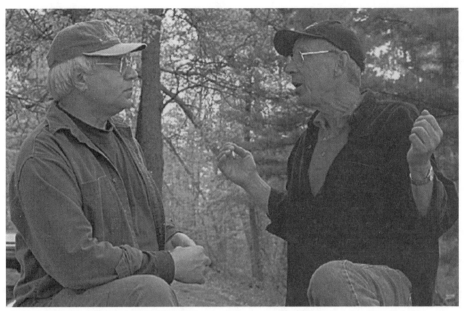

Strong, positive relationships with people around you can benefit your overall well-being.

Social Wellness: Beyond Self

For the purpose of this discussion, we define **social wellness** as the way we deal and communicate with other people. This generally involves the way we express our feelings and the manner in which we communicate with those around us. It also gauges our ability to get along with a variety of people and to demonstrate concern for the welfare of our community.

Too often the fast pace of our daily schedules does not allow time for positive interactions with others, even those very close to us. Strong, positive relationships with people around us can benefit our overall well-being, not only making our lives much more enjoyable, but many times improving our physical health as well. Those who help others through community involvement and other assistance programs report lower levels of stress.

> **SOCIAL WELLNESS:**
> The way we deal and communicate with other people.

■ Gauging Your Influence

A high percentage of our waking time reportedly is spent relating to and communicating with other people. These interactions can involve family members, peers, or work associates with whom we speak daily. They also can involve individuals we meet infrequently in a social or business situation. An important goal of social wellness is to be able to relate and communicate in a positive, effective manner. Every contact we have with another person can potentially influence that person's life. With that in mind, consider these questions:

- What type of influence are you bringing into this contact?
- Is it a negative influence or is it a positive influence?
- Does your contact add in a positive way to that person's day?
- Do you influence that person in such a way that you detract from the quality of this individual's day?

If you have taken a communication class or attended a workshop to improve your communication skills, you have probably come across these key points:

- The foundation of good listening
- The importance of body language
- Conflict management
- Assertiveness

While understanding these principles may improve communication skills, they do not necessary ensure alignment with wellness principles. You can be an effective communicator and still not have the other person's best interest at heart. This chapter focuses on wellness principles as they relate to effective, positive communication. The goal is facilitating positive, effective relationships.

■ "Caring" Communication

Social wellness relies on "caring" communication. Hallmark Cards is known for its motto: "When you care enough to send the very best." That is essentially how we should view all of our contacts with others. If we care about and are aware of how we are interacting with others, our actions and behaviors will reflect positive communication.

Excerpt 6.2, How to Get Along With People

- Keep a chain on your tongue. Every unspoken word should pass through three doors: (1) Is it true? (2) Is it kind? (3) Is it necessary?
- Make promises sparingly and keep them faithfully.
- Never let an opportunity pass to say a kind or encouraging word to or about somebody.
- Be interested in others, interested in their pursuits, their welfare, their homes and families.
- Be cheerful.
- Preserve an open mind on matters of opinion. Hold fast to matters of faith, but do so in a loving spirit.
- Let your virtues speak for themselves, and refuse to talk of others' vices.
- Be careful of another's feelings.
- Pay no attention to ill-natured remarks about you. Live so that nobody will believe them.
- Do not be anxious for what is due you.
- Forget self and you will be rewarded.

Source: "How to Get Along with People," *Winning the Race—A Publication of the Indy Racing League Ministry* 4, no. 10 (October 2000).

The Golden Rule

One meaningful and often-used communication guideline has been around for a long time. **The Golden Rule** offers a key standard for evaluating how to interact with others. The Bible states the Golden Rule twice:

> *"Do for others what you want them to do for you."* Matthew 7:12

> *"Treat others as you want them to treat you."* Luke 6:31

THE GOLDEN RULE:
A rule of ethical conduct based on Matthew 7:12 and Luke 6:31; a maxim to treat others as you would want to be treated.

The Golden Rule can provide both an important foundation and a worthy goal for relating to other people in a positive way. In using the Golden Rule to evaluate how well you "measure up" to its principles, ask yourself the following questions:

- How well would *you* interact with yourself?
- How would *you* like to be treated if you were answering the same question you are asking someone else?

- How would *you* expect to be treated if you were a team member or coworker who was working with you?
- If *you* were dealing with yourself, would you like to be treated in the same way you treat others?

Sadly, individuals often do not put themselves in the shoes of others. When it comes to interacting and communicating with others, the Golden Rule most often is ignored today.

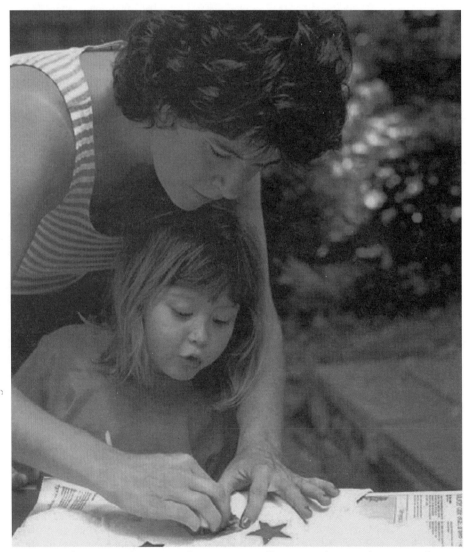

One way to demonstrate love is to make a conscious effort to spend time with someone else.

■ The LOVE Principle

The foundations that direct how we deal with others can arise from many different and sometimes negative sources, some of which are these:

- The mood we are in at the time of the contact
- The way someone else has recently treated us
- The amount of time we have available at the time of the interaction

It is important to look for these subtle influences and to circumvent them when we notice that they are guiding our conversations and interactions in undesirable ways. We do not want these factors to negatively influence those who are communicating with us. It is also important to remember the concept of choice. We can

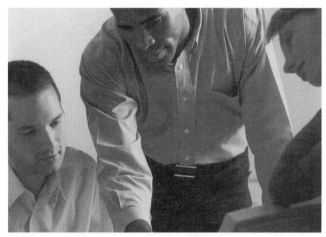

We can choose how we interact with others.

choose how we interact with those around us. Along with that choice comes responsibility—we take responsibility for our actions.

Denis Waitley has developed the acronym LOVE to describe a positive foundation for communication. Each letter describes actions that project and foster positive communication:

L – is for **listen**. To love is to listen to someone unconditionally, to listen to the needs and values of others without prejudice or judgment.

O – is for **overlook**. None of us are perfect. To love someone is to overlook the flaws and the faults in favor of looking for the good.

V – is for **voice**. To love is to voice approval and encouragement on a regular basis. There is no substitute for honest encouragement, a positive "stroke," and words of praise.

E – is for **effort**. To love is to make a constant effort to spend the time, to make the sacrifice, or to go the extra mile to show your interest.[2]

Waitley describes this type of love as an act of "demonstrating value in and looking for the good in another person . . . [it] is one of the few experiences in life that can be kept best by giving it away."[3]

The Building Blocks of Caring Communication

To develop goals for caring communication, we first need to look at the three general areas of communication that influence individual well-being:

- Communication with self
- Communication with others
- Communication with God

■ Communicating with Self, Caring for Self

A key factor in how well we communicate with other people is often how positively we communicate with ourselves. What do we say to ourselves? What is our "self-talk"?

What we say and think to ourselves, consciously or subconsciously, can become our reality. This reality can then influence how we act and react to the people and situations we encounter. Whether we realize it or not, we are almost constantly saying or thinking something to ourselves concerning our value as an individual, our personal abilities, or our ability to deal with a situation or individual. What we communicate to ourselves can influence the attitudes and the behaviors we carry into our interactions. If we do not think positive thoughts about ourselves, we can find it difficult to interact with others in a positive manner. Consider these options and think about your focus when interacting with others:

> What we say and think to ourselves, consciously or subconsciously, can become our reality.

- Are you thinking of the skills and abilities you already possess, as well as the new skills and abilities you wish to develop?

OR

- Are you thinking of the skills and abilities you believe others have, and focusing on the skills and abilities you believe you lack?

- Are you thinking of and planning for the positive opportunities available to you in the future?

OR

- Are you focusing on opportunities you believe passed you by or were never made available to you in the past?

- Are you looking for the positives in the people you meet, giving them words of encouragement?

OR

- Are you looking for the negatives and imparting words of criticism?

Your position on these and other related attitudinal options can indicate the type of communication you have with yourself. Is it caring and supportive, or is it critical and self-defeating? Patterns in thoughts and outlooks are important clues to the kind of self-talk or self-communication we experience.

■ Building Self-Esteem

You are probably familiar with the popular term **self-esteem,** which we can define as self-respect or your level of satisfaction with yourself. As we consider the thought patterns above, we find that self-communication generally reflects the way we think of ourselves. Thus, our self-esteem can be the beneficiary or the victim of our self-talk.

> **SELF-ESTEEM:**
> Self-respect; your level of satisfaction with yourself.

How strong and how positive do you generally rate your current self-esteem? The way you talk to yourself influences how you perceive yourself and your abilities. If you feel positive and optimistic about yourself and the efforts you are making, you usually find it easier to feel positive toward other areas of your life. Thus, you probably have positive contacts with those you encounter, communicating effectively and listening with interest.

On the other hand, if you think negatively and pessimistically about yourself and your abilities, you most likely will carry a negative attitude into other areas of your life, including your interactions with others.

In *Seeds of Greatness*, Denis Waitley lists key steps to building positive self-esteem. These actions or outlooks can help provide an inner sense of positive well-being that can positively direct the way you interact with others. Examine this summary of some of Waitley's key suggestions:[4]

- Always greet people with a smile. If you do not feel like smiling, the act of smiling can soon help you feel like smiling.

- Listen to inspirational tapes and radio shows while traveling. Listen to positive messages of self-improvement.

- Invest in personal self-development and pursue opportunities for personal and professional growth.

- Accept compliments when they are offered and always say "thank you."

- Do not brag. Your actions will speak for themselves.

- Do not tell your problems to people unless they are involved in the solution. Speak positively about your progress and the steps you are taking.

- Pattern yourself after successful "role models." Find someone who has conquered any fears you may have.

- Look at mistakes as learning experiences. Look at rejection as related to the performance, not the performer.

- Spend some spare time each week doing something you really want to do.

- Spend some time on an important priority: you!

We've often heard the saying that you must first take care of yourself before you can effectively care for others. Suggestions such as Waitley's can elevate self-esteem and help us become more sensitive to those around us. These are also important steps to developing long-term goals for building self-esteem and learning to exercise caring communication with others.

A wellness perspective of self-communication also involves the pursuit of positive goals for developing the body, mind, and spirit. This development builds personal confidence that will influence both internal and external communications in a positive way. What steps can you take to help increase your self-esteem?

■ An Unwavering Foundation

No discussion of self-esteem is complete without examining self-esteem's *true* foundation. Authentic self-esteem should be strongly related to spiritual wellness and to one's personal spiritual infrastructure. God lovingly creates every human being. He gives each of us a definite purpose and gives us unique skills and abilities. Being aware that we are God's special creations is the true foundation of positive self-esteem. People often get caught up in what they think are the building blocks of self-esteem—annual income, physical appearance, a job title, or other measures of power and prestige. These worldly measures of self-esteem lack permanence and substance; they can change or disappear in an instant. God's love and support will always be present and is an unwavering foundation of true self-esteem.

■ Communicating with Others, Caring for Others

Excerpt 6.3, The Eight Emotional Needs of People

1. The need to be loved.
2. The need to make a significant difference.
3. The need to be admired.
4. The need to be recognized for who you are as a person.
5. The need to be appreciated.
6. The need to be secure.
7. The need to be respected.
8. The need to be accepted.

Source: Bobb Biehl, *Weathering the Midlife Storm*: *Map a Successful Course through Your Middle Years* (Wheaton, IL: Victor Books, 1996), 68. Used by permission.

■ Alone in a Crowd

Lack of communication or contact with other individuals can create one of the most serious problems to individual well-being—loneliness. Psychiatrist Harry Stack Sullivan states that the greatest problems in today's society are loneliness, isolation, and difficulty with a positive sense of self-esteem.[5]

SOLITUDE:
The choice to be temporarily set apart from society; generally viewed in a positive light.

LONELINESS:
Imposed isolation, real or imagined; often viewed in a negative light.

There are two types of "aloneness." **Solitude** is aloneness by choice, a desire to be temporarily set apart from society. Solitude can be a time of creativity and replenishing of body, mind, and spirit—a kind of battery charging that adds to one's positive development. But **loneliness** is imposed aloneness. It carries with it sadness, desolation, emptiness—a sense of being involuntarily cut off from others. Robert Bolton reports that if an individual is not really in touch with him/herself or others, this sense of loneliness can occur even in the middle of a crowd.[6] Some of the reasons he gives for the loneliness rampant in today's society include:

- Materialism – taking comfort from things (worldly objects) rather than from people
- Mobility – the common uprooting of families
- Inadequate methods of interpersonal communication

In examining the last of these three reasons, interpersonal communication, ask yourself these questions:

- Do you really communicate with others in the way you *want* to communicate, or do you communicate with others in the same way *they have communicated* with you?
- When you are communicating with someone, who really provides the focus and the direction of the communication?

■ Getting Real or Getting Even?

If a person is nice and kind to us, usually we will respond in a nice and kind manner. On the other hand, if someone is rude and unkind to us, we may want to "one up" that person by being more rude and unkind in return. Our goal becomes one of getting even. That type of response or focus does not foster a positive and caring communication process, one that aligns with wellness communication. Further, we often can forfeit control of our caring communication goals as we seek "revenge" for being treated poorly. In the heat of the moment, we lose track of the Golden Rule.

To keep emotion from eclipsing control and facilitating negative results, focus on positive traits. Frequently review and model these traits, especially as they impact someone else—no matter how this person may communicate in return. Two passages from the Bible provide excellent summaries of the traits we should model to others:

> *"But when the Holy Spirit controls our lives, he will produce this kind of fruit in us: love, joy, peace, patience, kindness, goodness, faithfulness, gentleness and self-control."* Galatians 5:22

> *"And whatever you do, do it with kindness and love."* 1 Corinthians 16:14

Those key passages mention very important traits to remember as we interact with the people around us. What do others see in us when we interact and communicate with them? What traits do they see and learn from us? Many people are watching—what are they seeing and learning? Is it what we want them to see and learn?

■ Communication Ground Rules

When you communicate, how do you express your values and the points you wish to share? Do you push too hard, asserting your view of things above anyone else's? Or do you hold back from honestly and assertively expressing your values and your beliefs? *The Wellness Book* examines four methods of communication and the ground rules implied in expressing oneself:[7]

1. **Assertive Communication:**
   I count and you count. All participants are allowed to openly express their values and feelings, and are assured that everyone is listening.
2. **Aggressive Communication:**
   I count, but you do not count. One participant dominates the others by repeatedly expressing his or her values and feelings, with little concern or interest in the values or feelings of the other participants.
3. **Passive Communication:**
   I do not count, but you count. A participant accepts another participant's values and feelings as fact, without offering his or her own values and feelings for consideration.
4. **Passive-Aggressive Communication:**
   I count and you do not count, but I am not going to tell you this.

Where we are located within these options tells a lot about our self-image and our ability to communicate effectively with others. Our goal should be to strive for assertive communication—where listening is key and all involved can openly and honestly exchange their values and feelings.

■ Encourager or Discourager?

In ranking your communication style, ask yourself if you are an *encourager* or a *discourager*. When you communicate with others, do you encourage them or discourage them? How do they feel about the way you communicate to them? Do people generally feel better about themselves after interacting with you, or do they leave that interaction feeling somewhat negative? Look over an example of each communication type below:

1. **Convicted of "Discouraging":**

   During the Boer War (1899-1902), an individual was convicted of a rather unusual crime. He was found guilty of being a "discourager." When the South African town of Ladysmith came under attack, this person moved up and down the front line of soldiers who were defending the city, doing everything he could to discourage them. He pointed out the enemy's strength, the difficulties of defending against the enemy, and the inevitable capture of the city. He did not use a physical weapon in his attack—his weapon was the power of discouragement.

2. **Affirmed and Encouraged:**

   On the other hand, poet Robert Burns was an encourager. At a gathering of famous writers, he was impressed with a picture that hung on the wall of the host's home, especially a beautiful excerpt of verse beneath the picture. Burns asked who had written the verse, but no one seemed to know. Shyly, a teenager who had been left weakened and lame from a childhood illness spoke up. He not only knew the writer's name, but he even quoted the rest of the poem. Burns was impressed. He laid his hands on the young man's head and said, "Ah, my boy, I am sure you will be a great man in Scotland someday." That young man grew up to be Sir Walter Scott. Because of his physical problems, most people thought he would never amount to anything. But that brief conversation with Robert Burns provided an affirmation that helped Scott along the road to greatness.[8]

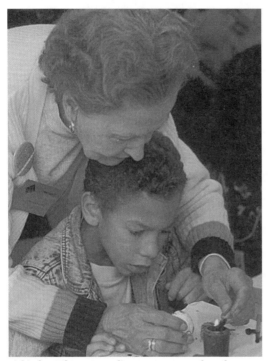

A kind word or a compliment can strengthen the weak and give wings to the soul.

Encouragers and discouragers can be found in every church, family, or community. A put-down or critical words can sear a person' soul. Yet a kind word or a compliment can strengthen the weak and give wings to the soul. An encourager:[9]

Listens:	Just listening can provide a strong sense of support. Not listening can rapidly drain enthusiasm.
Accepts:	An encourager is not judgmental. An encourager accepts an individual at face value.
Compliments:	It is the norm to receive more complaints than compliments. An encourager goes against the norm, knowing that everyone can use and will appreciate some kind words.
Laughs:	A sense of humor helps an encourager focus on the brighter, more positive aspects of life and pass that perspective on to others.
Uplifts:	An encourager is there for people during special times of need. Simple things like letters and notes can help others get through difficult times.

Excerpt 6.4. How to Get People to Like You: Ten Practical Rules

1. Learn to remember names. Inefficiency at this point may indicate that your interest is not sufficiently outgoing. A [person's] name is very important to that person.

2. Be a comfortable person so there is no strain in being with you—be an old-shoe, old-hat kind of individual. Be homey.

3. Acquire the quality of relaxed easy-goingness so that things do not ruffle you.

4. Don't be egotistical. Guard against giving the impression that you know it all. Be natural and normally humble.

5. Cultivate the quality of being interesting so that people will want to be with you and get something of stimulating value from their association with you.

6. Study to get the "scratchy" elements out of your personality, even those of which you may be unconscious.

7. Sincerely attempt to heal, on an honest Christian basis, every misunderstanding you have had or now have. Drain off your grievances.

8. Practice liking people until you learn to do so genuinely. Remember what Will Rogers said, "I never met a man I didn't like." Try to be that way.

9. Never miss an opportunity to say a word of congratulation upon anyone's achievement, or express sympathy in sorrow or disappointment.

10. Get a deep spiritual experience so that you have something to give people that will help them to be stronger and meet life more effectively. Give strength to people and they will give affection to you.

Source: Norman Vincent Peale, *The Power of Positive Thinking* (New York: Fawcett Columbine, 1996), 198-99.

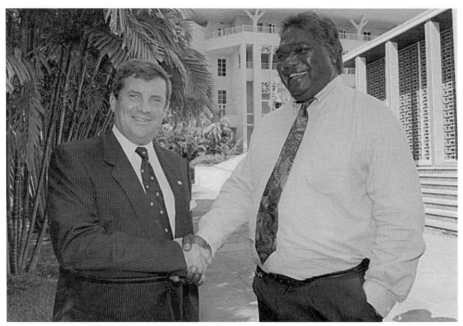

To communicate effectively, try to understand other cultures and backgrounds.

■ Looking Through a Cultural Lens

One of the most rapidly changing aspects of communication in today's world is the variety of backgrounds, values, languages, and traditions that individuals bring into an interaction. A common error is to assume that everyone sees and understands things in the same way we do. An expression of kindness in one culture may be interpreted differently in another culture. To communicate effectively, we must understand the culture and background of the individual(s) with whom we are interacting.

In *Living Well*, authors Curtis Byer and Louis Shainberg offer the following guidelines for communicating and interacting with individuals from different cultures:

- Develop an understanding of your own cultural values and biases. Most of us tend to be somewhat ethnocentric, assuming that the ways of our own culture are "best" and judging other cultures by how well they approximate our own.

- Develop an understanding of the cultural values, beliefs, and customs of other ethnic groups with which you interact.

- Be respectful of, interested in, and nonjudgmental about cultures other than your own. When two cultures are different, it is not necessary to judge which one is "better" or "right"; you can simply accept them as being different. You can learn to enjoy and appreciate the richness that ethnic diversity brings into your classroom and your community.

- Speak in a way that promotes understanding and shows respect for someone from a different ethnic group. Be especially careful to avoid statements such as, "She's really (smart/tall/beautiful/etc.) for a (fill in the ethnic group)." Even though the intention may be good, such statements are certain to offend the subject and to reveal the speaker's biases.

- Avoid using slang or idioms that might be misunderstood by someone from a different ethnic group. Many of the everyday phrases instantly understood within one ethnic group may have no meaning or a totally different meaning to someone from a different group.

- Remember that the same gestures can carry different meanings in different cultures. Avoid body language that might be offensive or misunderstood. Observe closely the use of gestures by people in different cultures; it could save a major embarrassment.

- Do not assume that someone who speaks less-than-perfect English or speaks English with an accent is not intelligent or has nothing to say. Remember that he or she speaks at least two languages, even though one is spoken with an accent.[10]

As we communicate with those around us, our personal goal of implementing positive attitudes, words, and actions can provide a positive foundation for the way we interact with others. How we interact with others is *our* choice, not that of the situation or the other people involved. By establishing guidelines for our behavior and holding ourselves accountable to those guidelines, our interactions will be well intentioned and well received.

■ Communicating with God, Knowing He Cares for You

Our discussion to this point should lead to a better understanding of how personal attitude and outlook on life are foundational to the way we communicate and interact with others. Do you strive to cultivate a positive and open outlook? Your ability to do so is tied to another important building block of caring communication—your personal spiritual values.

A Christian worldview places a high priority

on communicating with God and striving to meet human needs in God's way. Christians primarily communicate with God in two ways: by prayer and by reading God's Word in the Bible.

■ Why Pray?

To answer the question of why we should pray, look at what Psalm 116:1-2 has to say: *"I love the Lord because he hears my prayers and answers them. Because he bends down and listens, I will pray as long as I breathe!"*

If there is one "constant" in this life, it is, ironically, change. The situations we face change constantly, as do the people with whom we interact. Our bodies change, along with our health. Everything changes. But change does not have to overwhelm and dominate our lives. In the midst of change, we can hold onto an unchanging constant, an unwavering source of strength and comfort: God. The Psalm above tells us that we can always go to Him in prayer for support, love, and peace because *He is always there to listen*. Loneliness and stress are intensified when one's outlook is framed by the sense that no one cares and no one ever listens. Those with a Christian worldview, however, don't have those kinds of concerns—they know that God is always there for them and will always listen to them.

How should we pray? Some excellent guidelines also can be found in the Bible:

- *"And so, dear brothers, now we may walk right into the very Holy of Holies where God is, because of the blood of Jesus."* Hebrews 10:19

- *"You can get anything—anything you ask for in prayer—if you believe."* Matthew 21:22

- *"Don't worry about anything; instead, pray about everything; tell God your needs and don't forget to thank him for his answers."* Philippians 4:6

To pray effectively, first of all you must believe. You must have faith in the Word of God and remember that God's answers to prayer are better than any worldly answers that we could ever develop. The foundation of prayer comes from the realization that God sent His only Son, Jesus Christ, to die on the cross for *our* sins and that through Jesus we now have a way to reach God through prayer. Second, pray about any and every issue or question in your life. No problem or concern is too large or too small for God. Third, trust God's judgment. What you may think is the best solution for a problematic situation in your life may not be what God has in mind at all. He alone knows what is truly best for you. You also need to be aware of the answers He provides and open to their implications. It is not uncommon to ask for direction through prayer, but then ignore the answers God provides. It takes personal responsibility to listen and to act.

When should you pray? Establish a regular prayer time every day and find a private place where you will not be disturbed. The best way to establish a healthy habit is to develop a routine and then commit to maintaining that routine. This will not happen by waiting to "find time" to pray. Make a commitment and "make time" in your daily routine to communicate with God. Many less important priorities will somehow wedge their way into your day and push out the more meaningful priorities, unless you make a commitment to communicate daily with God. Refer back to chapter 5 for some suggestions on when to pray.

■ Why Read the Bible?

The second way Christians communicate with God is by reading the Bible, which Christians see as God's revealed Word. Many good resources are available today on how to read the Bible. This form of communication is critical to learning God's mind-set and perspective. The Bible defines God's principles for right living, shows us how godly men and women modeled those principles, and explains the consequences of wrong living. Most important, the Bible offers us God's plan of salvation and gives us a pattern in Jesus Christ upon which to model our lives.

■ Equal in God's Eyes

Realizing that we and all the people we encounter daily are equal—equal in that we are all creations of God—can strengthen our spiritual foundation of communication. Focusing on this inherent equality can help eliminate negative labeling, typecasting, and stereotyping others as either superior or inferior. Such labels seriously damage honesty, sincerity, and caring in wellness communication.

Remember also the importance of caring about yourself, so that you can care about others in positive ways. The bedrock for all of this is that God always cares about you.

Family Wellness: Love without Condition

Thus far in this chapter, the focus has been on the social aspects of wellness and caring communication. In no environment could this be more important and possibly more needed than in the family environment. Charles Swindoll states that generally in our society the concept of family

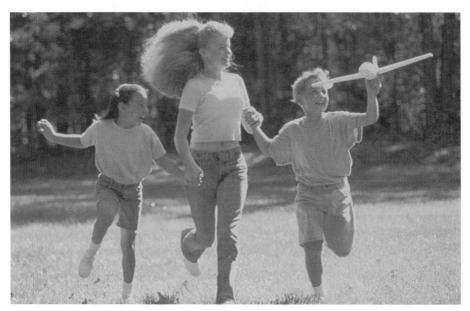

It is our responsibility to counteract the social forces seeking to erode the concept of family.

is disintegrating.[11] As in all other areas of wellness, it is our personal responsibility to take steps to help protect our family environment against this disintegration.

What does the term family mean to you at this time? The term **family** can mean different things to different people. Your definition could include the people in your current and immediate family, or it could include plans for the development of a future family. Family may include those living under the same roof, or family may be in various geographical locations and in various homes. As you can see, the term family can have many definitions. Commonly, it is the people in our life who are important to us and for whom we care deeply.

FAMILY: Traditionally, the basic unit of society; a group of people related to one another or united by a common purpose; any of various social units differing from but regarded as equivalent to the "traditional" family. In the context of this book, it is the people in your life who are important to you and for whom you care deeply.

■ What Do You Value?

A number of years ago at a church service, a retired corporate officer told his story. This gentleman stated that he had established some lofty goals when he began his career in an organization several years earlier. He then explained that he did all the right things to follow up on those goals: taking on additional responsibilities, working overtime, attending functions—all the things expected of an up-and-coming young man looking to advance within the organization. After many years of prioritizing time for these activities, he finally accomplished his goal. He was what he wanted to be, a high-ranking officer within a large national organization.

> It is all too easy in today's hectic world to succumb to responsibilities that demand more time or a higher ranking than one's family.

He then sadly noted that there was only one problem when he reached his ultimate career goal—he arrived at that pinnacle alone. By the time he had achieved his goal, his family had left him. He had been so focused on his career that time with his family was never a priority. He arrived at the pinnacle only to discover that his career goal was a very misdirected priority in his life after all. In working to provide material possessions for his family, he was not able to provide the one commodity they wanted the most—his time.

Unfortunately, this story is not that uncommon. Family (or the individuals we consider as family) can be one of the most important priorities and values in our lives. On the other hand, family also can be taken for granted; time for family can

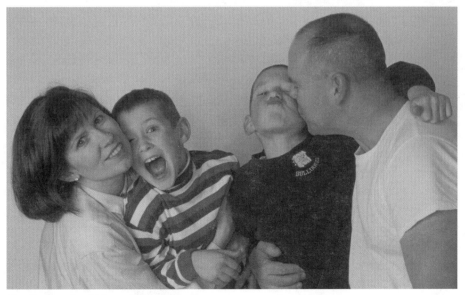

Family time should be a constant priority.

be cut or rearranged to accommodate other areas of responsibility in our lives. It is all too easy to get caught up in worldly priorities and goals, only to forget the real priorities in life: husbands, wives, children, sisters, brothers, mothers, fathers, and the other family members God has placed into our care and responsibility. It is all too easy in today's hectic world to succumb to responsibilities that demand more time or a higher ranking than one's family. It is all too easy to elevate career, education, and/or community involvement above the people we care most about because we mistakenly assume they will always be there. That is not to say these other responsibilities are unimportant or irrelevant. However, we need to be aware of all of our true priorities in life, making sure that these priorities are in proper and positive balance to our other responsibilities.

■ Developing a Positive Family Environment

Modeling, or learning from observation, is an important and very powerful part of the learning process. To **model** means to serve as a pattern, to typify or exemplify an ideal. Modeling as a teaching tool essentially means that individuals learn through the behavior of those in the environment around them. Learning and education do not begin in preschool, kindergarten, or the first grade. Learning begins as soon as someone comes into contact with others. Commonly our first contacts are with the members of our immediate family.

■ What Values Do You Model?

What values are you now modeling to your family members? What examples are you providing to those around you? Are you modeling love, kindness, patience, and other traits mentioned in the biblical passages found earlier in this chapter? How do you really want to interact with the people who are a priority in your life? Is it by caring, by sacrificing, by providing time with them?

> **MODEL:** To serve as a pattern; to typify or exemplify an ideal.

What others see us doing is what makes an impression on them—for good or for bad. They do not hear as clearly what we say *they* should be doing because they are observing and learning from what they see *us* doing.

In the work environment, it is not uncommon for an organization to have a strategic plan to organize and direct people. This can involve goal-setting sessions, time management seminars, workshops on how to deal with people in various work-related situations (conflict management, enhancing communication, developing listening skills), or how to interact with various personality styles.

However, all of that training is often forgotten when we enter the front door of our homes and confront the all-too-frequent chaos of family relationships! Very few families have a strategic plan. It is uncommon for a family to set aside time to decide on goals, organize schedules, solve personality conflicts, and develop communication skills. But a positive family environment doesn't just "happen." It has to be *developed*, just as painstakingly as a corporation—and for much more important reasons.

■ Positive Guidelines

In attempting to develop a positive family environment, Charles Swindoll offers six guidelines:[12]

1. Be committed to the family.
2. Spend time with the family.
3. Develop good family communications.
4. Express appreciation for each other.
5. Develop a spiritual commitment.
6. Strive to solve problems in a crisis situation.

Naturally, how we carry out these guidelines will be a personal decision tailored to our individual family needs. The most important point for family wellness is simply to consider how to implement these guidelines and then follow through on the plan.

Key to implementing these guidelines is not just how well they can be discussed around the kitchen table, but how well they can be modeled. Other modeling behaviors that will strengthen the family environment include:

- **Prayer** – Do you pray regularly with your family? Do family members see you pray and study your Bible regularly? Can they tell from your behavior that this is a priority? After praying, does your behavior express that you have been communicating with God, or do you automatically sink into an attitude of criticism and irritation?

- **Kindness** – Are you as kind to your family members as you are to complete strangers? What is your normal tone of voice with family members? Is it as upbeat and courteous with family members as it is with friends and work associates? Or is it toneless, uninterested?

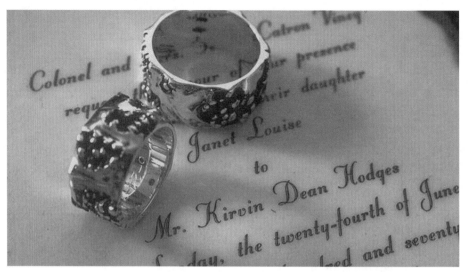

The institution of marriage is one of the most important bonds and relationships in life.

- **Unconditional love** – Are you as forgiving with family members as you are with others? Are you willing to listen honestly to a family member's "side" of things? Do you feel that a family member is disappointing you or embarrassing you, or do you try to see the world through that family member's eyes?

- **Patience** – Do you demonstrate the same level of patience with family members as you do with a group of Sunday school students you teach? Do you have reasonable expectations of family members based on their abilities and perceptions, or do you try to mold them to the expectations of others?

In his sermon, "Steps to a Healthy Family," Pastor Steve Poe offered several "action steps" to help develop a positive family environment:[13]

- **Make fun**—Do you make a conscious effort to have fun with your family? It is all too easy to get caught up in the seriousness of work and the world's priorities. We sometimes forget the importance of planning enjoyable family activities together or simply joining in spontaneous fun activities with family.

- **Give attention**—Don't you like to receive positive attention? So does everyone else. Plan time with individual family members on a regular basis. Make it a priority to inquire consistently about family members, asking how their day went, and taking time to listen and support them.

- **Capture memories**—Want to see the family album? Even if that does not seem like an exciting event right now, family memories become more priceless over time. Establish family traditions and record family times together. Share stories of the family's history and experiences. Today's developments in technology make "capturing memories" more fun and creative than ever before.

- **Verbally inspire**—Do you praise those you care about? Sadly, the people to whom we are closest are the ones we most take for granted. Look for positive reinforcements to pass on to family members. Let them know why you appreciate them and why they are important to your life.

- **Love without condition**—Can you love the sinner? Jesus does. It is important to separate the person from a behavior. You may not agree with a family member's behavior or action, but you can still love that person and remind him or her of your unconditional love.

- **Yield to God**—Can you let go? Are you unconsciously trying to control the actions and decisions of family members? At all times, pray for family decisions and your family's well-being. Seek God's direction and purpose for your family.

All of these action steps and guidelines require a commitment of time. That is the most valuable resource we can offer our families as we seek to improve communication and facilitate family wellness.

■ What God Has Joined Together: The Marriage Bond

The institution of marriage is one of the most important bonds and relationships in life. Whether you currently are married or single, looking at wellness through the lens of marriage can help you evaluate your current or future family relations.

■ The Benefits of Marriage

A strong marriage bond seems to provide many benefits. Several studies have shown that married people tend to be healthier than their unmarried counterparts. One theory is that being married encourages healthy behavior. A recent study comparing more than 4,400 married and widowed people over sixty-five years of age seems to confirm this theory. Results indicate that married people are more likely to wear seat belts, to be physically active, to have their blood pressure checked regularly, to eat breakfast, and not to smoke than those whose spouses had died. A strong, loving marriage also is reported to bring not only better health, but also more happiness.[14] One source even reported that the benefits of marriage were greater for men than for women.[15]

■ Negative Begets Negative

There is a correlation between the type of marriage relationship and the results or consequences of that relationship. As in other areas, positive relationships seem to foster positive results (benefits). The same is true of negative relationships. Some negative consequences of a negative relationship include these:

- Marital strife increases the risk for depression.
- Couples going through a separation suffer more illness and face a greater risk for automobile accidents than do happily married couples.
- When couples attack each other maliciously during an argument, they exhibit deep declines in immune functioning.[16]

It is easy to see from these negative aspects how important it is for married couples to develop positive goals for their marriage, goals that will foster their mutual well-being.

■ Marriage Reinforcers

Though often neglected, the techniques for preserving intimacy and warmth in a marriage are quite simple. They are based on one basic principle: *"We love people who make us feel good about ourselves."*[17] Two ways to achieve this principle are: (1) to provide positive reinforcement to your spouse, and (2) to work to solve common problems. Dr. Ellen Wachtel offers these insights:[18]

Positive Reinforcements:
- Praise your spouse for traits you appreciate or admire.
- Save your criticism for what is really important.
- Practice kindness.
- Do not take your spouse for granted.
- Do not pigeonhole [categorize] yourself or your spouse.

Solving Problems:

- Explain why you feel the way you do.
- Recognize the signs that an argument is getting out of control.
- Do not bring up difficult subjects when you are angry.
- Set a date to revisit the issue.
- Start with the positive.
- Listen for areas of agreement.

■ Marriage Barriers

In his book, *Love for a Lifetime*, Dr. James Dobson refers to barriers to a positive marriage as "marriage killers."[19] These barriers include many factors that relate to overall personal well-being, among them:

- Overcommitment and physical exhaustion
- Excessive credit and conflict over how money will be spent
- Selfishness
- Interference from in-laws
- Unrealistic expectations

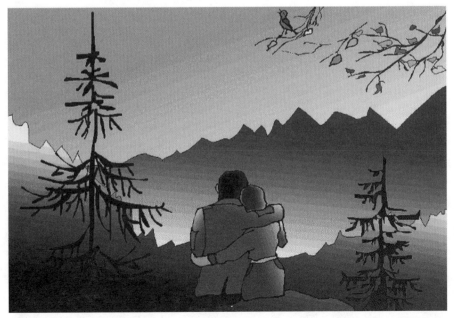

Meaningful touch is a powerful way to demonstrate caring.

- Space invaders
- Alcohol or substance abuse
- Pornography, gambling, and other addictions
- Sexual frustration, loneliness, low self-esteem, and the greener grass of infidelity
- Business success
- Business failure
- Getting married too young

How do you rate yourself and your marriage according to these barriers? What changes do you want to make in any of these areas? A personal awareness of current habits, while not always what we want to see or hear, can be foundational to positive change in the present and positive goal-setting for the future.

■ Positive Modeling Behaviors

The Bible is an excellent blueprint for building a strong marriage and family. Two especially pertinent Scriptures regarding marriage are these:

"And you husbands, show the same kind of love to your wives as Christ showed to the church when he died for her." Ephesians 5:25

"A man must love his wife as a part of himself; and the wife must see to it that she deeply respects her husband." Ephesians 5:33

Earlier, we stressed the importance of modeling the values we wish to instill in our family. In *Leaving the Light On*, Gary Smalley and John Trent offer the following teaching and modeling behaviors to help build family harmony and cohesiveness.[20] Notice how many of these are relevant to both marriage and general family well-being:

- **Provide Affirmations**—Provide positive statements of support and encouragement. Be consistent in this form of support.
- **Build Character**—External image and physical appearance are often a primary focus of the marriage/family. It is more important to build integrity and conform life to one's internal values.

- **Make Time for Listening**—Be available to listen to others. God provided us only *one* mouth but *two* ears for a definite reason. If you do not take time to listen, meaningful times of communication can be lost.

- **Value Differences**—Although God created all of us to be equal, He created each of us with differing skills, interests, and likes, along with the power of choice over how we apply those gifts. Rather than focus critically on a marriage partner or family member's differences (as they relate to what you perceive as valuable), value these differences because they express the infinite variety of your Creator.

- **Resolve Conflicts**—Focus on the facts of a situation and try to remove emotions from the discussion. Forgiveness can be a key to resolution, keeping in mind we all make mistakes. A spirit of forgiveness also can help to remove any unrealistic expectations of self or of others.

- **Provide Meaningful Touches**—Hugs can provide a sense of caring and unconditional love. The true strength of a hug can never be overestimated and may be more powerful than we can imagine.

■ Not Too Young to Know

Regarding meaningful touch, the story is told of newborn twins who were placed in separate incubators, primarily because one of the twins was in poor physical health. The ill twin's condition continued to deteriorate. Although it was against hospital regulations, a nurse decided to place the healthy twin in the same incubator with his ill sibling. After being placed in the incubator, the healthy twin edged close to and placed his arm around the shoulders of his ill sibling. Almost immediately, the vital signs of the ill twin started to return to normal and his overall condition improved dramatically. Within a few days, both twins were well enough to go home with their parents. Not only is meaningful touch a powerful way to demonstrate caring, but its benefits can be acknowledged at a very young age.

■ Single, But Not Alone

Some people choose to remain single. Others become single for different reasons at various stages in their life. It is important to keep in mind that marriage may not be right for everyone. Singleness also can provide opportunities to devote more time in serving those individuals and/or populations who are important in one's life.

Developing relationships is also important in the life of a single person. Single people should establish goals in their efforts to develop and/or strengthen relationships. Relationship development can focus on family time and contacts, involvement in a church or church group, participation in community service organizations or community singles groups, or possible involvement with a specific support group.

Support group participation often is a priority for individuals who have recently become single due to the death of a spouse or through divorce. Support groups can assist with the grieving process, help with acceptance of a current life situation, or focus on the need for forgiveness. Singleness is described in the Bible as a gift from God, just as marriage is described as God's gift.

> *"We are not all the same. God gives some the gift of a husband or wife,*
> *and others he gives the gift of being able to stay happily unmarried."*
> 1 Corinthians 7:7

Both marriage and singleness can at times be burdensome. The responsibilities of each family and family situation are different from those of other families and situations. We can cope more positively with those burdens as they occur if we keep in mind that our current family situation is a gift from God and part of the plan God has for our life *at that time*. While the family environment or any related situation may not be what we consider to be ideal, remember to implement a key wellness activity during those stressful times: Pray to God for wisdom, strength, and direction for coping with the situation and developing goals for future change.

■ Caring for Children

The wellness perspective stresses that meeting individual needs is important to individual growth, development, and well-being. Nowhere is this more important than in the care of the most cherished gift God can offer a family—a child. It is important to remember that unlike young animals, children take a long time to reach maturity. They are dependent on their families to provide for their needs. Those needs go beyond food, shelter, clothing, security, and socialization. We sometimes forget that a small child has meaningful needs, just as adults do.

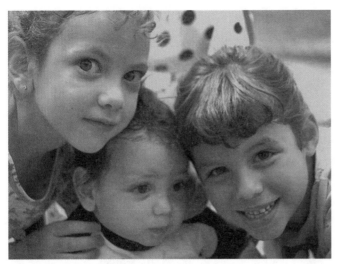

The most cherished gift God can offer a family is a child.

Meeting those needs is not only critically important to a child's development, it is a primary responsibility of family members. Among those meaningful needs are these:[21]

- **Compassion**—Caring and demonstrating through your actions that a child and the child's needs are important.

- **Counsel**—Teaching and modeling a value system that will guide a child's future attitudes and behaviors. Willingness to discuss this value system with the child.

- **Correction**—Providing discipline to help direct a child's understanding of right from wrong and to help direct future decision making. Learning to distinguish between punishment (to penalize) and discipline (helping a child learn and develop).

- **Confidence**—Helping a child develop belief in the child's abilities and

Excerpt 6.5, Cultivate a Child

If a child lives with criticism, he learns to condemn.
If a child lives with hostility, he learns to fight.
If a child lives with ridicule, he learns to be shy.
If a child lives with shame, he learns to feel guilty.
If a child lives with tolerance, he learns to be patient.
If a child lives with encouragement, he learns confidence.
If a child lives with praise, he learns to appreciate.
If a child lives with fairness, he learns justice.
If a child lives with security, he learns to have faith.
If a child lives with approval, he learns to like himself.
If a child lives with acceptance and friendship, he learns to find love in the world.

Source: Charles Swindoll, *Growing Wise in Family Life* (Portland: Multnomah Press, 1988), 82, quoting Dorothy Nolte.

the value of "if at first you don't succeed, try, try again." Building the child's self-esteem and self-motivation.

- **Celebration**—Recognizing important milestones in a child's development. Fostering fun and enjoyment in life. Demonstrating the importance of laughter and humor as a way to relieve stress.

- **Challenges**—Providing opportunities for learning and growth. Helping a child develop positive independence. Reinforcing the satisfaction of a job well done in all areas of responsibility.

- **Consistency**—Demonstrating the correlation between word and deed. Stressing the importance of core values and modeling them on a daily basis in a variety of situations.

The Bible provides wise counsel for teaching and dealing with children. In seeking ways to positively impact your child's well-being, remember this advice:

> *"And now a word to you parents. Don't keep on scolding and nagging your children, making them angry and resentful. Rather, bring them up with the loving discipline the Lord himself approves, with suggestions and godly advice."* Ephesians 6:4

■ Summary

Family—whatever that term means to us and the individuals involved—is a gift from God, a meaningful and important priority in our lives. As we become more comfortable with the people we care about, we often take them for granted, pushing aside time and activities devoted to them. It is a responsibility of overall wellness to keep family as a priority in life and to "make time" for family contacts. Achievements and goals accomplished at the expense of family commitments often, in retrospect, seem very hollow.

We often view the term "sacrifice" in a negative light. Giving up something we value is hard to do. To sacrifice family time and commitments in pursuit of other goals will erode the foundation of the family and result in negative consequences for the family environment. To make a personal sacrifice in order to have more time with one's family will almost always result in positive benefits for the family environment. Which sacrifice will you make?

KEY CONCEPTS

family
the Golden Rule
loneliness
model
self-esteem
social wellness
solitude

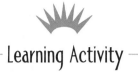

Learning Activity

1. This chapter has examined the three main foundations of caring
    communication as they pertain to social and family wellness. How do
    you currently evaluate yourself in each of these areas? What goals can
    you pinpoint to increase your communication in each area?

    Communication with Self:
    Rating:

5	4	3	2	1
High				Low

    Goals:

    _____

    _____

    _____

    Communication with Others:
    Rating:

5	4	3	2	1
High				Low

    Goals:

    _____

    _____

    _____

    Communication with God:
    Rating:

5	4	3	2	1
High				Low

    Goals:

    _____

    _____

    _____

Positive traits you wish to model in your communications with others:

_____

_____

2. In reviewing the suggestions for positive teaching and modeling to family members, what steps can you initiate in order to increase your level of family wellness?

Activities or types of contacts you wish to begin with your family:

_____ date to begin:_____

_____ date to begin:_____

_____ date to begin:_____

_____ date to begin:_____

_____ date to begin:_____

Steps or changes required in order to "make time" for these contacts:

_____

_____

_____

_____

Possible barriers that could inhibit your family goals and actions:

_____

_____

_____

_____

Actions you can take to overcome your perceived barriers:

_____

_____

_____

_____

_____

Additional Activities and References

1. How can you better apply the Golden Rule in your interactions with others? Can you think of situations/contacts for which you believe the Golden Rule would not apply?

_____

_____

_____

_____

_____

_____

2. What steps or actions can you take to become more of an "Encourager" to people?

_____

_____

_____

_____

_____

_____

3. Review the following resource for additional information on various perspectives of family wellness:

www.kidshealth.org

Endnotes

1. Charles Swindoll, *Growing Wise in Family Life* (Portland: Multnomah Press, 1988), 35.
2. Denis Waitley, *Seeds of Greatness: The Ten Best-Kept Secrets of Total Success* (Old Tappan, NJ: Fleming H. Revell, 1983), 40-41.
3. Ibid., 134.
4. Ibid., 40-41.
5. Robert Bolton, *People Skills* (New York: Simon and Schuster, 1979), 5, quoting Harry Stack Sullivan.
6. Ibid., 5.
7. Herbert Benson and Eileen M. Stuart, *The Wellness Book* (Secaucus, NJ: Carol Publishing Group, 1992), 250.
8. Delores Bius, "The Ministry of Encouragement," *Holiness Digest* (n.p., n.d.).
9. Ibid.
10. Curtis O. Byer and Louis W. Shainberg, *Living Well: Health in Your Hands* (New York: Harper Collins, 1995), 29.
11. Charles Swindoll, *Growing Wise in Family Life*, 20.
12. Ibid., 36.
13. Steve Poe, "Steps to a Healthy Family," a sermon delivered at Northview Christian Life Church, Carmel, Indiana, on November 5, 2000.
14. Ellen Wachtel, "A Good Relationship Is Good for Your Health," *Bottom Line Health* (March 1999): 5.
15. "Wellness Facts," *University of California-Berkeley Newsletter* 15 (February 1999): 5.
16. Wachtel, 5.
17. Ibid.
18. Ibid., 5-6.
19. James Dobson, *Love for a Lifetime: Building a Marriage That Will Go the Distance* (Portland: Multnomah, 2001), 103-06.
20. Gary Smalley and John Trent, *Leaving the Light On: Building the Memories That Will Draw Your Kids Home* (Sisters, OR: Questar, 1994), 25-115.
21. Steve Poe, "Seasons of Parenting," a sermon delivered at Northview Christian Life Church, Carmel, Indiana, Summer 2001.

7

OCCUPATIONAL AND EDUCATIONAL WELLNESS

"You are free to choose, but the choices you make today will determine
what you have, be, and do in the tomorrows of your life."

—Zig Ziglar[1]

Personal growth and professional development are important aspects of life satisfaction and overall well-being. Higher levels of education have been associated with lifestyle choices that promote positive well-being. To continue to develop and enhance our God-given skills and interests, applying those abilities within our circles of influence, is to fulfill our life purpose. Author Richard Bolles captures the essence of purpose-driven wellness by explaining that we have three missions during our time on earth. These three missions are:

OBJECTIVES

- Explore decision-making models for career and educational fields.

- Identify future career and educational goals.

- Evaluate career change options.

- Discuss alternative programs for obtaining educational training.

- Recognize the importance of lifelong learning.

1. To seek to stand hour by hour in the conscious presence of God, the One from whom your mission is derived.

2. To do what you can, moment by moment, day by day, step by step, to make this world a better place, following the leading and guidance of God's Spirit within you and around you.

3. To exercise that particular talent which you particularly came to earth to use—your greatest gift which you most delight to use, in the places or settings which God has caused to appeal to you the most, and for those purposes which God needs to have done in the world.[2]

A Matching Process

Occupational wellness and educational wellness are strongly related. One area often will provide a focus or bearing to help direct decisions related to the other. In this chapter we will explore aspects of both occupational and educational goal planning and decision making.

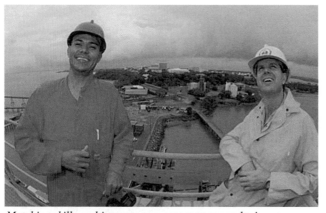

Matching skills and interests to a career area results in more personal satisfaction.

We can look at this study of occupational and educational wellness as a "matching process." This term refers to matching individual skills, interests, values, needs, and personality traits to either a career area or an area of educational training. A proper match is important for the desired end results of personal satisfaction and fulfillment with the career area or educational field selected. A satisfactory outcome to the matching process does not "just happen." A process involves steps or stages. Two important aspects of good decision making are exploration and planning. However, these two aspects often are overlooked. Many people make career and/or educational decisions without adequately researching information about specific career or educational areas of interest. Even worse, they sometimes base their decisions on what areas happen to have openings at the time or what areas offer the greatest potential for financial gain. There is more than a kernel of truth to the saying that many people put more planning into a Christmas or birthday party than they do into their own career or educational search process. Does that saying reflect any of your past decision-making efforts in these areas?

As we look at the matching process for occupational and educational planning, we will focus on five steps:

1. Developing personal awareness

2. Establishing initial priorities

3. Exploring and evaluating these initial priorities

4. Developing action steps toward a priority goal

5. Appraising progress

The decisions we make in both occupational and educational planning will influence our overall sense of wellness. If we derive little satisfaction from our careers and/or fields of education, that frustration and lack of satisfaction can negatively impact our actions and perceptions in all other areas of our lives. Frustration at work can lead to stress. Stress can negatively affect our home life and family interactions, as well as cause us to develop negative personal physical habits and emotional outlooks.

Keep in mind the implications of the "matching process" as you examine the relationship between occupational and educational wellness.

- Career interests are pivotal in determining what educational and training programs are right for each person.
- Educational interests are foundational for determining an individual's career areas of interest.

With an eye to the positive aspects of this relationship and realizing that individual situations will determine which area directs the other, we will turn first to a discussion of occupational wellness.

Occupational Wellness: A Sense of Personal Purpose

"Whatever you do, do well . . ." Ecclesiastes 9:10

In defining occupational wellness, we want to focus on its part in helping to attain a positive sense of purpose and self-satisfaction through work responsibilities. God places every person on this earth for a purpose. A job can provide a vehicle for that purpose. It is a function of occupational wellness to match a personal sense of purpose to a specific career area in order to provide a sense of personal career satisfaction. To find a good match, we must ask ourselves: How and where can I best use the gifts God has given me?

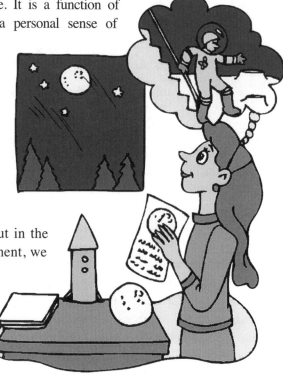

■ Career Search

A career search may not be a personal priority at this time. But in the ever-changing world of employment, we never know when we might need to initiate a voluntary or involuntary career search. Even in a worst-case scenario (sudden, unexpected job loss), planning possible career options should have a positive focus at any stage of our lives. If you are currently pursuing an educational degree or taking courses to enhance your education, consider how this can positively affect your future career choices, improve your standing in your current career, or prepare you for a career change.

> It is a function of occupational wellness to match a personal sense of purpose to a specific career area in order to provide a sense of personal career satisfaction.

The career search process is a method to positively match your personal and career purposes. Earlier we listed a five-step process to help implement this match. In the next section, we will discuss in more detail that five-step process as it relates to a career search.

■ Step One: Personal Awareness

"God has given each of you some special abilities; be sure to use them to help each other, passing on to others God's many kinds of blessings." 1 Peter 4:10

Personal awareness in career planning involves a personal assessment and understanding of traits and characteristics that are important to career satisfaction. These traits and characteristics should reflect an individual's purpose as it relates to a career field. To define purpose:

- Identify your skills—what you do well.
- Identify your interests—what you enjoy doing.
- Identify your needs—as they relate to career satisfaction.
- Identify your values—what you consider to be your personal core beliefs.

Matching one's purpose-driven personal traits and characteristics to career areas and responsibilities that utilize those qualities is an effective way to begin a career exploration and search process. Among personal matches to consider are these:

- Career responsibilities that involve your personal interests and likes
- Career responsibilities that involve your strongly held personal values
- Career responsibilities that fulfill needs you believe are meaningful
- Career responsibilities that involve skills you enjoy utilizing

You will probably never find a "perfect" career match for these personal qualities, but the closer you can match these qualities to the responsibilities of a particular career area, the better your chance of locating a career that provides satisfaction. Your focus, then, should be to locate career areas that match a high percentage of your personal qualities.

Consider these personal traits in relationship to one another. You may excel in a particular skill, but this does not necessarily mean that you also have an interest in consistently applying that skill in a career setting. You may find a career field that successfully meets your financial expectations but does not reflect your important personal values or interests. As much as possible, match your personal traits with any career areas you are considering.

John Holland developed a career model that matches personal interests to possible career options (see Exhibit 7.1). His model lists career options categorized by the personal characteristics necessary to fulfill the responsibilities of various careers. He divided career fields into six categories, with each category featuring the personal characteristics of individuals who might best fit those career fields.

Exhibit 7.1. Holland's Typology of Personalities and Occupations

Realistic:

Personal Interests: Likes to work with objects, tools; enjoys using physical abilities and working outdoors.

Personal Characteristics: Shy, genuine, materialistic, persistent, stable.

Sample Occupations: Mechanical engineer, skilled tradesman, police officer, forester, military, or air traffic control.

Investigative:

Personal Interests: Likes to investigate and solve problems, work with abstract problems, and understand how things work.

Personal Characteristics: Analytical, cautious, curious, independent, introverted.

Sample Occupations: Economist, physicist, physician, engineer, mathematician, or computer programmer.

Artistic:

Personal Interests: Likes to use imagination, work in unstructured environments, and create using artistic abilities.

Personal Characteristics: Disorderly, emotional, idealistic, imaginative, impulsive.

Sample Occupations: Journalist, advertising manager, drama teacher, interior decorator, composer, photographer, or author.

Social:

Personal Interests: Likes to assist and support people, train, teach; has a concern for the welfare of others.

Personal Characteristics: Cooperative, generous, helpful, sociable, understanding.

Sample Occupations: Counselor, social worker, clergy, teacher, personnel director, therapist, or dietitian.

Enterprising:

Personal Interests: Energetic, likes to assume leadership and persuade others; has a desire to achieve power and status.

Personal Characteristics: Adventurous, ambitious, energetic, domineering, self-confident.

Sample Occupations: Attorney, sales person, purchasing agent, real estate agent, market analyst, recruiter.

Conventional:

Personal Interests: Likes well-ordered activities and well-defined tasks; enjoys office work, working with data, and applying clerical skills.

Personal Characteristics: Efficient, obedient, practical, calm, conscientious.

Sample Occupations: CPA, office manager, computer operator, credit manager, or court reporter.

Adapted from *Career Management,* 1st edition by Greenhaus. © 1987. Reprinted with permission of South-Western, a division of Thomson Learning: www.thomsonrights.com. Fax 800 730-2215.

To demonstrate how the self-awareness process might work, let's create a hypothetical career search for a woman named Holly. Holly's personal interests, needs, skills, and values revolve around helping others, teaching, serving, and persuading. If we try to match Holly's traits to the Holland Model, we find that she probably would do well in the career areas of teaching, counseling, sales, marketing, law, medicine, and/or ministry.

The personal awareness stage of a career search is a time to develop as many options and areas of interest as possible. Expand your horizons at this point. Try to think of any and every career area that might involve your valued, personal characteristics. Some of the career options you target may have specific job titles, while others may involve general areas or career clusters. While at this point in the search process these are only options to consider, remember that in matching your interests to career fields, any thoughts and options at this stage are positive and useful. Explore and evaluate these options carefully before making a final decision. The more thorough you are at this stage of exploration, the more informed your decision will be.

■ Step Two: Establish Initial Priorities

"Help me to do your will, for you are my God. Lead me in good paths, for your Spirit is good." Psalm 143:10

After establishing a comprehensive list of future career options, it is important to develop a priority ranking for the options you have developed. Consider a few questions concerning your career future to help focus on personal priorities.

- Careerwise, what do you want to be doing five years from now? Why does this type of work appeal to you?
- What kinds of job responsibilities interest you? Why do these responsibilities appeal to you?
- In what geographical region do you wish to live? Why does this area appeal to you?

As you answer these questions, consider the list of career options you developed in step one. Avoid a common career development barrier often referred to as "tunnel vision." **Tunnel vision** occurs when people eliminate possible career options solely because they have no previous experience in that area or do not at this time have the training or education required for that specific career area.

To downplay unnecessary tunnel vision, consider these two points. First, every individual has obtained numerous skills through past work experiences and/or various training and educational programs. Focus on the skill areas you *can* bring to a career area of interest. Focus on the positive. Sadly, most people see only the skills they do *not* have, or they focus on why they would *not* be a good match for a position.

> # TUNNEL VISION:
> A career development barrier that causes people to eliminate career options because they feel unqualified.

Second, turn that awareness of a possible shortcoming into a goal for future development. In what way(s) are you not qualified for a certain position of interest? This foundation of awareness can provide positive direction for your future actions. Look at what you believe to be your possible shortcomings and then use this determination to develop goals to obtain the necessary experience, education, and/or training you will need. Turn your perception of negative barriers into a positive perception by developing methods to overcome these potential barriers.

Once you have developed a list of future career options, it is then important to prioritize your career possibilities. Ask yourself this question: Of all the career options I have listed, if I could begin working immediately in any of these fields, what would be my first choice?

> Turn your perception of negative barriers into a positive perception by developing methods to overcome these potential barriers.

To prioritize, review the list you have developed and circle your top choice, according to your abilities and perceptions *at the present time*. Continue to prioritize your list until you have five or six options in which the job responsibilities seem to provide a good match for your personal characteristics.

If we return to Holly, you will recall that her personal traits aligned with career options in teaching, counseling, law, marketing, medical service, and sales. Following step two, she considers these career fields and some of the options available within these fields. She then prioritizes her list in this order: elementary education teacher, lawyer, special education teacher, nurse, and retail selling. She feels that these career options best match her interests in helping, serving, persuading, and teaching others.

An important part of the process now is to find more specific information about each career option. A problem could arise if Holly decides only to become a lawyer and ignores her other options. Since at this point she is still in the decision-making process, she could be circumventing the process by making a hasty decision to enter a career field. The most important stages of this process have not yet occurred. What she now knows about these career areas is probably just the tip of the iceberg. If she is to be thorough, she needs to acquire as much information as possible about her career areas of interest, as well as to be certain of the accuracy of the information upon which she originally based her decision to choose a particular career area. She also needs to evaluate these areas to affirm a good match with her personal characteristics.

Exhibit 7.2 offers several career information sources through which people can gather information and make informed decisions.

Exhibit 7.2. Career Information Sources

Friends and Family:
> Those working in organizations or career areas of interest
> Those who know people in organizations or career areas of interest
> Those who know people with contacts

Written Sources:
> Career libraries
> Career placement offices
> Bookstores
> Computerized career informational services
> The World Wide Web
> *Occupational Outlook Handbook* (Department of Labor)
> Corporate annual reports
> Investment analysts' reports
> Trade publications and directories
> Journal articles about companies
> Recruiting brochures
> Advertisements
> Newspaper articles
> Industry – company case studies

People in Industry and Professions:
> Alumni
> Trade associations
> Professional societies
> Visiting speakers
> Chamber of Commerce

Social, Religious, and Political Organizations:
> Church groups
> Political parties
> Kiwanis, Rotary, etc.

People with Contacts:
> Bankers
> Doctors, dentists
> Lawyers
> Accountants
> Insurance agencies
> College instructors
> Personnel directors
> Investment analysts

Adapted from Manuel London and Stephen A. Stumpf, *Managing Careers* (Reading, MA: Addison-Wesley, 1982), 51, Table 3.6. Reprinted with permission of the authors.

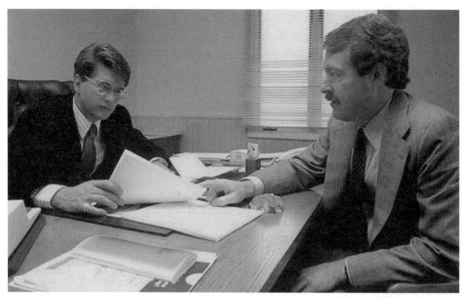

Personal "information interviews" are an excellent way to learn more about a career area of interest.

■ Step Three: Explore and Evaluate Initial Career Priorities

"Show me the path where I should go, O Lord; point out the right road for me to walk." Psalm 25:4

After determining priority career areas of interest, it is important to find out as much as possible about these specific areas. The more information you obtain, the more confidence you can have in your decision. Consider the following questions as you explore and evaluate career options:

- What are the daily responsibilities of this career area?
- How can you best prepare to enter this career area?
- What are the chances and prerequisites for advancement?
- Are future local and national job markets promising?
- What changes are foreseen in the next five to ten years?
- What other career areas involve similar responsibilities?
- What are the benefits of this career, both financial and nonmonetary?

It is important to remember as you progress through this stage of career exploration that there is no perfect career field. Every field will have positive and negative factors. Do not let either the positives or the negatives stop your exploration. We can cite numerous examples in which people cut short the career exploration process based only on their positive findings. Thus, they never realized the negative factors of a particular career field until they had already made a final decision. The opposite is also true. Some people have halted their search after finding a few negative factors about a particular career field, instead of waiting to see if the positives would outweigh the negatives.

Exhibit 7.2 details a number of ways to explore career options. Two especially helpful methods are career reference materials—available both in hard copy and online—and informational interviews with people knowledgeable about a career area.

Two common print reference sources of career information include the *Occupational Outlook Handbook* and the *Encyclopedia of Careers and Vocational Guidance*.[3] These resources contain a wealth of information related to job responsibilities, necessary preparation, job outlook, salary ranges, and additional career areas that may involve responsibilities related to a career area of interest. However, it is important to remember that the information available in these printed reference materials may have taken two years or more to compile—before printing. Since printed resources are updated every two to three years, some of the information may already be three to four years old at the time of your research. In addition, job outlooks and salary ranges listed in these resources are taken from a national research database. That information may vary greatly one way or another from the actual situation in a particular region of the country.

Personal "information interviews" are an excellent way to learn more about a career area of interest. An informational interview involves someone employed in a career area of interest or someone who may be responsible for hiring in a particular career area of interest. These interviews can be classified as "warm" contacts or "cold" contacts. A "warm" contact is someone the interviewer knows personally or who can introduce the interviewer to someone else in a career area of interest. A "cold" contact is acquired by calling an organization and asking for the name of a person who works in or oversees a certain career area of interest. Be sure to explain to these contacts that the purpose for the informational interview is to gather information about the career field, not to interview for a job.

Let's return to Holly. At this point, she has established initial career priorities in the fields of elementary education, law, special education, nursing, and retailing. She then begins to read reference materials and talk to people in these various career areas. Part of her exploration includes "shadowing" a nursing unit and visiting nurses in a local hospital. Through these contacts she discovers that she does not like the amount of science she would have to study to earn a nursing degree. She also finds that she is not completely comfortable with some of the specific daily responsibilities required of nurses.

She turns next to the legal field. After extensive reading, she talks to a pre-law academic advisor. She learns that the legal area in which she is interested requires a graduate degree before she can even enter the field. She also discovers that this field will not provide the type of people-oriented service in which she is interested. Turning to retail sales, Holly obtains part-time employment in a local retail clothing store. While she enjoys the work for the short term, she realizes that it will not be a "good fit" for her long-term goals.

Holly then visits the elementary school she attended as a child, interviewing some of her past elementary instructors. She also takes a class in experiential teaching, which reinforces her belief that education is the field for which she is best suited. She thus narrows her choices to elementary education and/or special education.

The purpose of step three is to gather as much information as possible about career areas of interest. Following the exploration phase, evaluate the information you have obtained in order to establish a priority career goal. From informational interviews, independent research, and even "field experience," you are able to evaluate your initial options and make a well-informed decision on the priority career field or title that best fits you.

■ Step Four: Develop Action Steps toward Your Priority Goal

"Be sure that you do all the Lord has told you to." Colossians 4:17

Having established a priority career goal, it is important to develop action steps both to realize this goal and to continue the exploration of this career field. Action steps will help you focus on what is needed to become a strong candidate for a specific career area. This means developing short-term preparation goals to help move you toward your long-term career goal. The purpose of action steps is to make sure you are well prepared when the time comes to apply for a position in a desired career area. Sample action steps might include these:

- Researching required training and/or educational courses
- Enrolling in specific training or educational courses
- Pursuing a degree related to the career area of interest
- Researching ways to obtain work experience in or related to the career area of interest
- Pursuing volunteer work experience in related work areas

Short-term action steps can be some of the most difficult steps to take. It is often easy to discuss and plan long-term goals that are months or even years from being fulfilled. With long-term goals, you may feel a sense of relief at having made a decision, knowing you are not under pressure to produce immediate results. However, when you commit to short-term action steps, you realize that it is time to take a risk, to visibly move toward a goal. This step can be a true test of motivation and commitment to that goal.

The risk is related to the willingness to make a commitment—either a financial commitment, a commitment of time, and/or a sacrifice of some other personal commitments and contacts. Risk is also involved when asking a supervisor or employer for an opportunity to obtain related work experience in some way, either through volunteer work, internships, a transfer to a different area, or involvement with a community or organizational group or committee. This is the time that the easy discussion of future goals suddenly becomes more complex—intricately connected to your commitment to action steps that are meant to prepare you for that ever-nearing future.

In step four, Holly takes the action step of enrolling in an elementary education program at a local college. By taking introductory courses in elementary education and continuing her contacts with the teachers she interviewed during her initial exploration, she is preparing to enter the field of elementary education by learning more about the field. While her decision is fairly certain, she continues to thoroughly explore and evaluate all aspects of her chosen career field.

■ Step Five: Appraising Progress

"I will instruct you . . . and guide you along the best pathway for your life; I will advise you and watch your progress." Psalm 32:8

As you move through your selected action steps, you will need feedback to help assess your progress. Are you comfortable with the steps you are taking—not in the sense that they are necessarily easy, but are you meeting the challenges in a positive way? Do you continue to sense that this career is a good match for your personality traits? As you make additional contacts and gain more experience within an area of interest, your interest level can move in one of two directions.

Your contacts and the information you gain may strengthen your resolve to enter this field, solidifying your decision to continue. Or, you may find through additional contacts and experiences

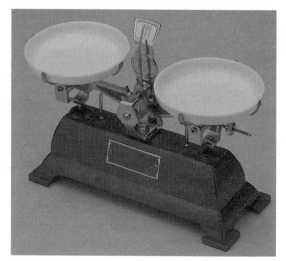

Before making a decision, always compare at least two alternatives.

that this career area is not as appealing as you first thought. If the second option is the case, it may be necessary to return to step two of the process, reestablish priorities, and begin to explore another priority area. Evaluating your satisfaction with the career area you are currently pursuing is the best way to determine whether to continue with your action steps or go back to step two. Do not consider the second option a failure on your part. Be persistent and keep the process in motion until you find a positive career match.

In *Career Management and Survival in the Workplace*, authors Manuel London and Edward Mone reiterate this aspect of commitment in their career decision-making model.

This model involves five steps:

1. Identify the problem; evaluate the need for change.

2. Explore alternatives; survey the available alternatives.

3. Evaluate alternatives; weigh and compare the alternatives.

4. Make a choice; establish a point of decision.

5. Make a commitment; implement and adhere to the plan.[4]

Fred J. Hecklinger and Bernadette M. Black offer a decision-making model based on the possible obstacles someone may encounter. They advise comparing two alternatives in the evaluation process before making a decision.

> Their model involves six steps:
>
> 1. Define the decision you need to make.
>
> 2. Identify any obstacles and then deal with them.
>
> 3. Get adequate information before making a decision.
>
> 4. Before making a decision, always compare at least two alternatives.
>
> 5. Know your most important personal values and rank them in terms of their importance to you.
>
> 6. When it is time to make a decision, *you* make the decision. Do not let other people or circumstances decide for you.[5]

You will always confront obstacles to your personal goals. As you learn to recognize these obstacles, please remember that being aware of future barriers allows you time to address and overcome those barriers. Do not let the term *barrier* impede your progress. Explore ways to prepare for and deal with any real or perceived obstacles. This does take effort, but career fit and satisfaction are long-term outcomes well worth the effort you will expend.

Combining the various components we have just reviewed, we come up with a career decision-making model that includes these important elements:

> 1. Develop a list of personal skills, interests, and values.
>
> 2. Considering that list, develop a list of career interest areas.
>
> 3. Explore and compare these career areas of interest.
>
> 4. Study the requirements for entry into priority career areas of interest.
>
> 5. Identify and address possible obstacles.
>
> 6. Make your decision—establish a priority career area of interest.
>
> 7. Develop an action plan and a commitment to your goal.
>
> 8. Evaluate your progress at regular intervals.

No matter which model you select or which steps you believe to be the most relevant to your situation, the important thing is to continue to plan, prepare, and take action toward your career goals. Be proactive as you explore your options and evaluate your progress. The primary goal is to match your unique skills and interests to the career area that will offer you professional growth, career satisfaction, and life purpose.

NETWORKING: Sharing career goals with other individuals, exchanging information and services, and being open to new ideas, relationships, and/or opportunities in a career field.

■ Career Networking

Career networking is similar to the informational interviewing process we discussed earlier in this chapter. While informational interviewing is useful during the career exploration stage, networking generally occurs once you have selected a career area of interest and have determined to enter that field. We will define **networking** as sharing career goals with other individuals, exchanging information and services, and being open to new ideas, relationships, and/or opportunities in a career field. You can network with anyone you contact on a regular basis or with individuals you know or meet in conferences, professional organizations, community groups, church, your neighborhood, on a trip, or on any occasion that brings you into contact with

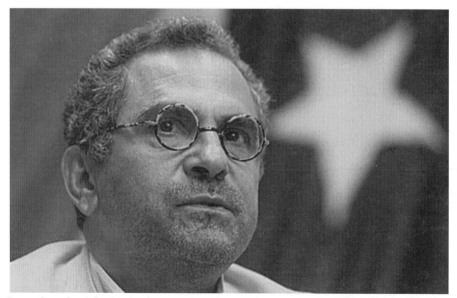

Career fit and satisfaction are long-term outcomes well worth the effort you will expend.

other people. Each networking contact you make may provide you with names for future contacts. Networking is a reciprocal process. As you make and expand these contacts, you learn more about the people that you meet, as well as the career field in which they are employed. Your networking contact also learns more about you, your goals, and your background. Your networking contacts may be able to provide important information, feedback, and additional contacts for your career search. You even may meet people who someday could be in a position to hire you.

In *The Career Adventure*, author Susan Johnston suggests the following questions to ask a networking contact:

1. What are the specific duties associated with your position?

2. How did you obtain your present job?

3. How could I prepare myself to enter this field?

4. Where do you see this field going during the next five to ten years?

5. What do you like most about your job?

6. What do you like least about your job?

7. Who else would you recommend I speak with who knows about this field?[6]

■ Career Stress

Earlier in this text, we looked at emotional wellness as it relates to stress and stress management. One's work environment, as we learned, can be a major cause of stress. Some factors involved in job-related stress are:

- Change
- Personal appraisals
- Daily hassles

The work environment in today's world is constantly changing and fiercely competitive. Particular work conditions or situations can result in negative personal appraisals. The sheer complexity of work demands coupled with the hectic pace of events often can rank high on your list of daily hassles.

Another primary source of stress is recognizing that your career or the specific responsibilities in your career do not involve or match your personal values. We have seen the importance of this match earlier in this chapter as it relates to career decision making. One list includes these stress factors:

- Role conflict
- Person/role conflict
- Role or task overload
- Role or task underload
- Role ambiguity
- Discrimination
- Stereotyping
- Marriage/work conflicts
- Social isolation[7]

Another list includes these stress factors:

- Organizational characteristics
- Working conditions
- Career transitions[8]

Whatever the cause of work-related stress—and these stress factors are different for different people—anticipating and being aware of personal factors of stress at work are important beginning steps to dealing with the stress. That awareness must be followed up with positive coping responses. After determining personal factors of work stress, it can be helpful to return to the chapter on stress management and review the "change, accept, or leave" model. Remember that the "change, accept, or leave" choice related to the cause of stress will help in determining the type of coping action to pursue:

- Change—focus on changing the stressful situation.
- Accept—focus on positive methods to strengthen your body, mind, and spirit in order to cope.
- Leave—focus on distancing yourself from the situation.

■ Burnout

"Burnout" is a term often associated with career stress. **Burnout** can be defined as a type of stress reaction in jobs that involve negative emotional contacts with other people, negative work environments, negative perceptions of the work environment, and/or a perceived lack of control over these

BURNOUT: Exhaustion of physical or emotional strength or motivation, usually as a result of prolonged stress.

situations. Continual contact with these influences can drain a person to the point of emotional exhaustion. Several organizational conditions and personal traits can be factors in the presence of burnout.

1. Organizational conditions influencing burnout can include:

   - Lack of recognition, rewards, and feedback
   - Lack of control over the work environment
   - Lack of clarity of job responsibilities
   - Lack of support

2. Personal traits that can influence burnout are:

   - Idealistic/perfectionistic expectations of outcomes
   - Assuming personal responsibility for failure[9]

As has been common in our study of wellness, burnout at work can negatively influence other areas of life. Personal physical care and your relationships with others seem to suffer the most during periods of burnout. Your best recourse is to anticipate stress factors and develop positive coping methods *before* you reach the point of burnout.

■ Coping with Stress

"Let him have all your worries and cares, for he is always thinking about you and watching everything that concerns you." 1 Peter 5:7

To repeat, effective coping methods for career stress can be found in the "change, accept, or leave" model of stress management.

In dealing with career stress, Jeffrey Greenhaus addresses specific action steps. These action steps focus mainly on the "change" option of stress management, which involves the attempt to change the stressful situation or the factors related to the stressful situation. He suggests these steps:

- Attempt to eliminate burdensome parts of the job.
- Attempt to add or better utilize staff to help relieve pressures.
- Attempt to build more challenge or responsibility into the job.
- Seek clarification of job duties.
- Seek clarification of career prospects.
- Seek feedback on job performance.
- Seek a more flexible work schedule.
- Seek a job transfer.
- Seek a different organization or career field.
- Seek the advice of others.
- Attempt to upgrade job skills through education and/or experience.
- Attempt to resolve conflicts with supervisors, peers, and/or subordinates.
- Participate in a career-planning program.[10]

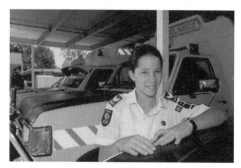

Dual-career families are common in today's society.

It is important to keep in mind that you always have a choice regarding what to do about the cause of stress. It then becomes your personal responsibility to follow up and act upon the available choices.

■ Dual-Career Families

Dual-career families are common in today's society. A dual-career family is one in which both marriage partners pursue career goals and responsibilities. Dual-career families can encounter either positive benefits or negative consequences of this situation. Benefits include fulfilling individual purpose, career satisfaction, financially adding to the quality of family life, and/or adding a greater balance of power to the relationship.

On the other hand, dual-career responsibilities also can be a factor of stress in the family relationship. Common sources of stress in a dual-career family include:

- Conflict regarding work, family, and leisure roles
- Identity problems
- Competition and jealousy
- Career priorities
- Impact on career achievement[11]

Some helpful ways to cope with stress in dual-family environments are to develop flexible schedules, support one another through shared responsibilities at home, and commit to social, recreational, and/or family time together.

■ Career Satisfaction

"The thief's purpose is to steal, kill and destroy. My purpose is to give life in all its fullness." John 10:10

Research studies report that between 40 to 80 percent of the workforce is unhappy at work.[12] For whatever reason, these individuals do not find contentment or a sense of purpose in their work. As you consider a career change or initiate a career search, it is important to consider options that provide a sense of satisfaction in your life. Authors Lee Ellis and Larry Burkett offer four guidelines to achieve a sense of career satisfaction and contentment through career responsibilities:

1. True fulfillment is not accomplished through work.
   Our primary need cannot be filled by the process or the results of work, but from a spiritual relationship with God.

2. Work should enable us to fulfill our overriding life purpose. God has placed all of us on earth for a purpose and we have been provided with a desire to do something that has meaning. Since most of our waking hours are spent at work, it seems logical that work serves as a focal point for carrying out our personal purpose and mission.

3. Work can fill many of our needs. Important needs that can be provided through a career include:

   - Survival – providing food, shelter, and other necessities of life.
   - Creativity – opportunities to express personal characteristics.

- Achievement – seeing the results of our efforts.
- Recognition and Reinforcement – receiving feedback regarding our work efforts.
- Order – understanding the structure, rules, and policies of the organization.
- Variety – opportunities to expand skills and responsibilities.
- Fellowship – providing a sense of belonging and ability to build relationships.

4. Maximum fulfillment from work comes from using our God-given personal interests and talents.[13]

Career satisfaction is meaningful to personal fulfillment. The importance of career satisfaction hinges on your awareness and consideration of personal interests, skills, needs, and values when you make career decisions. Without that match of personality traits and career responsibilities, career satisfaction is difficult to achieve.

Exhibit 7.3. The Five Stages of Career Development

1. Preparation for Work. Age Range: 0 – 25 years
   - Major Tasks: Develop occupational self-image, assess alternative options, develop initial occupational choice, pursue necessary education.

2. Organizational Entry. Age Range: 18 – 25 years
   - Major Tasks: Obtain job offer(s) from desired organization(s), select appropriate job based on accurate information.

3. Early Career: Establishment and Achievement. Age Range: 25 – 40 years
   - Major Tasks: Learn job, learn organizational rules and norms, fit into chosen occupation and organization, increase competence, pursue dream.

4. Mid Career. Age Range: 40 – 55 years
   - Major Tasks: Reappraise early career and early adulthood, reaffirm or modify dream, make choices appropriate to middle adult years, remain productive in work.

5. Late Career. Age Range: 55 – Retirement
   - Major Tasks: Remain productive in work, maintain self-esteem, prepare for effective retirement.

Adapted from *Career Management,* 1st edition by Greenhaus. © 1987. Reprinted with permission of South-Western, a division of Thomson Learning: www.thomsonrights.com. Fax 800 730-2215.

■ Career Management: Preparing for Change

Career management involves the ongoing planning and preparation for future career decisions (whether voluntary or involuntary), along with striving toward meaningful career responsibilities.

Because of the constantly changing environment of organizations and employment status, it is important to prepare for change and to develop career options and alternatives. Even though you may have a sense of satisfaction and security in your present career, *change* has become the watchword of our society.

"Job security" has been replaced by "personal security." **Personal security** means planning and preparing for alternative career paths should you experience a voluntary or involuntary change in your primary career choice. If a situation should arise in which employment choices are made for you, it is important to have planned and prepared for that possibility by exploring optional choices ahead of time. In *Change Your Job, Change Your Life*, author Ronald Krannich speaks of the connection between educational preparation and career planning, referring to this continuous process as "re-careering." He states that **re-careering** is the process of "repeatedly acquiring marketable skills and changing careers in response to a turbulent job market."[14]

> **PERSONAL SECURITY:** Planning and preparing for alternative career paths should you experience a voluntary or involuntary change in your primary career choice.

> **RE-CAREERING:** Ronald Krannich's term for the process of "repeatedly acquiring marketable skills and changing careers in response to a turbulent job market."

Complacency in job security is dangerous. Many see the only re-careering option available after an involuntary change as that of leaving the current organization for a new company. If you wish to make a voluntary change in career responsibilities, it is important to remember your options for change. Common alternatives to consider include these:

- A new position within your current career field and organization
- A new position within your current organization but in a new career field
- A new position or career field within a new organization
- A different way of implementing your current position

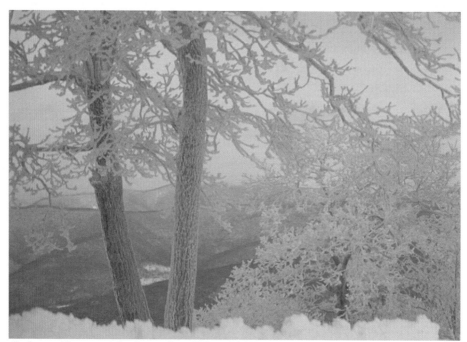

God meant for us to strive for quality of life and fulfillment of purpose every day.

There are various ways to involve yourself in different work responsibilities and career areas of interest. Explore new or changing interests and obtain additional work experience before you make career changes or decisions. This aspect of career development and preparation includes these options:

- Part-time employment
- Internships
- Volunteer positions
- Community groups
- Job shadowing

Can you use any of these options to gain experience, expand your abilities, or fulfill a personal sense of purpose at the same time that you explore additional areas of interest?

■ Retirement Planning

Another type of change for which we often do not prepare or manage well is retirement. Many factors are involved in one's decision to retire. The authors of *Aging in Good Health* report that retirement can take place for negative and positive reasons, as well as for health reasons. They categorize these reasons in this way:

1. Health reasons: Health will be improved or preserved by retiring.

2. Negative reasons:
   - Downsizing
   - Dissatisfaction with aspects of job
   - Family pressure
   - Compulsory retirement policy

3. Positive reasons:
   - To enjoy life while healthy
   - To pursue a second career or other interests
   - More time with family
   - Financial benefits[15]

Naturally, the cause of retirement will influence one's outlook toward retirement status. To assist in cultivating a positive outlook about retirement, purposefully consider and plan options before deciding to retire. Options for retirement time and outlets can include:

- Involvement in volunteer activities
- Part-time involvement in past career responsibilities
- Involvement with new career responsibilities using current skills and experience
- Education or training to enter new career areas
- Travel, recreation, and family contacts

While the final option—recreation, travel, and more time with family—is a meaningful and fulfilling one, it is often difficult for many to make the adjustment. After so many years of building their identities through their careers, many new retirees find themselves bored and feeling a loss of identity. That is all the more reason to plan ahead about how to spend one's retirement years. We all need a sense of purpose in our lives—no matter how we personally define that purpose and no matter what stage of life we may currently be experiencing. We can fulfill this purpose in many ways, but we need to prepare ourselves and plan ahead as we consider the years following retirement. God meant for us to strive for quality of life and fulfillment of purpose every day.

Educational Wellness: A Sense of Personal Development

"Any enterprise is built by wise planning, becomes strong through common sense, and profits wonderfully by keeping abreast of the facts. A wise man is mightier than a strong man. Wisdom is mightier than strength." Proverbs 24:3-5

EDUCATION: The general knowledge base of information one can use for decision-making or problem-solving applications.

Educational wellness is closely associated with occupational wellness because in many career areas education is a foundational prerequisite. Educational planning can serve as a springboard for entering a desired career area. It also can serve as a "stand alone" goal, providing specific training and/or a degree that may or may not be related to career options. We will use the terms *education* and *training* to refer to choices for personal and professional development. **Education** refers to the

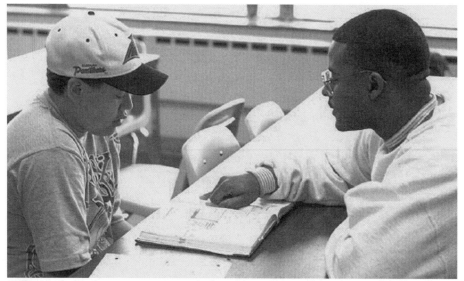

Educational planning can serve as a springboard for entering a desired career field.

general knowledge base of information one can use for decision-making and/or problem-solving applications. **Training** usually refers to the development of specific skills necessary for personal or professional growth.[16] When we discuss educational wellness in this text, we are including options for either education or training.

> **TRAINING:** The development of specific skills necessary for personal or professional growth.

■ A Matter of Growth

The specific career goal being considered will determine the type of education or training needed. Educational preparation can relate to any of the following career goals:

- To help someone initially enter a career area of choice
- To help someone advance in a present career area
- To help someone change to a different career field or to a different level of responsibility in a current career field

A career change or advancement may not be the main focus of one's educational/training endeavors. Instead, a person may wish to focus on individual development through these options:

- Selecting a degree program of interest
- Selecting a certification program of interest
- Selecting a course or courses to increase knowledge/skill level
- Selecting a course or courses for personal development

The overall goal of any of these options—and the primary goal of educational wellness—is to continue to plan and pursue goals for personal and/or professional development and growth. Having completed an initial goal, the next goal is to evaluate personal and/or professional status at that time and begin the developmental process again. A barrier to this developmental process is a mind-set that believes educational development and skill training should or can be accomplished only in the early years of life. However, wellness is based on the principle that growth is a continual process. For personal satisfaction and professional achievement, continued development (lifelong learning) should be a process that is evaluated and maintained throughout one's entire life.

Exhibit 7.4. Holland's Typology of Personalities and Occupations

Note: adapted to include educational options

Realistic:
Personal Interests: Likes to work with objects, tools; likes using physical abilities and enjoys working outdoors.
Personal Characteristics: Shy, genuine, materialistic, persistent, stable.
Sample Educational Programs: Construction trades, surveying, geology, law enforcement, landscaping, engineering technology.

Investigative:
Personal Interests: Likes to investigate and solve problems, work with abstract problems, and understand how things work.
Personal Characteristics: Analytical, cautious, curious, independent, introverted.
Sample Educational Programs: Chemistry, biology, pre-med/pre-dental, mathematics, computer information.

Artistic:
Personal Interests: Likes to use imagination, work in unstructured environments, and create with artistic abilities.
Personal Characteristics: Disorderly, emotional, idealistic, imaginative, impulsive.
Sample Educational Programs: Architecture, interior design, writing, music, art, photography, commercial design.

Social:
Personal Interests: Likes to assist and support people, train, teach; has a concern for the welfare of others.
Personal Characteristics: Cooperative, generous, helpful, sociable, understanding.
Sample Educational Programs: Psychology, social work, counseling, education, nursing, ministry.

Enterprising:
Personal Interests: Energetic, likes to assume leadership and persuade others; desires to achieve power and status.
Personal Characteristics: Adventurous, ambitious, energetic, domineering, self-confident.
Sample Educational Programs: Pre-law, marketing, communications, management/ supervision, public relations, sales.

Conventional:
Personal Interests: Likes well-ordered activities and well-defined tasks; enjoys office work, working with data, and using clerical skills.
Personal Characteristics: Efficient, obedient, practical, calm, conscientious.
Sample Educational Programs: Accounting, finance, office management, computer technology, investment management.

■ Educational Decision Making

Like the career selection process we reviewed earlier in this chapter, the process of selecting an educational or training goal involves self-awareness and the right match of personal interests, values, and abilities to educational and training options. Instead of developing options for career exploration, however, educational/training options target general courses and/or educational programs

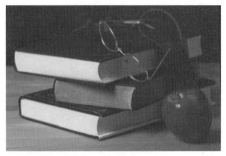

Select courses that match your interests and skill areas.

that people are interested in exploring. The decision-making process involves:

- Personal awareness of interests and skills
- Selecting programs/courses that match those interests and skill areas
- Exploring and evaluating those options
- Taking steps to enroll in a course or program
- Continuing to evaluate personal progress

Lee Ellis and Larry Burkett offer additional factors as one explores and evaluates alternatives for future educational courses, programs, and/or training:[17]

1. How much do you want? For your career area of interest, how much education/training do you need?

    - A few specific courses
    - A two- or four-year degree program
    - A graduate degree program
    - A program leading to a specific certification

2. What is your level of motivation? What is the level of commitment you are willing to make at the present time and your purpose for obtaining additional education?

    - Personal awareness of long-term benefits
    - Personal understanding for maintaining a balance of priorities in life while pursuing education
    - Personal commitment to calling upon various support resources, if needed

3. What is your level of financial commitment? What financial assistance options are available? Are you willing to explore and accept financial assistance?

- Personal financial resources needed
- Availability of grants, scholarships, and/or loans
- Availability of assistantships or internships
- Availability of employer tuition assistance programs

It is important to assess personal needs for continued learning, as well as to evaluate personal commitment and motivation to take the required action steps.

Networking

As with career research, an excellent way to explore and obtain information about various educational options is to talk with other individuals who have

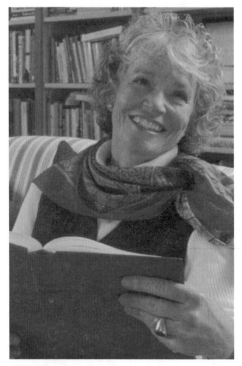

Wellness is based on the principle that growth is a continual process.

experience in your interest area. To repeat, career networking involves interviews or discussions with people who are involved in your career areas of interest. Educational networking involves discussions or interviews with instructors, academic advisors, counselors, and/or current students or graduates who have knowledge about the educational or training areas in which you have an interest. Questions for this networking process should focus on the types of courses involved, methods for taking those courses, entrance requirements for taking a course or entering a degree program, career placement options, placement success, and any other questions relevant to the decision-making process.

■ Lifelong Learning: Benefits and Barriers

The pursuit of continuing education and/or training has many benefits and can influence all other areas of individual well-being in positive ways. Improving a personal skill or increasing one's level of knowledge can bolster personal confidence and self-worth. These positive outlooks can reinforce positive perceptions and actions toward total wellness development: body, mind, and spirit. A sense of positive growth in one area of life often will result in positive growth in other areas of life. Naturally, an important benefit is that additional skills and knowledge can be used for career change and/or development.

As in any endeavor, barriers can hinder educational development by either blocking someone from initiating the process or preventing that person from completing a goal. A common barrier to progress can be

> Fears are learned behaviors and, therefore, can be changed and overcome.

a negative attitude toward learning in general or toward a specific topic due to negative results or experiences in the past. As we have pointed out numerous times, a lack of success or motivation in the past is not an accurate evaluation of one's chances for success in the future. Personal commitment, effort, and motivation change over time, offering one the opportunity to anticipate more positive outcomes. Look to the past not to label efforts or abilities negatively, but to help in planning and preparing for positive changes ahead.

Another barrier that can prevent individuals from even considering educational/training goals is being unaware of the many options available today. Even a cursory investigation will reveal many options in both the types of courses and programs available and the various methods for taking these courses and programs.

Fear of change and fear of failure are very real barriers to one's attempts to enhance personal development, even when these changes can produce positive results. Anticipating personal fears can keep them from sabotaging educational development efforts. Fears are learned behaviors and, therefore, can be changed and overcome. Address personal fears and be open to support resources and people who can assist in overcoming those fears. The personal benefits of overcoming fear include increased motivation for personal development efforts.

Adding a new commitment to an already tight schedule is another common barrier. Educational programs do take a commitment of time and effort. These commitments can mean sacrificing time with other priorities in one's life (family, recreational time, personal time, etc.). In considering this commitment, review the benefits that educational development can provide. At the same time, focus on maintaining a positive balance with other personal priorities and

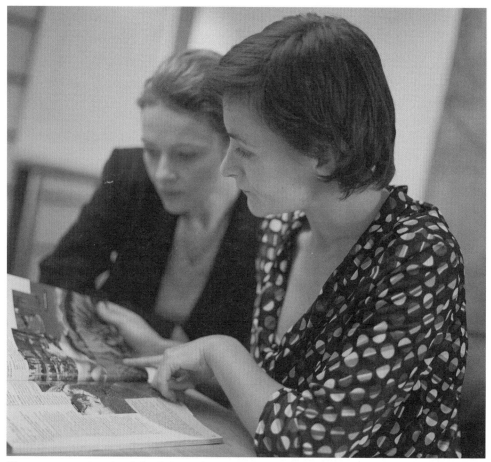

You can pursue educational development through self-directed learning.

values. Balance means to guard against allowing new educational goals to push aside current priorities.

Educational well-being is an important portion of overall well-being and a means of fulfilling a personal sense of purpose. However, it is just as important to address overall well-being in satisfying ways. We do not realize the overall goal of balance if we obtain a new degree and the promise of career enhancement at the cost of personal health and/or family relationships.

■ Pursuing Your Educational Goal

We can pursue individual courses, educational programs, and training in many different ways. Institutions and organizations provide a variety of educational and training alternatives to fit anyone's schedule. The presence of multimedia technology has added to the many available options. We can pursue our educational development through such alternatives as these:[18]

- Self-directed learning:

  Reading journals, books, and magazines, asking questions, getting involved with groups that help provide information and/or upgrade skills in an area of interest

- On-the-job training:

  Training programs offered in-house for employee skill development

- Apprenticeships-Internships:

  Methods to obtain hands-on experience and training in a work environment or occupational field of interest

- Co-op education:

  Programs that alternate between terms of structured instruction and terms of work experience

- Military:

  Leadership and training programs provided by all branches of the military while an individual serves the country

- Vocational schools:

  Programs that offer specialized training; day and evening classes are usually available.

- Community colleges:

  Programs provided within close proximity of one's geographic location; programs are focused on occupations available in that specific area.

- Four-year colleges and universities:

  Institutions providing four-year educational degrees and/or graduate degrees that may be required for entry into certain occupational areas

- Churches:

  Programs dealing with many areas of personal growth and skill development that can be transferable into many occupational areas

- Distance learning:

  Many of the providers mentioned above will offer courses or degree programs to learners separated by physical distance. They offer options such as educational radio, television, computer, and other multimedia technologies.

Consider occupational and educational goals in selecting the method that best meets personal needs. The provider offering the courses or programs most closely related to specific goals for growth can provide a list of options to research. Evaluate the methods through which these programs are provided and focus on the methods that best meet personal geographic location and time demands. An important factor in the final decision will be matching individual needs and schedules to the provider most closely aligned with personal program goals.

KEY CONCEPTS

burnout
education
networking
personal security
re-careering
training
tunnel vision

Earlier in this text we noted that without physical activity, the heart cannot function at its highest potential capacity. We can make the same point about the brain and its potential. Without the continuous activities of learning and acquiring new knowledge, the brain will not receive stimulation for growth. Continuous, lifelong learning can keep the brain functioning at a high level, can provide opportunities for possible career changes or advancements, and can provide many benefits to overall wellness. Be open to learning opportunities. They are all around us if we remain open to their existence.

Learning Activity

1. Future planning:

   Richard Bolles states that we all have a definite mission to use our God-given skills in the best way possible and in the best environments possible.

   At the present time, what career areas seem to be the best match for your skills and interests?

   _____

   _____

   _____

   _____

   _____

   _____

   What educational or training areas sound the most interesting to you at this time?

   _____

   _____

   _____

   _____

   _____

   Whom can you contact (network) to gain additional information about your career area(s) of interest?

   _____

   _____

   _____

   _____

   _____

Whom can you contact (network) to gain additional information about your educational/training areas of interest?

_____

_____

_____

_____

_____

_____

I will make my first networking contact by_____
                                                    Date

2. Present Planning:

What steps can you take to improve yourself in your current position or organization?

_____

_____

_____

_____

_____

What are some actions you can take to help increase your current level of career satisfaction?

_____

_____

_____

_____

_____

What steps can you take to help reduce any stress you may be experiencing from your job or career environment?

_____

_____

_____

_____

_____

In what courses or programs could you enroll to provide additional education or training for your current job or career area?

_____

_____

_____

_____

_____

Additional Activities and References

1. How will you use the degree you are currently pursuing to enhance your personal career development?

   _____

   _____

   _____

   _____

   _____

   _____

2. What major issues do you need to consider as you develop your future career goals?

   _____

   _____

   _____

   _____

   _____

   _____

3. Review the following resources for additional information related to occupational and educational development:

   http://stats.bls.gov:80/ocohome.htm   Career information

   www.petersons.com/   Educational programs

Endnotes

1. Zig Ziglar, *Top Performance* (Old Tappan, NJ: Fleming H. Revell Co., 1986), 23.
2. Richard Nelson Bolles, *What Color Is Your Parachute?* (Berkeley: Ten Speed Press, 2001), 244-54.
3. The *Occupational Outlook Handbook* and the *Encyclopedia of Careers and Vocational Guidance* are produced by the Department of Labor, Bureau of Labor Statistics. See the Additional Activities and Resources on the previous page for the Department of Labor Web site.
4. Manuel London and Edward M. Mone, *Career Management and Survival in the Workplace: Helping Employees Make Tough Career Decisions, Stay Motivated, and Reduce Career Stress* (San Francisco: Jossey-Bass Publishers, 1987), 27.
5. Fred J. Hecklinger and Bernadette M. Black, *Training for Life: A Practical Guide to Career and Life Planning*, 7th ed. (Dubuque, IA: Kendall/Hunt Publishing, 2000), 123-25.
6. Susan M. Johnston, *The Career Adventure: Your Guide to Personal Assessment, Career Exploration, and Decision Making*, 3rd ed. (Upper Saddle River, NJ: Prentice Hall, 2002), 79.
7. London and Mone, *Career Management and Survival in the Workplace*, 150-51.
8. Jeffrey H. Greenhaus, *Career Management* (New York: Dryden Press, 1987), 193.
9. Ibid., 201.
10. Ibid., 203.
11. Ibid., 218-20.
12. Lee Ellis and Larry Burkett, *Your Career in Changing Times* (Chicago: Moody Press, 1993), 91.
13. Ibid., 91-95.
14. Ronald L. Krannich, *Change Your Job, Change Your Life: High Impact Strategies for Finding Great Jobs in the Decade Ahead*, 7th ed. (Manassas Park, VA: Impact Publications, 1999), 26.
15. Sue E. Levkoff, Yeon Kyung Chee, and Shohei Noguchi, eds., *Aging in Good Health: Multidisciplinary Perspectives* (New York: Springer Publishing Co., 2001), 124.
16. Ellis and Burkett, *Your Career in Changing Times*, 231.
17. Ibid., 241-42.
18. Ibid., 235-40.

8

WELLNESS AND NUTRITION

"We [now] devote more attention to the patient's diet and habits, and more often send him away with good advice than with hastily-written prescriptions."

—Robert Hall Babcock, 1901[1]

In considering optimal wellness, one of the most important topics is maintaining proper nutrition. The food and drink we consume or avoid will undoubtedly affect the functioning of our bodies and brains. We need sustained energy and stamina to meet the varied demands of life. Good nutrition is essential for doing our best and getting the most out of our work, family life, recreational activities, and social life. In addition to providing energy for optimal performance, food and liquids are paramount to how we feel physically, emotionally, and even spiritually.

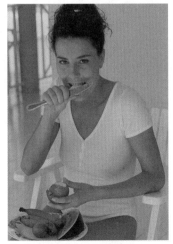

Optimal wellness includes maintaining proper nutrition.

Nutrition and Well-Being

Nutrition scientists now generally agree that diet is directly and causally related to the development of certain diseases, such as diabetes and heart disease. Because of health concerns or worry over physical appearance, many people often are willing to try any dietary regimen to improve health or attain weight loss. Some may go beyond common sense and develop dietary habits that harm the body. Less than desirable nutrition habits often begin when life changes include moving away from home to begin college or employment. In addition to a new environment and lifestyle, young people come in contact with an abundance of misinformation about food and nutrition, thus compounding the problem. These factors add to the difficulty of making knowledgeable food choices. In order to make healthy choices that lead to personal well-being, we need to know and understand the basics of proper nutrition and how to recognize nutritional misinformation.

As you continue to read this book (including this chapter on nutrition), you will gain wisdom. With this gain in wisdom, you will have more tools for a satisfying life, one that helps you fully realize your potential. Caring for your body, expanding your mind, and nurturing your soul will help you understand more completely the mission God has for your life.

■ Nutrition Awareness

The Bible tells us that we should care about our bodies. The body contains the mind and soul. In addition, the body is a temple of the Holy Spirit (1 Corinthians 6:19). Our bodies are "in process" until we return to God. Therefore, we should continue to seek answers to a true and God-honoring understanding of our body's capacity for maximal wellness.

Nutrition awareness is important because it affects eating style, which in turn affects almost every aspect of one's life: appearance, energy, stamina, resistance to illness, mental outlook, stress levels, susceptibility to substance abuse—even academic and social success. The relationship between what we eat and our health and behavior is so subtle that we may overlook connections that could change our lives for the better.

■ "Freshman 15"

A common tag given to first-year college students is "Freshman 15." This number is not a reference to credit hours, but rather the average number of pounds a freshman usually gains in the first year of college! First-year students generally experience independence for the first time. Caring for themselves is

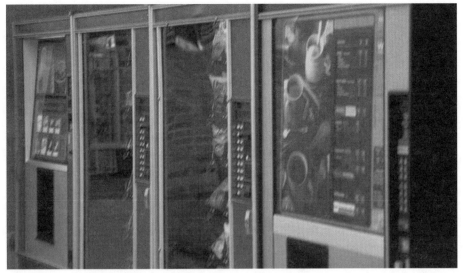

Along with a first-year student's new independence comes a vast array of temptations.

a new responsibility. Along with this new independence comes a vast array of temptations. With no one to tell them what or when to eat, they easily consume excess food—especially food that adds fat weight. Excess consumption of food can happen at meals or simply through "mindless snacking" while students are studying or socializing with friends. Add to this picture a decrease in physical activity due to studying, part-time work, or partying, and the pounds can add up more quickly and in higher amounts.

■ The Calorie Connection

One way to understand this phenomenon better is to realize the connection between calories consumed and calories expended. A **calorie** is the unit used to measure the energy-producing value of food. The body needs calories but, more important, it needs the right type of calories. All of the calories the body uses originate from dietary protein, carbohydrates, fat, or alcohol. If you consume more calories than your body needs to produce energy, those calories will be converted into fat until needed at a later time. An increase of 3,500

> **CALORIE:** A unit used to measure the energy-producing value in food when oxidized in the body.

calories will result in one pound of fat stored in the body. If you added around forty potato chips to your daily diet, the extra calories—approximately 500—would add one pound of fat by week's end! This gives you an idea of how easy it is to gain fifteen pounds in one year.

■ Good Nutrition: God's Plan

Food and water are vital to energy and stamina. Energy from food is created from the absorption and metabolism of carbohydrates, fats, and proteins. When we eat plants and/or animals that have consumed plants, we obtain energy from the sunlight that was originally captured by the plants. By consuming the foods God has provided us, both plant and animal, we follow His plan to sustain our bodies. The Bible tells us of God's instructions to freely take of both seed-bearing plants and trees, in addition to animals for nourishment and sustenance.

> By consuming the foods God has provided us, both plant and animal, we follow His plan to sustain our bodies.

The Bible also tells us that water is even more important than food. In fact, it is the most important nutrient of all, but often is not regarded as such. The body can survive for weeks without food, but death will result much sooner if the body does not have water. Adequate intake of water is essential for:

- All energy production in the body
- Temperature control
- Transportation of all nutrients and waste products in and out of the body
- Lubrication of joints and other structures

Failure to consume adequate water, sixty-four ounces each day (think of drinking eight, eight-ounce glasses), will result in fatigue, fluid retention, and faulty regulation of body temperature (which can lead to heat illnesses).

■ Building Disease Resistance

Proper nutrition is vital to building resistance against viruses and bacteria that are plentiful in our environment. If your body is lacking vitamins, minerals, and nutrients, either from lack of food or improper eating—for instance, processed snack foods instead of fruits, vegetables, and animal foods—you will be more susceptible to colds and infections. Other concerns that are related to poor eating habits include the risk of developing cardiovascular disease, cancer, diabetes, hypertension, osteoporosis, and other degenerative diseases. The statistics are alarming:

- One out of every two Americans will die from heart disease.
- Cancer strikes three out of every four families.

- Almost twelve million Americans have diabetes.

- Fifty-eight million people have hypertension.

Factors that increase the risk for developing cardiovascular disease include excessive intake of fatty foods and foods that are high in cholesterol. An excessive amount of body fat (**obesity**) is also associated with this chronic disease. Likewise, obesity is associated with hypertension and

OBESITY: A condition characterized by an excessive amount of body fat.

diabetes. While cancer is not caused by diet, it is influenced by the foods we eat. Research continues to show a connection between high-fat diets and certain cancers such as colon and breast cancer. Well-balanced nutrition is also necessary for reducing the risk of osteoporosis, a condition in which bone mass decreases and susceptibility to fracture increases. Women are particularly susceptible to this disease, in which inadequate dietary calcium plays a major role.

■ Optimizing Function

The proper balance of nutrients aids the function of the brain, as well as the organs. Not only does the brain control mental tasks, but it also controls moods, thoughts, feelings, behaviors, and emotions. For example, consider how you feel immediately after you have consumed a high-sugar food or liquid. Then consider how you feel one to two hours later. Upon digestion of this food or liquid, your blood sugar rises rapidly and you feel a burst of energy. However, shortly thereafter, your pancreas secretes insulin in large amounts, which makes your blood sugar fall dramatically. This in turn produces feelings of fatigue, lightheadedness, and irritability. You also notice an increase in your hunger level, perhaps signaling the need for even more of the same sweet food or liquid!

The answer to this unhealthy cycle is a balanced diet that lends itself to diminished cravings for high-sugar or high-starch foods and drinks, as well as processed foods. Think more of the foods that God has provided. Remember that animal food is as important as plant food. The Bible does not depict animal food as inferior to plant food, but affirms that they both nourish us similarly. Manufactured food was obviously not available to those who lived during biblical times. Rather, the food from plants and animals gave men like David and his warriors mental acuity and physical strength to defeat the enemies of Israel (1 Samuel 17:17-18; 25:18; 2 Samuel 17:28-29). Likewise, balanced nutrition from grains, fruits, vegetables, meats, and dairy products will help individuals function optimally at all levels—mentally, physically, spiritually, and socially. This will lead to excellence in academic endeavors, career, personal life, and most important, our work for Christ.

Nutrition Basics

Most of us have considerable freedom over what we eat and when or how often we eat. As we saw earlier, those who make a transition to a different life phase—college, new job—realize this rather abruptly. Whether you are a college student experiencing independence for the first time, or someone who is seeking to improve personal nutritional wellness, there is no better time than the present to learn the basics of nutrition.

■ Creating Energy: The Process

A basic principle of healthy nutrition, one that leads to a greater state of wellness, is balance. Balance is a familiar concept, one that appears in other areas of health and wellness. In reference to nutrition, the balance we strive for includes consumption of the six classes of nutrients: carbohydrates, proteins, fats, vitamins, minerals, and water. Further described in Table 8.1, these six classes of nutrients are a part of the essential nutrients necessary for human function.

METABOLISM: In the human body, the process of converting food into compounds and chemicals, deriving energy for the body's functions.

The physiological functions of the body occur after the breakdown of food during digestion. As food and liquid are delivered through the gastrointestinal tract, they are broken down into compounds. This allows the body to absorb the nutrients and use them to provide energy, build and repair tissue, and regulate functions of the body. The first and foremost function upon completion of this process is the provision of energy.

METABOLIC RATE: The amount of energy the body uses at any time.

We refer to the energy that is derived from the food we eat as a kilocalorie. This unit of energy is more frequently referred to as a calorie. Calories are either used immediately for fueling metabolic processes or stored as fat or glycogen (sugar). **Metabolism** is the process of converting food first into compounds and then into chemicals which the body will use to facilitate its functions. Metabolism is a constant process, providing energy while we study, walk, exercise, eat, and even sleep. The amount of energy the body uses varies not only from person to person, but from day to day. We refer to this energy as the **metabolic rate.** Metabolic rate is partly affected by the food we eat and our activity levels.

The Macronutrients

Three of the six nutrient categories supply energy for the body. These nutrients, also referred to as **macronutrients,** are carbohydrates, protein, and fat.

Table 8.1, The Six Classes of Nutrients and Their Functions in the Human Body

Nutrient	Function	Major Sources
Proteins	Form important parts of muscles, bones, blood, enzymes, some hormones, and cell membranes; repair tissue; regulate water and acid-base balance; help in growth; supply energy.	Meat, fish, poultry, eggs, milk products, nuts, legumes
Carbohydrates	Supply energy to cells in brain, nervous system, and blood; supply energy to muscles during movement and activity.	Grains (breads, cereals), fruits, and vegetables
Fats	Supply energy; insulate, support and cushion organs; substance supplied for absorption of fat-soluble vitamins.	Saturated fats (mostly animal sources), palm and coconut oils and hydrogenated vegetable fats; unsaturated fats (fish, vegetables, grains)
Vitamins	Promote specific chemical reactions within cells.	Fruits, vegetables, grains, meat, and dairy products
Minerals	Help to regulate body functions; aid in growth and maintenance of body tissue; facilitate the release of energy.	Found in most food groups
Water	Provides approximately 50-70 percent of body weight; substance supplied for chemical reactions; transports chemicals; regulates temperature; eliminates waste products.	Fruits, vegetables, and other liquids

Carbohydrates

Carbohydrates are the body's primary source of energy. As the body breaks down and metabolizes carbohydrates, it forms glucose. Some glucose is used immediately for energy, while the rest is

MACRONUTRIENTS: Three of six essential nutrients that provide energy to the human body. They are carbohydrates, protein, and fats.

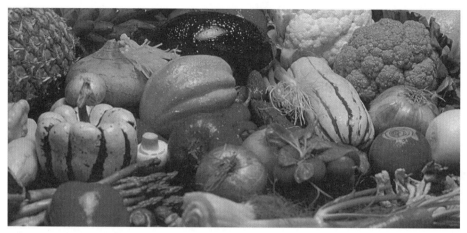

When considering a balanced diet, think of the foods that God has provided.

stored in the liver for later use. There are two types of carbohydrates: simple and complex.

Simple carbohydrates include refined sugars and naturally occurring sugars. Examples of refined sugars are table or brown sugar, corn syrup, and honey. Natural sugars, which are found in healthy foods such as milk and fruit, contain vitamins, minerals, protein, or fiber.

Complex carbohydrates are starches and fibers, and include vegetables, fruits, beans, pasta, rice, grains, and breads. Complex carbohydrate foods have greater nutritional value than simple carbohydrate foods, due to the significant amounts of protein, vitamins, and minerals they contain. Generally, the fat content of complex carbohydrates is low, unless the food has been prepared with fat (fried, buttered, or creamed). Recommendations for most average adults is 50 to 100 grams daily. (See Table 8.2 for the carbohydrate content of some foods.)

Table 8.2, Carbohydrate Content of Sample Foods

Fruits, Vegetables, Legumes	Carbohydrate (grams)	Bread, Cereal, Rice, Pasta	Carbohydrate (grams)
Banana, 1 medium size	26	Whole wheat bread, 1 slice	14
Apple, 1 medium size	20	Pita pocket bread, 6" round	33
Orange, 1 medium size	18	Oatmeal, 1 cup, regular/quick	25
Carrots, 1 cup	11	Brown rice, 1 cup	45
Corn, 1/2 cup	17	White rice, 1 cup	35
Baked potato, 1 medium size	50	Macaroni, 1 cup	40
Beans/peas (navy, lima, green) 1 cup	20-50	Spaghetti, 1 cup	40

Complex carbohydrates also provide fiber or roughage, which aids in digestion and helps to protect against disease. High-fiber diets have been shown to lower the risk of heart disease and colon cancer. Nutritionists recommend that adults consume 20 to 35 grams of fiber daily. (See Table 8.3).

Table 8.3, Fiber Content of Sample Plant Foods

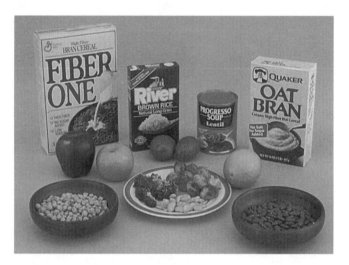

Only plant foods contain fiber. The following fruits, vegetables, grains, cereals, and legumes are examples of high-fiber food items.

Food item/size	Fiber/grams
Apple (with skin), 1 medium size	4.0
Orange, 1 medium size	3.8
Pear, 1 medium size	4.8
Prunes (uncooked), 5 average size	3.9
Raspberries, 1/2 cup	3.0
Bread (whole wheat), 1 slice	2.5
Oatmeal (cooked), 2/3 cup	3.0
Garbanzo beans (cooked), 1/2 cup	4.9
Kidney beans (cooked), 1/2 cup	4.6
Lima beans (cooked), 1/2 cup	4.3
Artichoke (cooked), 1 medium size	4.0
Green beans (cooked), 1/2 cup	2.0
Corn (cooked), 1/2 cup	4.6
Peas (cooked), 1/2 cup	3.5
Potato (baked with skin), 1 medium size	5.0

■ Protein

The second macronutrient, protein, is a complex nutrient that is necessary for all aspects of the growth and repair of body tissues, including muscles, skin, organs, blood, hormones, and enzymes. It also can be a source of energy when your food intake lacks needed carbohydrates or fats for energy expenditure. Derived from both animals and vegetables, protein is made up of amino acids. Twenty amino acids are found in animal food, but only eight are essential for health. These essential amino acids are required because the body cannot manufacture them, nor can they be stored in amounts sufficient for growth and maintenance of body tissues. Daily consumption of protein, about 50 to 60 grams, can be obtained from animal tissue such as meat, fish, eggs, and dairy products. (See Table 8.4 for some sources of protein.)

The protein found in vegetables is typically deficient in essential amino acids. Therefore, people who are strict vegetarians (no intake of meat, eggs, or dairy products) must eat a variety of foods that allow each vegetable protein to make up for the amino acids missing in the other. For example, when you combine legumes (peas, peanuts, lima beans) with grains (rice, wheat, corn) or nuts and seeds at the same meal, you obtain the amino acids you need without eating protein from an animal source.

Table 8.4, Sources of Protein

The foods below are good sources of protein. From this chart you can determine if you are getting the daily amount recommended (50-60 grams). Low-fat protein sources (30 percent or less calories from fat) are annotated with double asterisks (**).

Meat and Fish	*Protein (grams)*	*Dairy and Eggs*	*Protein (grams)*
Cod, 4 oz. (broiled/grilled)**	26	Cottage cheese, 1/2 cup (low fat)**	14
Tuna, 4 oz. (water-packed can)**	22	Milk, 1 cup (low fat)**	8
Chicken, 4 oz. (white, broiled)**	30	Yogurt, 1 cup (low fat)**	12
Hamburger, 4 oz. (grilled)	30	Cheddar cheese, 1 oz.	7
Sirloin steak, 4 oz. (grilled)	31	Egg, 1 medium size (boiled)	6

Legumes	*Protein (grams)*	*Grains*	*Protein (grams)*
Black-eyed peas, 1/2 cup **	7	Spaghetti, 1 cup (cooked/plain)**	7
Kidney beans, 1 cup **	13	Brown rice, 1 cup (cooked/plain)**	5
Soy nuts, 1/4 cup **	12	White rice, 1 cup (cooked/plain)**	4
Cashews, 1/4 cup	5	Oatmeal, 1 cup (cooked/plain) **	6
Peanut butter, 2 Tbsp.	8	Whole wheat bread, 1 slice **	3

■ Fats

Fats, also referred to as lipids, are the most concentrated source of energy. In addition to providing energy to the body, they help with the absorption of fat-soluble vitamins, assist certain body regulations (blood pressure), insulate the body, and cushion the organs. The four dietary fats are cholesterol and three forms of fatty acids—saturated, monounsaturated, and polyunsaturated.

The Cholesterol Factor

Cholesterol is a form of fat that is made primarily in the liver and then secreted into the blood. The body uses cholesterol to make essential body substances such as cell walls, cell structures, and hormones. However, if there is too much cholesterol in the blood, the excess will be deposited in the arteries, narrowing them and increasing the risk for heart disease. Cholesterol can be found in animal sources such as meats, egg yolks, milk, and butter. Saturated fats, such as lard, animal fat, and coconut oil, tend to be more dense and solid, whereas unsaturated fats (most oils) are more liquid in substance. The difference between saturated and unsaturated fats is important because a diet high in saturated fats increases blood cholesterol and the associated risk of heart disease. A diet that is high in saturated fat also increases the body's susceptibility to certain cancers.

Far superior to saturated fats are the polyunsaturated and monounsaturated fats, which usually come from plants. Certain exceptions are tropical oils, such as coconut and palm oil, which contain a higher proportion of saturated fats. (See Table 8.5.) The American Heart Association recommends keeping the daily consumption of fat below 30 percent of the total calories each day (including $\leq 10\%$ saturated fat). However, typically, people consume as much as 35-40 percent of their total calories as fat on a daily basis. This is one of the reasons obesity is such a problem in today's society!

The total amount of fat necessary for body functions is equivalent to only one tablespoon of vegetable oil. In addition to monounsaturated and polyunsaturated oils, omega-3 polyunsaturates are another form of healthy fat. This particular fat has been shown to reduce the risk of heart disease. It can be found in many kinds of fish, such as salmon, mackerel, whitefish, herring, oysters, and lake trout.

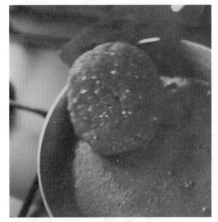

A diet high in saturated fats increases your risk for heart disease.

Table 8.5. Saturated and Unsaturated Fats	
Saturated Fats:	Butter, beef tallow, vegetable shortenings, coconut/palm oil; also found in whole milk, cream, egg yolks, meat/meat fat, chocolate, regular margarine, and lard.
Polyunsaturated Fats:	Safflower, cottonseed, corn, soybean, and sesame oils; fatty fish.
Monounsaturated Fats:	Olive and canola oils and some nuts.
"Fat Facts":	Margarine and butter are both 100 percent fat, with the same number of calories (100 per tablespoon), but butter contains cholesterol and margarine does not. Foods with "hidden" dietary fats include avocados, olives, egg yolks, nuts, and seeds.

■ The Micronutrients

The remaining three nutrients necessary for the body's daily functions are vitamins, minerals, and water. Referred to as **micronutrients,** they are as essential as the macronutrients for helping the body create energy. Most nutrition scientists believe that without taking supplements we can obtain the vitamins and minerals necessary for good health from a well-balanced diet. In fact, certain vitamins in high doses can harm the body. For example, excessive intake of vitamin B-6 can cause neurological damage. Excessive vitamin C can lead to urinary stones. Too much vitamin D can cause irreversible kidney and heart damage. Because vitamins and minerals are sold without a prescription, it is especially important to know individual needs and, better yet, to consult a physician or registered dietitian before purchasing them.

> **MICRONUTRIENTS:** Three of six essential nutrients the body needs to create energy. They are vitamins, minerals, and water.

■ Vitamins

Vitamins do not provide energy. Rather, they facilitate and regulate energy stored in carbohydrates, proteins, and fats. In addition, they assist with the structure and preservation of body tissues. The human body needs thirteen vitamins, most of which can be obtained from food. Four vitamins—A, D, E, and K—are fat-soluble, meaning they can be absorbed only in the presence of fat. The remaining nine vitamins—C and the eight B-complex vitamins—are water-soluble. They do not need fat to aid in their absorption by the body. Vitamins are present in vegetables, fruits, and grains. Just as mega-dosing with vitamins can lead to illness, so can depriving the body of necessary vitamins through an inadequate diet. For example, vitamin B-6 deficiency can cause seizures, vitamin B-12 deficiency can cause anemia, and vitamin A deficiency can cause blindness.

■ Minerals

Minerals are compounds that help to regulate bodily functions. They are essential for cell membrane maintenance, nerve impulse conduction, and muscle contraction. Minerals are found in many foods, especially fruits and vegetables. Just as a well-rounded diet facilitates the absorption of vitamins, a wide variety of foods will give most people the minerals they need. The most common mineral deficiencies today are iron and calcium. Children and women often need higher amounts of both iron and calcium. Iron-rich foods, such as eggs, lean meats, beans, whole grains, and green leafy vegetables, are recommended for those with calcium and iron deficiency, especially those who have developed the blood disorder anemia.

Much information is available on the recommended daily allowances (RDA) of vitamins and minerals appropriate for one's age and lifestyle. One such source is the U.S. Food and Drug Administration's Web site, listed in the reference section at the end of this chapter.

In order to obtain the most nutritional value possible from the foods we consume, we must prepare and store them properly. Otherwise, vitamins and minerals will be lost or destroyed. The following recommendations will help to keep food nutrient value high:

1. Consume or process vegetables shortly after purchase.
2. Prepare lettuce salads just before eating them.
3. If storing vegetables, keep them in the refrigerator in covered containers or plastic bags.
4. For longer storage, freezing will preserve nutrients better than canning.
5. Don't thaw frozen vegetables before cooking.
6. Avoid soaking vegetables in water.
7. Bake, steam, microwave, or boil vegetables.
8. When boiling vegetables, use a tight-fitting lid to reduce water evaporation.
9. Cook vegetables such as potatoes in their skins.
10. Cook in as little water as possible, and cook as little as possible.

▪ Water

Of all the nutrients we have described, water is the most important. The body is about 60-70 percent water by weight, making it the body's primary component. Water is necessary for digestion, elimination, maintenance of bodily fluids, joint lubrication, body cooling, and disease prevention. Water is found in almost all foods, especially fruits and vegetables. In addition to consuming foods and other drinks that contain water, we need to remember to drink plain, pure water.

Even though the general recommendation is eight, eight-ounce glasses of liquids per day, we can take several things into consideration. Sweet drinks, such as sodas and juices, will reduce the amount of water in the bloodstream and body tissues by diverting fluid to the digestive tract. Caffeine and alcohol are diuretics, and thus will increase water loss. Also important is the fact that we lose several quarts of fluid every day through perspiration, elimination, and even breathing. If the weather is hot and humid, and especially if we are working or exercising in this type of environment, we will lose even more water through perspiration. In such situations, we should consume extra water in advance and then eight ounces about every fifteen minutes thereafter. Continue to consume water after completing the activity.

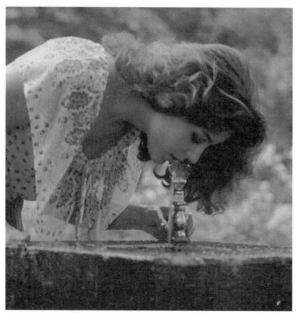

Of all the nutrients, water is the most important.

▪ Destructive Habits

Alcohol is not a nutrient because it does not contribute to growth, maintenance, or repair of any body tissue. Furthermore, it may damage tissues if consumed in even moderate amounts or for long periods of time. Often those who indulge in heavy and/or frequent drinking of alcohol neglect more

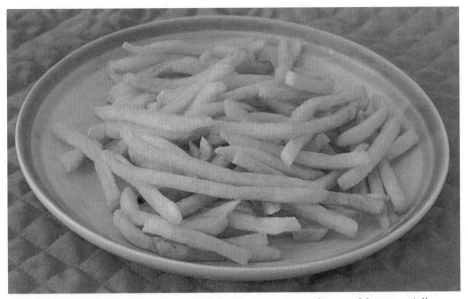

The diet of Americans is generally too high in calories, sugar, sodium, and fat—especially saturated fat.

nutritious foods, which in turn lowers their health status. In addition, alcohol can add extra calories and ultimately extra body fat. Alcohol is converted to fat when the total intake of calories from other foods along with alcohol exceeds daily needs. Drinking alcohol excessively has become one of the most destructive habits that Americans have developed over the years.

Along with alcohol excess, Americans have increased their intake of fat, sugar, and overall calories, which has led to higher incidence of diseases associated with such overconsumption. Many health-related organizations and associations recommend and agree on dietary guidelines for promoting health and wellness, in addition to preventing chronic diseases such as heart disease, cancer, and diabetes. These groups include the American Heart Association, the American Cancer Society, the American Diabetes Association, and the National Cholesterol Education Program.

■ Dietary Guidelines

In 1977, the Senate Select Committee on Nutrition and Human Needs determined that the diet of Americans was too high in calories, sugar, sodium, and fat (especially saturated fat). In addition, they found that we were eating too little fiber and complex carbohydrates. As a result of the evaluation, this committee created a set of recommendations titled "Dietary Guidelines for Americans." It includes the following recommendations:

1. Decrease consumption of foods high in fat: (a) oils, shortening, and margarine, (b) fatty meats and dairy products, and (c) convenience or prepared foods that are high in fats and oils.
2. Limit consumption of meat; choose only extra-lean cuts and substitute with skinned poultry, fish, and plant proteins.
3. Decrease consumption of cholesterol-rich foods, such as eggs and organ meats.
4. Decrease consumption of refined sugars and processed foods high in sugar.
5. Decrease consumption of salt, sodium-containing additives, and salty foods.
6. Increase consumption of fresh fruits and vegetables, whole-grain breads and cereals, and cooked dried beans and peas.
7. If you consume alcoholic beverages, do so in moderation.
8. Consume only enough calories from nutrient-dense foods to maintain a healthy body weight. At least 48 percent of the calories you consume should be complex carbohydrates, with no more than 30 percent of calories as fat, approximately 12 percent in protein, and no more than 10 percent in refined and processed sugars.

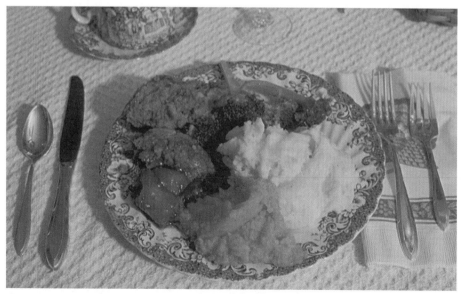

It is important to learn how to put together a healthy food plan.

Nutrition Balance

■ The Food Guide Pyramid

Having been introduced to the basics of nutrition, it is important to learn how to put together a healthy food plan. The Food Guide Pyramid developed by the U. S. Department of Agriculture and published in 1992 was created to replace the previously used "four food groups." The Food Guide Pyramid is intended to serve as a guide for daily food choices that will ensure a balanced intake of essential nutrients. (See Figure 8.1.)

Figure 8.1, The Food Guide Pyramid

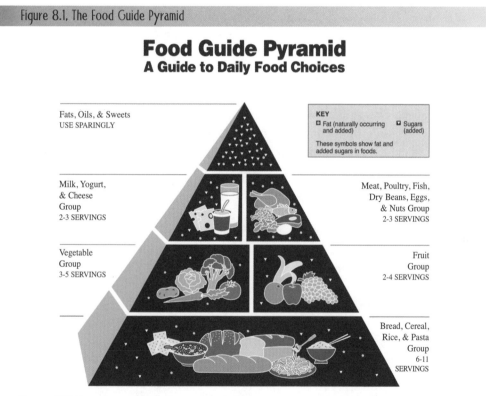

Food Guide Pyramid
A Guide to Daily Food Choices

Fats, Oils, & Sweets
USE SPARINGLY

KEY
□ Fat (naturally occurring and added)   ■ Sugars (added)
These symbols show fat and added sugars in foods.

Milk, Yogurt, & Cheese Group
2-3 SERVINGS

Meat, Poultry, Fish, Dry Beans, Eggs, & Nuts Group
2-3 SERVINGS

Vegetable Group
3-5 SERVINGS

Fruit Group
2-4 SERVINGS

Bread, Cereal, Rice, & Pasta Group
6-11 SERVINGS

Source: U.S. Department of Agriculture and the U.S. Department of Health and Human Services.

■ At the Base

Following the Food Guide Pyramid is relatively simple, as it summarizes the foods we need every day and the amounts of those foods. The basic premise is to eat more foods at the base of the pyramid (grains, fruits, vegetables) and fewer at the top (meat, dairy products, sugars, fats). The Food Guide Pyramid is based on a recommended number of servings from six food groups. Six to eleven servings a day should come from breads, cereals, rice, and pasta. These foods are a good source of complex carbohydrates and are filled with vitamins, minerals, and nutrients. A typical serving could be one slice of bread or one-half cup of cooked rice, pasta, or cereal.

■ Vegetables

We should select three to five servings of vegetables a day. These foods are high in fiber, low in fat, and contain necessary vitamins and minerals that are conducive to good health. Both vegetables and fruits have been found to protect against certain diseases, such as colon and breast cancer. A serving from this category would include one cup of raw leafy vegetables, one-half cup of other raw or cooked vegetables, or three-quarters of a cup of vegetable juice.

■ Fruits

We need two to four servings of fruit a day. Similar to vegetables, fruits provide necessary vitamins and minerals, are low in fat, and are high in fiber. A serving consists of one medium size banana, apple, or orange, one-half cup of chopped, canned, or cooked fruit, or three-quarters of a cup of fruit juice.

■ Meat, Beans, Eggs, Nuts

The Food Guide Pyramid recommends two to three servings of meat, poultry, dry beans, eggs, and nuts each day. In addition to containing high amounts of vitamins and minerals, these foods are excellent sources of protein, which we need for tissue growth and repair. A serving would include approximately two to three ounces of cooked meat, fish, or poultry. Think of a serving as about the size of a deck of cards. Another serving would consist of one egg or one-half cup of cooked (dry) beans.

■ The Dairy Group

We are advised to consume two to three daily servings of milk, yogurt, and cheese. Young adults up to age twenty-four and women who are pregnant or breast-feeding need three servings of these dairy products. Most dairy products are excellent sources of protein, vitamins, and minerals, especially calcium. Milk and yogurt provide the most calcium, but also can provide extra fat calories unless we select low or nonfat products. A serving in this category consists of eight ounces of milk, one cup of yogurt, or one and one-half ounces of hard cheese.

■ At the Top

The Food Guide Pyramid gives no recommended servings for fats, oils, and sweets, which are found at the very top of the pyramid. These food items have few vitamins or minerals, if any, yet they contain ample calories. Besides obvious fats, oils, and sugars, many foods contain "hidden" amounts as well. For instance, one can of regular soda contains nine teaspoons of sugar. A pork or beef hot dog is more than eighty-percent fat! Because fats, oils, and sugars are found in many foods, we should include them sparingly in food preparation or consumption.

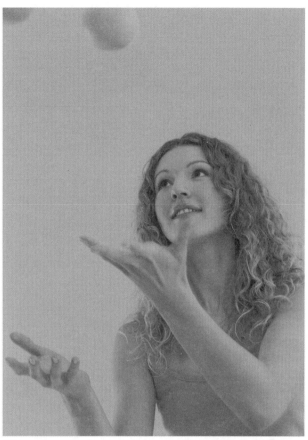

We need sustained energy to meet the various demands of life.

■ Recommended Dietary Allowances

Another tool available to help us put together a healthy food plan is the guide for Recommended Dietary Allowances (RDAs). Contained in the RDAs are specific recommended values for protein, eleven vitamins, and seven minerals that are considered adequate to meet the needs of most healthy people. (See Table 8.6.) Knowing RDAs and planning a diet that follows them can help to prevent certain deficiencies that may be subtle, but that over time may create problems. For example, someone may develop iron-deficiency anemia after prolonged, inadequate intake of foods that contain iron. Perhaps a college student who eats poorly is prone to frequent respiratory infections. In the latter example, we could conclude that cell damage from a poor diet diminished this student's immune system, subsequently lowering the body's resistance to viruses. We can determine if our diet contains the RDA of certain nutrients by referencing tables listing the composition of foods, or by reading the nutrient composition labels of packaged foods.

Table 8.6. Recommended Dietary Allowances[a]

Category or Condition	Age (years)	Weight (kg)	(lb)	Height (cm)	(in)	Protein (g)	Vita-min A (μgre)[c]	Vita-min D (μg)[d]	Vita-min E (mg αTE)[e]	Vita-min K (μg)	Vita-min C (mg)	Thia-min (mg)	Ribo-flavin (mg)	Niacin (mg NE)[f]	Vita-min B6 (mg)	Fo-late (μg)	Vitamin B12 (μg)	Cal-cium (mg)	Phos-phorus (mg)	Mag-nesium (mg)	Iron (mg)	Zinc (mg)	Iodine (μg)	Sele-nium (μg)
Infants	0.0–0.5	6	13	60	24	13	375	7.5	3	5	30	0.3	0.4	5	0.3	25	.03	400	300	40	6	5	40	10
	0.5–1.0	9	20	71	28	14	375	10	4	10	35	0.4	0.5	6	0.6	35	0.5	600	500	60	10	5	50	15
Children	1–3	13	29	90	35	16	400	10	6	15	40	0.7	0.8	9	1.0	50	0.7	800	800	80	10	10	70	20
	4–6	20	44	112	44	24	500	10	7	20	45	0.9	1.1	12	1.1	75	1.0	800	800	120	10	10	90	20
	7–10	28	62	132	52	28	700	10	7	30	45	1.0	1.2	13	1.4	100	1.4	800	800	170	10	10	120	30
Males	11–14	45	99	157	62	45	1,000	10	10	45	50	1.3	1.5	17	1.7	150	2.0	1,200	1,200	270	12	15	150	40
	15–18	66	145	176	69	59	1,000	10	10	65	60	1.5	1.8	20	2.0	200	2.0	1,200	1,200	400	12	15	150	50
	19–24	72	160	177	70	58	1,000	10	10	70	60	1.5	1.7	19	2.0	200	2.0	1,200	1,200	350	10	15	150	70
	25–50	79	174	176	70	63	1,000	5	10	80	60	1.5	1.7	19	2.0	200	2.0	800	800	350	10	15	150	70
	51+	77	170	173	68	63	1,000	5	10	80	60	1.2	1.4	15	2.0	200	2.0	800	800	350	10	15	150	70
Females	11–14	46	101	157	62	46	800	10	8	45	50	1.1	1.3	15	1.4	150	2.0	1,200	1,200	280	15	12	150	45
	15–18	55	120	163	64	44	800	10	8	55	60	1.1	1.3	15	1.5	180	2.0	1,200	1,200	300	15	12	150	50
	19–24	58	128	164	65	46	800	10	8	60	60	1.1	1.3	15	1.6	180	2.0	1,200	1,200	280	15	12	150	55
	25–50	63	138	163	64	50	800	5	8	65	60	1.1	1.3	15	1.6	180	2.0	800	800	280	15	12	150	55
	51+	65	143	160	63	50	800	5	8	65	60	1.0	1.2	13	1.6	180	2.0	800	800	280	10	12	150	55
Pregnant						60	800	10	10	65	70	1.5	1.6	17	2.2	400	2.2	1,200	1,200	300	30	15	175	65
Lactating	1st 6 months					65	1,300	10	12	65	95	1.6	1.8	20	2.1	280	2.6	1,200	1,200	355	15	19	200	75
	2nd 6 months					62	1,200	10	11	65	90	1.6	1.7	20	2.1	260	2.6	1,200	1,200	340	15	16	200	75

[a]The allowances, expressed as average daily intakes over time, are intended to provide for individual variations among most normal persons as they live in the United States under usual environmental stresses. Diets should be based on a variety of common foods in order to provide other nutrients for which human requirements have been less well defined. See text for detailed discussion of allowances and of nutrients not tabulated.

[b]Weights and heights of Reference Adults are actual medians for the U.S. population of the designated age, as reported by NHANES II. The median weights and heights of those under 19 years of age were taken from Hamill et al. (1979). The use of these figures does not imply that the height-to-weight ratios are ideal.

[c]Retinol equivalents. 1 retinol equivalent = 1μg retinol or 6μ β-carotene. See text for calculation of vitamin A activity of diets as retinol equivalents.

[d]As cholecalciferol. 10 μg cholecalciferol = 400 IU of vitamin D.

[e]a-Tocopherol equivalents. 1 mg d-a tocopherol = 1 a-TE. See text for variation in allowances as calculation of vitamin E activity of the diet as a-tocopherol equivalents.

[f]1 NE (niacin equivalent) is equal to 1 mg of niacin or 60 mg of dietary tryptophan.

Source: Food and Nutrition Board, National Academy of Sciences, *National Research Council Recommended Dietary Allowances,* 10th ed. (Washington, D.C.: National Academy Press, 1989).

■ Other Recommendations

In applying the Food Guide Pyramid principles and RDAs to the daily intake of foods, consider these additional recommendations for achieving a more balanced diet.

1. Choose various foods within each category to allow for the full range of different vitamins, minerals, and nutrients available. For instance, if you only ate apples, you would miss the higher amount of vitamin C found in oranges and the higher amount of potassium in bananas.

2. The foods you select should be as wholesome as possible. When foods are processed, such as potatoes into french fries or potato chips, they lose a great deal of their original vitamins, minerals, and fiber. Furthermore, processing adds fats and other additives such as salt that can contribute to health problems.

3. Plan your meals so that they are low in cholesterol and fat, especially saturated fat. Select dry beans, fish, poultry, and lean meat as your protein sources. In preparing meat, trim the fat and boil, broil, grill, or bake your selection instead of frying it. When selecting dairy products, look for the low or nonfat items.

4. Use sugar, salt, and sodium in moderation. Many processed and prepared foods, such as lunch meats, canned soups, crackers, cookies, and certain cereals, contain high amounts of salt and/or sugar.

5. In a cafeteria or restaurant, select foods that follow the Food Guide Pyramid recommendations and the RDAs. When your selection is limited to few healthy items, you have two options. Either eat less of the unhealthy food item or remove what makes it unhealthy; for example, scrape off heavy cream, butter, fried coating or skin. Remember moderation when you are eating out. Restaurants often provide a serving that is actually two to four times larger than a true serving size. Don't feel that you need to clean your plate! You can share with someone else, eat half and take the remaining half home, or simply throw the excess away.

6. Learn to slow down, relax, and enjoy food consumption. Eating more slowly will aid digestion and encourage moderation.

■ About Packaged Foods

Designing a healthy diet must take into consideration packaged foods. The federal government requires food manufacturers to provide nutritional information on the food item's label. The nutrient content is provided by weight, usually in serving sizes, and will include the amount of fat, carbohydrates, protein, cholesterol, sodium, and calories. Labels indicate the recommended levels of these items, except for protein, and the percentage each serving provides. These values are based on a 2,000-calorie food plan. Beneath the nutrition facts is a summary of suggested fat, saturated fat, cholesterol, sodium, carbohydrates, and fiber intake for both a 2,000-calorie diet and a 2,500-calorie diet.

The government also requires food manufacturers to include a list of ingredients on the package. The ingredient label lists the chemical composition of the food. Every substance in that food product is indicated by weight from the greatest amount to the least. These substances may include foods, water, natural and artificial sweeteners, fats, thickeners, flavorings, food colorings, and

Source: United States Department of Agriculture, Center for Nutrition Policy and Promotion: Available at www.usda.gov/dietaryguidelines.

preservatives. The ingredient label does not indicate the actual amount of these substances, only the amount as it compares to the others in descending order.

The U.S. government now stipulates that food manufacturers follow specific guidelines for health-related claims printed on the food label. The following examples provide definitions for specific claims:

- *calorie-free*: fewer than 5 calories per serving
- *fat-free*: less than 0.5 grams of fat per serving
- *reduced* or *less fat*: at least 25 percent less fat per serving than the higher-fat version
- *sugar-free*: less than 0.5 grams of sugar per serving
- *sodium-free*: less than 5 mg of sodium per serving, and no sodium chloride
- *low sodium*: 140 mg of sodium (or less) per serving
- *reduced* or *less sodium*: at least 25 percent less sodium per serving than the higher-sodium version
- *cholesterol-free*: less than 2 mg of cholesterol and 2 grams (or less) of saturated fat per serving

- *reduced cholesterol*: at least 25 percent less cholesterol than the higher-cholesterol version and 2 grams or less of saturated fat per serving
- *lean*: less than 10 grams of fat, 4 grams of saturated fat, and 95 mg of cholesterol per serving
- *high-fiber*: 5 grams of fiber (or more) per serving
- *good source of fiber*: 2.5 to 4.9 grams of fiber per serving

In order to follow a healthy diet, we certainly must have a basic understanding of labels, referring to them when we dine or shop for food. Make it a habit to compare items by labels in order to choose foods that better fit a wellness plan.

Nutrition: Misinformation, Misconceptions, and Myths

Today, nutritional myths and misconceptions abound. Most of this "misinformation" involves the idea that we can enhance our health through certain foods and supplements. This has become increasingly problematic as many people continue to seek "quick fixes" for weight loss and enhanced health, without following a nutritious dietary plan.

Nutritional Credentials

Some advice may seem credible because it is disguised as "scientifically proven" data. Pay attention not only to which organization makes a claim, but also to the person identified as the professional associated with the product or program. Regardless of qualifications, anyone can claim to be a nutritionist. Plenty of organizations provide certificates or diplomas that give the appearance of being education-based. In fact, they are not—but they *are* available for a price.

Reputable resources include literature supported by the American Dietetic Association and members of that organization. Registered dietitians have college degrees in nutrition and must pass a certification examination. When seeking a nutritional consultation, always choose professionals and nutrition experts with advanced degrees, including nutrition study.

Vitamin and Mineral Supplements

Vitamin and mineral supplements do not supply energy. Physically active people do not necessarily need more vitamin and mineral supplements than do sedentary people. Research has provided no evidence that vitamin and mineral supplements improve the athletic performance of people who follow nutritional guidelines for a healthy diet. Furthermore, supplements should not be taken to compensate for poor dietary habits. If you rely on supplements, you may not get all of the substances you could obtain in actual food.

In certain instances supplements are indicated for enhanced health. People who consistently consume less than 1,800 calories a day will not get the essential nutrients they need. Those who are allergic to certain foods or who cannot tolerate foods such as wheat or milk products may not receive important nutrients. Others who need nutritional supplementation include total vegetarians, heavy smokers or drinkers, persons with chronic illnesses, and women who are pregnant or breast-feeding. People in any of these categories need a physician or registered dietician to evaluate their specific needs and make the appropriate recommendations. Just as people can be adversely affected by excessive prescriptive medicines, they can suffer harm and even permanent organ damage from excessive dosing with supplements.

■ "Power" Food

As we saw earlier, no supplement will provide power or build larger muscles. Likewise, there is no food or "candy bar" that will do the same. Only exercise will help to build muscles and provide the body with increased power. Young people often take protein supplements because they believe this additional protein will improve physical or athletic performance. These supplements are unnecessary and actually may be harmful. Too much protein, either from foods or supplements, strains the liver and kidneys as they attempt to break down and eliminate the protein.

Another myth asserts that eating sugar before exercise will provide an extra boost of energy. Actually, sugar more than likely will diminish performance. Sugar is rapidly absorbed into the blood, which causes an increase in insulin secretion. The rush of insulin prevents fat from being metabolized by the muscles and forces muscles to utilize more glycogen stores. At the same time, insulin lowers blood sugar levels, which results in rapidly increasing weakness and fatigue. A far better choice is to consume complex carbohydrates several hours before exercise or athletic performance.

We do not recommend taking salt tablets to replace the salt lost from perspiring during heavy and long bouts of exercise. Because the sodium draws water out of the body's cells, their functions are impaired. In addition, salt tablets can irritate the stomach and cause nausea. To replenish sodium, rely on plain water and the salt already present in many foods.

■ Caffeine

No discussion about nutritional myths would be complete without mentioning caffeine. It is found in coffee, tea, chocolate, colas, and over-the-counter drugs. Caffeine is a stimulant to the central nervous system. It is also a diuretic and will contribute to fluid loss. The effects of caffeine differ from person to person, especially in how much is consumed. In small amounts it can lessen drowsiness, but in larger amounts or if consumed routinely, it can lead to psychological dependence. A tolerance to the stimulant may gradually develop. If discontinued, withdrawal symptoms such as headaches, irritability, and restlessness may follow. Those who take weight-control aids or "stay-awake" products often ingest higher doses, which can lead to nervousness, restlessness, tremors, and insomnia. In very high doses (10 grams or the equivalent of 60 cups of coffee), caffeine can produce convulsions and even death.

Nutrition and Weight Control

Earlier in this chapter, we mentioned the "Freshman 15" trait common among first-year college students. This refers to the fifteen pounds that many freshmen gain when they are away from home for the first time. We have known for years that overconsumption of calories and diminished expenditure

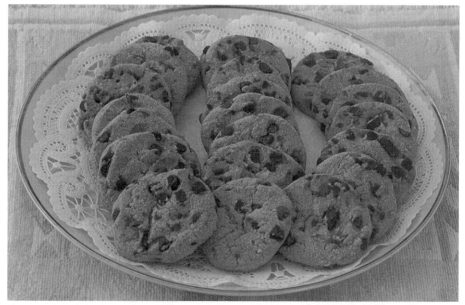

Overconsumption of calories and diminished expenditure of calories will ultimately add extra fat weight to the body.

of calories will ultimately add extra fat weight to the body. Eating and exercising are lifestyle behaviors, both of which generally change as people pursue higher education. Unfortunately, these behaviors often do not change for the better. Many college students may believe they are consuming the same amount of food as when they were at home, but the fat content could be higher. Also, their snacking habits may increase in frequency, amount, and fat content. Their activity levels also may be changing. They may not realize that because they no longer play racquetball or tennis or some other physical activity on a regular basis, their bodies are not getting the exercise they need to expend the extra calories they are consuming. Becoming aware of such changes is the first step toward changing their energy balance and controlling their weight.

■ Examine Your Diet

One of the best ways to determine and assess your current diet is to examine everything you eat for a specific time period. At the end of this chapter, you will find *Learning Exercise 1, A Daily Food Journal*. This journal will guide you toward evaluating your food intake and comparing it to recommended dietary goals. In addition to looking at what you have eaten, examine influencing factors as well; i.e., where you were at the time, what influenced your food choices, what your thoughts and feelings were at the time. This exercise will give you insight into certain eating practices that not only may be unconscious, but also may be culprits in weight gain.

Learning Exercise 2, Changes in Diet, is intended to help you identify different choices for the foods consumed and recorded in *Learning Exercise 1*. Look at the foods you have recorded and decide what could have been better choices. Take into consideration the recommended daily foods from the Food Guide Pyramid, and also the carbohydrate, protein, and fat allowances discussed earlier in this chapter. Finally, indicate how the changes could have improved your nutrition for the day.

■ Determine Your Proper Weight

As you learn more about your nutrition and eating habits, you may come to a number of conclusions. Perhaps you are happy with your weight, but want to change your diet to one that is more nutritionally sound. Or perhaps you believe your weight should increase, so you want to increase certain foods and calories. Perhaps you want to lose weight by reducing your consumption of fat and overall calories.

Regardless of your conclusion, knowing what approximate weight is appropriate for your gender and height will help in your decision. Several methods can determine proper weight. Among them are height/weight charts, body composition testing, and body mass index (BMI). A simple, but effective formula is as follows:

> Men start with 106 pounds for the first five feet of height and then add six pounds for every inch over five feet. Factor in ten percent (both plus and minus) for different body types, muscle mass, and bone structure. Example: 5'10" = 166 pounds +/- 10% = 149 - 183 pound range.
>
> Women start with 100 pounds for the first five feet of height and then add five pounds for every inch over five feet or subtract five pounds for every inch under five feet. Factor in ten percent. Example: 5'6" = 130 pounds +/- 10%= 117 - 143 pound range.

As we saw in chapter 3, body mass index (BMI) is a rough measure of body composition that is based on the concept that a person's weight should be proportional to height. Studies have shown that a high BMI (30 and above) is positively associated with hypertension, high blood cholesterol, and heart disease.

■ Weight Perfection or Weight Management?

With the help of such formulas, you have a better idea of the weight range that is most healthy and realistic for you. Keep in mind that the secret to weight happiness is not striving for what you see in magazines and promotional advertisements. Nor is it necessarily what others indicate is appropriate. For instance, height/weight charts do not take into consideration the differences between athletes with large amounts of muscle and others of the same gender, age, and height without the same muscle mass. Such athletes can actually fall into the category of those who are overweight—only because their muscle creates pounds that could be interpreted as fat (muscle is more dense than fat and thus weighs more).

> The most effective and permanent weight loss plans are those that involve making lifestyle changes that will continue beyond the weight loss you desire.

Likewise, the counterpart to this type of athlete could weigh normal on the height/weight chart, yet have much more body fat. In general, those of you who are athletic and muscular should not be concerned if your weight on scales moderately exceeds the pounds indicated as appropriate for your height. If you otherwise fall into your range on the chart, and you are comfortable in your clothing, everyday movement patterns, and other activities, strive more for weight management instead of weight perfection.

If you are thinking of weight loss as a goal, be aware that just as there are safe and effective programs, there also are dangerous and ineffective programs. If the success of a plan is based upon quick weight loss, very limited or special food intake, a fat loss pill, or something else that sounds "too good to be true," it probably is just that. The most effective and permanent weight loss plans are those that involve making lifestyle changes that will continue beyond the weight loss you desire. These safe programs do not involve rapid weight loss, but rather slow and progressive loss over a specified time period. Before we discuss some appropriate weight loss measures, let's look at two unsound plans that are popular today.

■ Doomed to Fail

A very low calorie or quick weight loss program is often doomed to fail, because most people are unable to maintain the lower weight. Once they begin to eat the way they did before the diet, they not only will regain the weight they lost, but they will gain it back more quickly than they lost it. Part of the failure is due to the type of weight that is lost, which is primarily water. If the diet has extended for some time, muscle also can be lost. Generally during this time frame, metabolism is greatly reduced, contributing to the addition of mostly fat during the rapid regain.

This type of dieter fails at making psychological and behavioral changes that could lead to weight management. Instead, the dieter may begin a cycle of losing and gaining weight referred to as "yo-yo" dieting. This form of weight cycling leads to a total reduction of resting metabolic weight, making weight loss more difficult and weight gain more likely as the loss/gain cycle continues. In addition to the obvious frustration that this causes among dieters, it also leads to an increase of risk for heart disease and death, as proven by scientific study.

Another popular diet that has gained a great deal of attention in recent years is the ***very restricted carbohydrate/very high volume protein diet***. Note the emphasis on "very." In this diet, the recommendation is to lower your carbohydrates to a level (as low as 20 grams per day) that limits the vitamins, minerals, nutrients, and fiber found in fruits, vegetables, and whole grain carbohydrates. Along with this deficit comes a recommended excess of protein, much of which is very high in fat. This diet prompts medical concern about high fat/high cholesterol intake, heart disease risk, and kidney stress. Digestion and elimination of protein in high volume will tax the kidneys. This should be of particular concern to those persons with kidney disorders or other chronic health problems that might influence disease or malfunction of the kidneys. As with the quick weight loss program, dieters who follow this program do not make behavior and lifestyle changes. Thus, their chances of long-term success are quite limited.

■ Effective Weight Loss Guidelines

When it comes to successful weight loss diets, follow a program that addresses:

- **Consumption of foods**—with respect to calories, fat content, serving size, frequency of intake
- **Exercise**—for the purpose of reducing body fat, along with increasing body metabolism

A calorie deficit is required to lose weight. A deficit of 3,500 calories is required to lose one pound of stored fat. Therefore, an individual who consumes an average of 2,500 calories per day and then reduces that daily consumption by 500 calories would lose one pound in a week. An additional fat pound would be lost if that same person walked at a pace and distance to burn 500 calories, daily, for one week.

■ Set a Realistic Goal

Most exercise professionals recommend setting a weight loss goal of one to two pounds each week. If people lose weight in this way, not only will they experience a greater likelihood of success, but they also will be more likely to maintain the necessary lifestyle changes.

■ Analyze Your Food Intake

A weight loss program is enhanced if the dieter addresses the behavioral aspects of weight gain. Keeping a food diary and monitoring diet changes, such as presented in *Learning Activities 1* and *2*, will help those interested in weight loss to better understand what foods limit their diet success. By analyzing your food intake and making decisions on how to substitute more nutritious foods that are lower in fat and calorie content, you truly gain control over your eating habits.

■ Seek Behavioral Assistance

Behavioral therapy is another adjunct that is helpful in successful weight loss. Those who are morbidly obese or who have been unsuccessful in previous attempts may find counseling to be the best intervention in conjunction with a weight loss regimen. Gaining family and social support also will increase the chances of success, just as a support system is advantageous to any other lifestyle change.

Nutritional Wellness: Commitment and Motivation

■ Interested or Committed?

Now that you have gained more knowledge about nutrition, weight management, and your own food intake, you have the necessary tools to make changes. To go beyond knowledge, however, requires commitment and motivation. Are you committed to change or merely interested in change? The outcome of "interest" generally means you will come up with good reasons *not* to work toward your health goal. Perhaps during a previous attempt you were attracted by the benefits, but found that the inconvenience and discomfort derailed your efforts to change.

Another trap you may have experienced is the tendency to rely on circumstances to direct the progress of your program instead of accepting personal responsibility. Sometimes circumstances are conducive to the efforts necessary to reach your goal and sometimes they are not. People in this trap "wait" for the right circumstances—a day when your effort seems reasonable, comfortable, manageable, and easy. Unfortunately, they are in for a long wait. Progressing toward your goal only when circumstances permit simply doesn't work.

Commitment is very different from interest. The outcome of commitment is the achievement of results. Committed people act to achieve desired results, no matter what difficulty is present. The perceived value of being healthy, well, and fit is so great that the difficulties of sticking to a daily plan seem insignificant—the goal becomes worth the extra effort.

■ A Clear and Compelling Purpose

In order to become committed, you must be motivated. Ask yourself the following questions:

- Do you want to go through life fatigued, uncomfortable, or perhaps even in pain due to your diet and lifestyle?

- Do you want to go through life feeling self-conscious, angry with yourself, and depressed because of your bad eating habits?

- Do you want to put your body at greater risk for disease, perhaps even shortening your life span?

The answer to all of these questions is undoubtedly "NO."

Develop a clear and compelling purpose for changing your eating behaviors. Express your purpose in a way that makes your behavior as essential and necessary as other daily habits. For example, if your purpose is to lose weight for medical reasons, then eating habits leading to that goal should fall into the same category as rest and sleep. If daily exercise is a goal, it needs to be classified as important as going to school or work.

After you have developed a purpose for eating behavior changes, develop a complete plan. Include in your plan all the steps necessary to reach your goal. Finally, include actions you will take to address slip-ups. Don't get stuck in the permanent failure trap by projecting that your goal is impossible due to your past failures. Instead, recognize that what happened before has nothing to do with what happens now. This is a new opportunity!

Remember the words of Proverbs 16:3: *"Commit to the LORD whatever you do, and your plans will succeed"* (NIV).

KEY CONCEPTS
calorie
macronutrients
metabolic rate
metabolism
micronutrients
obesity

Learning Exercise 1
Daily Food Journal

Name_____ Date_____ Day of week_____

Time	M/S	Food	Group	Serving size	# of servings	Location (where you ate the food)	What else were you doing?	What influenced your food choices?	What were your thoughts/ feelings?

M/S = Meal or snack

Learning Exercise 2
Changes in Diet

Name_____ Date_____ Day of week_____

Food Item	Substitute food item or different preparation	How this substitution or change could improve your nutrition

References

Webb, Denise, R.D. "Close-Up on Nutrition." *Advance for Nurse Practitioners*. (June 2001): 77-86.

American Cancer Society. *Cancer Facts and Figures—1993*. New York: American Cancer Society, 1993.

American Heart Association. *Heart and Stroke Facts*. Dallas: American Heart Association, 1993.

"The Truth about Dieting." *Consumer Reports* (June 2002): 26-31.

Food and Nutrition Board. *Recommended Daily Allowances*. Washington D.C.: National Academy of Sciences, n.d.

Lissner, L., et al. "Variability of Body Weight and Health Outcomes in the Framingham Population. *New England Journal of Medicine* 324 (1991): 1839-44.

Connelly, A. Scott. *Body Rx*. New York: Putnam, 2001.

Mayo Clinic Health Information. *Mayo Clinic on Healthy Weight*. Rochester, MN: Kensington Publishing, 2001.

McDrory, M., et al. "Dietary Variety Within Food Groups: Association with Energy Intake and Body Fatness in Men and Women." *American Journal of Clinical Nutrition* 69 (1999): 440-47.

Rodin, J., et al. "Weight Cycling and Fat Distribution." *International Journal of Obesity* 14 (1990): 303-10.

U.S. Department of Agriculture/U.S. Department of Health and Human Services. *Dietary Guidelines for Americans*. 5th ed. Washington, DC: U.S. Government Printing Office, 2000.

U.S. Department of Health and Human Services. *Healthy People 2010: Understanding and Improving Health*. 2nd ed. Washington, DC: U.S. Government Printing Office, November 2000.

Additional Resources
Nutrition Web Sites

American Dietetic Association (http://www.eatright.org/)

Fast Food Facts (http://www.olen.com/food/)

Food and Drug Administration (http://www.fda.gov)

Food and Nutrition Information Center (http://www.nal.usda.gov/fnic)

Government Nutrition (http://www.nutrition.gov)

Healthfinder (www.healthfinder.gov)

Healthy People 2010 or Healthy People 2010 documents
    (http://www.health.gov/healthypeople)

Mayo Clinic (http://www.MayoClinic.com)

Mayo Health Oasis (http://www.mayohealth.org)

National Institute of Health (www.nih.gov/health)

Tufts Univ. Nutri. Navigator (www.navigator.tufts.edu)

U.S. Department of Agriculture Food Composition Data
    (http://www.nal.usda.gov/fnic/foodcomp)

U.S. Food and Drug Administration Food Labeling Publications Page
    (http://www.fda.gov/opacom/campaigns/3foodlbl.html)

U.S.D.A. Food and Nutrition Services (http://www.fns.usda.gov/fns)

Endnote

1. Babcock, Robert Hall, "President's Address: The Limitations of Drug Therapy," *Trans Am Clin Climatol Assoc*. 17 (1901): 1-13.

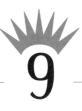

9

WELLNESS AND
EATING DISORDERS

"Fear is static that prevents me from hearing myself."

—Samuel Butler[1]

Eating disorders represent a wide spectrum of abnormal behaviors surrounding food and body image. High profile cases like the untimely death of singer Karen Carpenter have awakened us to the existence of eating disorders and their ever-increasing influence in today's society. Someone once quipped, "A person can never be too rich or too thin." Sadly, many people believe this saying. Those who suffer from an eating disorder struggle with another concern: to eat or not to eat. If they decide to eat, their next dilemma is what to do to compensate for their "failure." Wellness and eating disorders are mutually exclusive. In preparation for our discussion of eating disorders, let us first look at five case studies to determine some common denominators.

Eating Disorders: Case Studies

▪ Guilty and "Fat"

Susan is a twenty-one-year-old college senior. She has always done fairly well in school, but has never been quite satisfied with herself. No matter how well she does, she never feels good enough. She hopes to enter graduate school, but the program she is considering is highly competitive, accepting only the best. She wonders if she'll make it.

Through high school, she competed as a gymnast. She always felt too tall and too big, even though at 5'6" she never weighed more than 123 lbs. She dieted through high school, but never seemed to be able to get down to a weight that was "okay." Whenever she reached a weight goal, she wasn't satisfied. So, she would make a new, even lower weight goal, thinking that would make her feel better.

In college, her weight ranges between 95 and 100 lbs. She is rarely seen in the cafeteria, and always makes excuses that "she isn't hungry" or "just had a snack." People realize that they rarely see her eat. When asked how she manages to stay so thin, she replies that she "has a high metabolism." To deal with stress, she runs three miles a day. If she can't run, she feels very anxious and "fat." She lost a semester in her sophomore year due to illness. Her friends know that she was hospitalized, but she has never told them why.

Susan always seems to be very serious, goal driven, and somewhat isolated. Her roommates assume she doesn't eat much because of her stress level. Susan knows she doesn't eat much because she can't. Even a few bites make her feel guilty and "fat." Hunger feels like a weakness. It is important for her to get by with as little food as possible and to keep pushing herself.

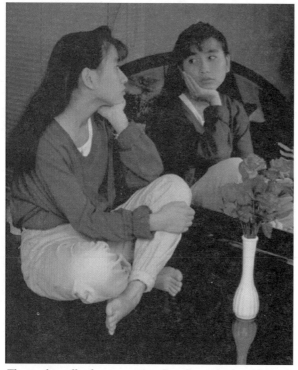

Those who suffer from an eating disorder struggle with a decision: to eat or not to eat.

■ A Mother in the Dark

Mrs. S. is forty-three years old and married. She homeschools her three children, is active in her church's women's ministry, and prides herself on a well-kept, nicely decorated home. Dinner is always ready when her husband comes home from work. Fast food is never an option for her family! She is taking courses to become a dietician because "healthy eating" has always been important to her. Her children aren't allowed to have sweets because "it's bad for them." She also worries because her husband is gaining a little weight now that he is in his forties. She continually reminds her thirteen-year-old daughter that if she's not careful, she'll put on weight during puberty. Mrs. S. believes that if she is a good role model for healthy exercise and healthy eating, her children will follow suit.

Yesterday, her world was shaken when she received a call from the church youth group leader. Mrs. S's daughter was found vomiting in the bathroom of the youth room. Her peers have been suspicious for a while that this was going on. When confronted, the daughter admits that she has to vomit anytime she lets herself eat "bad" food. Mrs. S is devastated by her daughter's behavior and remarks to the youth pastor, "How could she do this when I've worked so hard to teach her how to eat and properly manage her weight?"

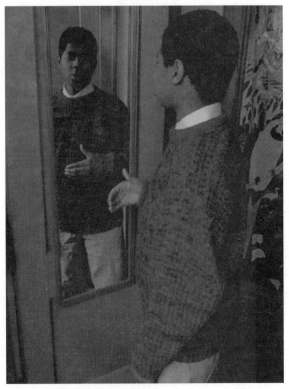

Many people with eating disorders look "normal."

■ "Defining" Himself

Andy is a twenty-four-year-old waiter at an expensive restaurant. His patrons are quite wealthy and his tips depend on the impression he makes. He has been trying to break into a modeling career, but has only managed to find a few low-paying jobs. Andy works out two to three hours a day, trying to achieve that muscular look that is so important to him. He even has considered plastic surgery, thinking that a stronger jawline might benefit his looks. Before important appointments, he fasts and takes over-the-counter water pills to better define his muscles. In high school, he was on the wrestling team. He is sure that the rapid weight loss tips he learned then will help him in his career goals.

Party Girl

Mary doesn't know why she can't get control of herself. Food is her best friend, but when she starts eating, she can't stop! In public, her eating is very restrained, even restrictive. Her friends comment that they don't understand why she carries around that extra ten pounds when they see her eat only carrots and diet soda. If they could only see her when she's alone! If they could only see her go from one drive-through to the next. If they could only see the floor of her car littered with the wrappers from cookies, candy, doughnuts, and anything else she can get her hands on! If they could only see how she loads the grocery cart with junk food, then smiles as she tells the checkout clerk that she's having a party at her place. If they only knew that the party is Mary and the food is her guest. If they could only see her vomiting out of control—then her friends would know her terrible secret. They would know that Mary hates herself. She hates her body. She believes that if her friends really knew what she was doing, they would hate her, too.

Worst Fear Confirmed

Ed has been steadily gaining weight. He has always been a large man, but over the past few years his weight has been climbing dramatically. During the day, he stays so busy that he doesn't eat very much. In the evening, he makes up for it. Once he starts eating, he can't stop. He is always surprised at how much food he can put away. He rationalizes that since he doesn't eat during the day, it's okay. Deep down, though, he is troubled by his behavior. This pattern has gone on for years. The more his weight goes up, the less active he becomes. Because of the decreased activity, he gains weight more rapidly. His physician informed him recently that he now has adult-onset diabetes. Ed is terribly upset. He has been afraid of this, and now his worst fear has been confirmed.

What Are Eating Disorders?

These case studies represent only a few of the ways eating disorders reveal themselves. These five situations may contradict some of our preconceived or stereotypical ideas of what people with an eating disorder "should" look like or how they "should" behave. Most of our ideas are wrong.

Many persons with eating disorders look "normal." They may be thin, average, or overweight. They may be rich, poor, or somewhere in the middle. They may be very intelligent and motivated, or they may struggle academically. They may come from a stable, two-parent home, or from a home affected by divorce, addiction, or mental illness. To recognize people with an eating disorder, you not only must look at the outside, but you must see what they are feeling about their bodies and how they relate to food. This is why the illness often is not recognized until serious medical or emotional

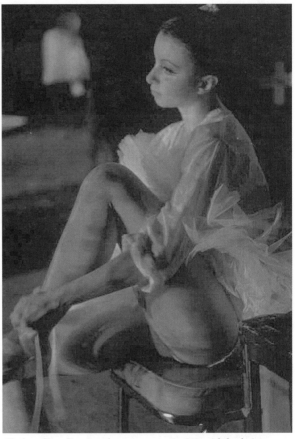

Eating disorders involve a preoccupation with body image.

consequences become evident. As you will see later in this chapter, early treatment and intervention are very important to success in recovery.

People with eating disorders often define their worth by their weight or size. Like looking in a carnival funhouse mirror, they do not see themselves as others see them.

An eating disorder is an abnormal relationship with food. Eating disorders involve a preoccupation with body image. People with eating disorders often define their worth by their weight or size. However, their view is often distorted.

Like looking in a carnival funhouse mirror, they do not see themselves as others see them. Food can be their best friend or their worst enemy. Eating is an event that is fraught with anxiety, or requires intense planning, or feels out of control. When eating gets out of control, the person often feels the need to somehow compensate to prevent weight gain. For those who do not compensate, chronic overeating leads to obesity.

■ The Scope of the Problem

Are eating disorders more prevalent today than at other times in history? Is it true that our culture and society have "pushed the envelope" and caused the current epidemic of eating disorders?

Case studies dating back to the 1800s describe women who went for long periods of time with no food or fluid. They were described as being almost saint-like, in that their bodies did not need the things average people required. In that society, women were expected to show restraint around food. It was "improper" to exhibit enjoyment of such physical pleasures as those associated with eating or sexuality.

In the development of American society, however, women were called upon to work to support an agrarian culture. A strong, solid body was the ideal for working the farm and bearing children. The frail and weak often succumbed to infection, illness, or death during childbirth.

Up until the late 1960s, the fuller female figure was considered the most appealing. Marilyn Monroe, the icon of the 50s and early 60s, probably would not get an audition in Hollywood today. Her curvaceous, size-14 figure would be too big by contemporary standards. Twiggy, the European model who hit the runway in the late 60s, introduced the standard of the shapeless, bone-thin supermodel we see today.

The average American woman today is 5'4" and weighs 135 lbs. The average model is 5'7" and weighs 108 lbs. For the current generation, this underscores a significant gap between what is normal versus what is "desired." Bombarded with media images of thin, sleek, glamorous models, many children, teenagers, and even adults feel inadequate and ashamed of their bodies. They begin to focus on the body types of a few perceived role models, assuming that this is the way they "should" look. This sets up the cycle of chronic body dissatisfaction and chronic dieting. To add to the paradox, we as a society are more overweight and out of shape than ever before! All of this focus on weight-loss products, programs, dieting, personal trainers, and supplements has resulted in a strange irony: we spend

Exhibit 9.1. Facts about Eating Disorders

Eating Disorder Are Widespread and Destructive
- Eating disorders cause immeasurable suffering for victims and families.
- Eating disorders have reached epidemic levels in America: all segments of society, young and old, rich and poor, all minorities, including African American and Latino.
- Eating disorders affect seven million women.
- Eating disorders affect one million men.
- Victims lose the ability to function effectively—great personal loss and loss to society.

Age at Onset of Illness
- 86% report onset of illness at the age of 20.
- 10% report the onset at 10 years or younger.
- 33% report the onset between ages of 11 and 15.
- 43% report onset between ages of 16 and 20.

Duration of Illness/Mortality
- 77% report duration from one to fifteen years.
- 30% report duration from one to five years.
- 31% report duration from six to ten years.
- 16% report duration from eleven to fifteen years.
- It is estimated that 6 percent of serious cases die.
- Only 50% report being cured.

Cost of Treatment
- Cost of patient treatment can be $30,000 or more a month.
- Many patients need repeated hospitalizations.
- The cost of outpatient treatment, including therapy and medical monitoring, can extend to $100,000 or more.

Source: The National Association of Anorexia Nervosa and Associated Disorders Web site. Retrieved 2-08-03 from http://www.anad.org/facts.htm

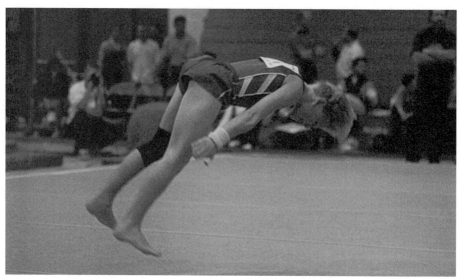

Many children and teenagers begin to focus on the body types of a few perceived role models, assuming that this is the way they also should look.

billions of dollars annually and, as a result, find ourselves fatter and with more health problems than ever before.

■ Disturbing Statistics

It is estimated that approximately 20 percent of females between fourteen and thirty years of age have an eating disorder. Another 20 percent are estimated to have subclinical eating disorders. This refers to patients with eating disorder symptoms who don't quite meet all the criteria for the full diagnosis. In females of all ages, the incidence of eating disorders is estimated to be 32 percent. Overall, the incidence appears to be increasing, but the largest increase is in women in the twenty- to forty-year-old age group. In teenage girls, the incidence appears to be relatively stable.

It also appears that the incidence is going up in males, although current estimates put eating disorders at 14 percent—considerably less than in the female population. Once thought to be a problem only in the gay male community, eating disorders are now extending into the heterosexual community. Males are now under more pressure to achieve a certain body type and look. Pressure to excel in athletic performance also continues to increase. In males, eating disorders are less about losing weight than they are about building more muscle and increasing muscle definition. This has resulted in a phenomena referred to as "reverse anorexia," in which a male feels that he can never be big enough and then goes to great lengths to build muscle and bulk. A related problem is the increased use of anabolic steroids to further the goal of increased muscle and bulk.

■ The Causes of Eating Disorders

From what you have read thus far in this chapter, it is obvious that cultural pressures play a part in eating disorders. What else causes eating disorders? This is a question that many families, patients, coaches, and medical professionals have asked. Families in therapy for eating disorders often want to know whose "fault" it is. Patients want a reason to justify their illness. This is a natural reaction.

For some, eating disorders stem from an obvious trauma or event. A situation involving rape or sexual abuse may lead a young girl or woman to attempt to change her body. In this way, she may think she will be less attractive and less vulnerable to attack. An adolescent whose parents are seeking divorce may restrict her eating, thinking that if she is sick, her parents might stay together. The eating disorder may give a person a sense of control in a world that feels out of control.

For some patients, eating disorder behaviors result from a culmination of multiple minor issues. A little brother makes a thoughtless remark, implying that his sister is fat. The sister initiates a diet that leads to an eating disorder. A coach comments that a student is overweight. The student begins a program to lose weight, then gets so caught up in changing her image, that she cannot stop losing weight.

Of course, many people have similar experiences, and *don't* develop an eating disorder. What is the difference? As with many other mental health problems, there are indications that a genetic predisposition can lead to the development of eating disorders. Some studies indicate that if the mother or sister has had anorexia nervosa or bulimia, the daughter is twelve times more likely to develop anorexia nervosa and four times more likely to develop bulimia. In studies of identical twins, findings disclose that if one twin has an eating disorder, there is a three to four times greater chance the other twin will develop one. The correlation between fraternal twins is much less, suggesting the genetic predisposition is stronger than environmental factors alone.

To summarize the causal factors, then, it is most likely that a person will develop an eating disorder according to unique environmental conditions in conjunction with a genetic predisposition. Recent research is focusing on a connection between infectious illnesses and the sudden onset of anorexia nervosa and other obsessive-compulsive disorders. While medical literature details documented cases, the outcome of this research is still unclear.

■ Types of Eating Disorders

Eating disorders are considered to be psychiatric illnesses. Of all the psychiatric illnesses, eating disorders carry with them the highest death rate. Death results not just from the physical consequences of the eating disorders. Due to the despair of living with an eating disorder, many patients eventually succeed at suicide. *The Diagnostic and Statistical Manual of Mental Disorders* (DSM-IV) is the text by which all psychiatric illness is diagnosed.[2] The purpose of this text is to standardize psychiatric diagnoses across the world, so that for research purposes, all physicians and researchers are speaking the same language. The DSM-IV categorizes eating disorders into three recognized diagnostic types:

- Anorexia Nervosa
- Bulimia Nervosa
- Eating Disorder - Not Otherwise Specified

While Binge Eating Disorder is considered by many to be part of the eating disorder spectrum, it is not yet included in the DSM.

As we review each of these categories and summarize the diagnostic criteria, remember that the DSM's primary purpose is to standardize diagnoses for research purposes. People do not fit into nice neat boxes, of course, so there may be variations—a symptom might express itself differently in different people. Keep this in mind, as well as the individual circumstances surrounding each person, before determining that someone has an eating disorder.

■ Anorexia Nervosa

The word derivation of **anorexia nervosa** tells us something of this eating disorder. In the original Greek, "an" means "without" and "orexis" means "appetite." Anorexia nervosa literally means nervous anorexia. This is not so much a literal loss of appetite as it is an irrational fear of food. A person diagnosed with anorexia nervosa usually exhibits four traits:

ANOREXIA NERVOSA:
A serious eating disorder characterized by a pathological fear of weight gain that leads to erratic eating patterns, malnutrition, and excessive weight loss.

1. Refusal to maintain body weight at a near normal weight for that person's height, or a loss of weight that brings the person to 85 percent or less of ideal body weight. For a child entering puberty, anorexia nervosa can be signaled by a failure to gain weight as expected during a growth phase, leading to a weight at 85 percent or less of ideal body weight.
2. Fear of gaining weight or becoming fat, even though the person is underweight.
3. Body image disturbance, denial of the seriousness of the low weight, or undue influence of body weight or shape on self-evaluation.
4. Failure to have a menstrual cycle for three months in a row in women whose menses has started. If a woman is on birth control pills or hormones, this criteria is not relevant, as the medication induces menses artificially and is not reflective of the woman's true hormonal balance.

Anorexia nervosa is generally broken down into two categories: binge-purge anorexia nervosa and restrictive anorexia nervosa. A person with binge-purge anorexia nervosa will at times restrict food intake, but at other times may binge and purge. A person with restrictive anorexia nervosa carefully restricts calories to continue to lose weight or to maintain an already low weight.

It might be surprising to learn that someone is anorexic (or anorectic), especially if we have seen this person eat "normal" food in the high school cafeteria, for instance. Our stereotypical view seems to declare that a person with an eating disorder would probably only eat celery and drink water. But an eating disorder is a very secretive and private illness. Patients often will go to great lengths to conceal their illness. If someone with an eating disorder feels she must eat in a social or public situation, she may spend time in advance fasting before the event, or she may plan extra exercise afterward to "work off" those calories.

Family members have described how a loved one with an eating disorder managed to fool them, so that they didn't realize she wasn't eating. Playing with or rearranging food, excessive cutting of food, and hiding food are common defenses the patient may use to hide the illness from the family. Once the illness is recognized, however, mealtime becomes a highly charged event. Family members may carefully watch the patient to be sure she is eating, at the same time the patient is working hard to preserve her eating disorder. If the

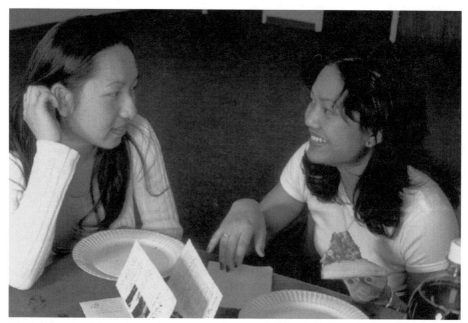

It might be surprising to learn that someone is anorexic, especially if we have seen this person eat "normal" food in the high school cafeteria.

patient feels that she has no choice but to eat, she may then begin purging behaviors to get rid of the calories.

Another issue common with anorexia nervosa is compulsive exercise. Some patients with anorexia rival an elite athlete training for the Olympics. To anorexics, the exercise is essential—they *have* to do it. Not working out restricts even more their ability to eat. If they are injured and cannot work out, anorexics may find themselves going over the edge emotionally. The need to exercise takes precedence over work, school, family, friends, or social activities. For some, the exercise regimen is not as rigorous, but their overall sense of well-being is tied to whether or not they can work out that day.

An obsessive activity common to anorexics is the careful monitoring of weight. They may hop on their bathroom scales multiple times a day to be sure they have not gained any weight. The number they see tells them whether they are "good" or "bad." Some focus on a certain size of clothing as an indicator. Others focus on a certain part of their body by compulsively measuring themselves. As with the number on the scale, the anorexic defines her sense of worth by the measurement she obtains. Failure to maintain a low weight or to continue to lose weight is often perceived as a great personal failure.

Exhibit 9.2, Warning Signs of Eating Disorders

Anorexia Nervosa

- Deliberate self-starvation with weight loss
- Intense, persistent fear of gaining weight
- Refusal to eat, except tiny portions
- Continuous dieting
- Excessive facial hair/body hair due to inadequate protein in the diet
- Compulsive exercise
- Abnormal weight loss
- Sensitivity to cold
- Absent or irregular menstruation
- Hair loss

Bulimia Nervosa

- Preoccupation with food
- Binge eating, usually in secret
- Vomiting after bingeing
- Abuse of laxatives, diuretics, diet pills
- Denial of hunger or of drug use to induce vomiting
- Compulsive exercise
- Swollen salivary glands
- Broken blood vessels in the eyes

Physical Repercussions from One or Both Diseases

Malnutrition	Intestinal ulcers
Dehydration	Ruptured stomach
Serious heart, kidney, and liver damage	Tooth/gum erosion
Tears or ruptures of the esophagus	

Psychological Repercussions from Both Diseases

Depression	Low self-esteem
Shame and guilt	Impaired family and social relations
Mood swings	Perfectionism
"All or nothing" thinking	

Source: The National Association of Anorexia Nervosa and Associated Disorders Web site. Retrieved 2-08-03 from http:// www.anad.org/warning.htm.

■ Bulimia Nervosa

The Greek for "boulimia" means "great hunger." A person diagnosed with **bulimia nervosa** usually exhibits the following traits:

1. Recurrent episodes of binge eating
2. Following the binge, recurrent purging
3. These behaviors occur with some regularity over a period of a few months.
4. Self-evaluation is unduly affected by body weight and size.

A **binge** is defined as eating in a two-hour period of time an amount of food that most people would consider excessive for that time and situation. (Overeating on Thanksgiving typically would not fall into this category.)

BULIMIA NERVOSA:
A serious eating disorder characterized by compulsive overeating, which is usually followed by self-induced vomiting, laxative, or diuretic abuse.

Purging describes the behaviors used to compensate for eating and bingeing; in other words, a way to rid the body of the food eaten or calories amassed in order to avoid weight gain. Usually accomplished through self-induced vomiting, purging also occurs through laxative use, diuretic use (water pills), or exercise. Some bulimics use so-called "fat burners" or "metabolism enhancers" to get rid of the unwanted calories. Sometimes after a binge the compensation may simply be a period of fasting or food restriction. Any of these behaviors qualify for a diagnosis of bulimia.

Substance abuse runs in approximately 30 to 37 percent of persons with bulimia. Bulimics may use drugs such as methamphetamine or cocaine—not necessarily for their ability to stimulate, but for their appetite-suppressing effects. Bulimics also may use alcohol to diminish anxiety associated with eating, or they may abuse many over-the-counter medications such as Ephedra and diet pills.

BINGE: Unrestrained and excessive indulgence or overeating.

Bulimia is often hard to recognize. Unlike the underweight anorexic, the bulimic may appear "normal" in weight and size. Bulimics often eat "normally" in public. Unless the person is caught in the act of purging, or unless laxatives or other such products are found, bulimics often escape notice. People with bulimia often have to take the courageous step of asking for help before others discover their problem.

■ Eating disorders - Not Otherwise Specified

This third category includes a number of eating disorder symptoms. A person in this category might exhibit low enough weight to categorize her as anorexic, but might still have a normal menstrual cycle. Someone else might have lost a tremendous amount of weight, but because she was quite overweight to begin with, she is not at less than 85 percent of her ideal body weight. Still another person might restrict her food sometimes, binge and purge at other times, then continue for a period of time in a normal pattern of eating. The thread tying these individuals together is an inordinate concern with weight and body image issues.

This category represents a large, unrecognized group who go unnoticed for long periods of time. They might suffer tremendous emotional pain and distress, but their concerns are never brought to the attention of health care or mental health professionals. They may have a lifetime of dissatisfaction with their bodies and may seem always to be looking for that next fad diet or miracle that will give them the bodies they want. When they hear of people with anorexia or bulimia and extremes of behavior associated with those disorders, they think, "I'm not like that." So they continue with lives of disordered eating, never confronting their body issues and missing out on the help they so desperately need.

■ Binge Eating Disorder

This eating disorder is characterized by bingeing and overeating, but not purging. Continuous eating or "grazing," as it is referred to, results in ongoing weight gain or the maintenance of an overweight condition. This disorder probably causes 25 percent of medical obesity cases. Often judged as just lacking control or willpower, these patients describe food as something "like a drug," and even consider themselves "food addicts." They constantly think about eating. Some former bulimics give up their purging efforts and become binge eaters, experiencing significant weight gain.

Exhibit 9.3, Eating Disorders Test

Researchers at St. George's Hospital Medical School in London have designed a simple questionnaire called SCOFF to help detect the eating disorders anorexia nervosa and bulimia nervosa that may afflict as many as one in ten Americans.

Anorexia is characterized by self-starvation and excessive weight loss, while bulimia nervosa is marked by a secretive cycle of binge eating followed by purging using vomiting, laxatives, and diuretics.

The London doctors tested the questionnaire on over 200 women, about half of whom suffered from an eating disorder. The quiz picked up 100 percent of anorexia and bulimia cases. While the questionnaire also indicated that some women suffered from a problem when they did not, the researchers said the false positive rate was an "acceptable trade off."

The SCOFF Quiz

1. Do you make yourself **S**ick because you feel uncomfortably full?

   Yes   No

2. Do you worry you have lost **C**ontrol over how much you eat?

   Yes   No

3. Have you recently lost more than **O**ne stone (14 pounds) in a three-month period?

   Yes   No

4. Do you believe yourself to be **f**at when others say you are too thin?

   Yes   No

5. Would you say that **f**ood dominates your life?

   Yes   No

If you answered "Yes" to two or more of these questions, this could indicate a possible case of an eating disorder.

If you have a positive result or think you suffer from an eating problem, please check with a doctor.

Source: Retrieved 2-08-03 from http://www.msnbc.com.modules/quizzes/loadquiz.htm. SCOFF questionnaire developed by J.F. Morgan, F. Reid, J.H. Lacey, "The SCOFF Questionnaire: Assessment of a New Screening Tool for Eating Disorders," *BMJ* 319 (1999): 1467.

Eating Disorders and Their Consequences

It is natural to think first of the physical complications that result from eating disorders: obesity, diabetes, malnutrition, etc. However, the consequences of eating disorders reach into all areas of the patient's well-being—emotional, relational, and spiritual, as well as physical. At the beginning of this chapter we noted that people with eating disorders have the highest death rate of those suffering a psychiatric illness. In this section, we will review some of these costly consequences.

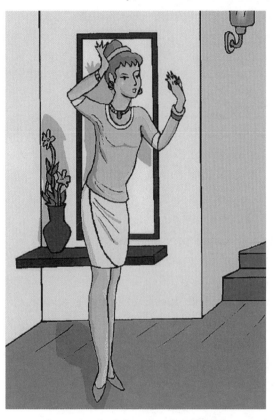

■ Medical Complications

Eating disorders have the potential to significantly compromise the health of the human body. Our bodies were designed to use food as a fuel source and to provide the things we need to stay healthy or to heal quickly when we are not healthy. Behaviors that deprive the body of its very basic requirements—energy (calories) and fluids—risk causing serious physical deterioration. Nearly every organ system is impacted in a negative way by an eating disorder (see Exhibit 9.2). To understand the potential medical complications, a health care provider must understand the behavior in which the patient is engaging. Since most eating disorder patients are secretive about their illnesses, many times the medical professional cannot achieve a true diagnosis.

LANUGO: Fine, downy hair seen on patients in later stages of physical starvation; thought to be the body's response to the loss of body heat.

■ The Body's Response to Starvation

Patients who are restricting food to the point of physical starvation may experience an overall slowing down of their physical functioning. The human body is designed to withstand periods of famine. The body does this by lowering the rate at which it uses energy (metabolic rate), so that it can continue vital functions until food is more readily available. Therefore, as the body adapts to the state of starvation, it exhibits bradycardia (low heart rate), hypotension (low blood pressure), and hypothermia (low body temperature). Other physical changes that occur include the following:

- The body grows fine, downy hair (especially on the arms and face) called **lanugo,** which is thought to help warm the body.
- Muscle, body fat, and liver tissue are broken down and used as an energy source, providing much-needed calories to keep the heart and respiratory functions going.
- The menstrual cycle stops and, in males, the testicles shrink.
- Calcium and phosphate in the bones are reabsorbed by the body, making bone tissue weaker and leading to osteoporosis.
- The brain function slows and brain tissue begins to waste away. CAT scans of the brains of adolescents with anorexia nervosa look similar to the elderly with dementia.
- The heart muscle becomes very small and unable to pump a normal amount of blood with each beat.
- Blood sugar drops, leading to chronic hypoglycemia.

In spite of these physical changes, patients with anorexia often will attempt to stay very busy and active, causing even more strain on an already stressed body. This is one characteristic that sometimes helps the doctor diagnosis the eating disorder. A person with low weight from cancer, HIV, or other serious medical illness generally has the appearance of one who is seriously ill. These patients look sick, act sick, and say they feel sick. Anorexics may look sick, but often act as if they have all the energy in the world. They might be shocked to learn that people are worried about them and reply that they feel fine. This is a part of the denial that is so much a part of this illness.

ELECTROLYTES: Electrically charged minerals which the cells of the human body use to maintain voltages across cell membranes and to carry electrical impulses to other cells.

■ The Results of Purging

Purging activity leads to many complications. In addition to the food that is lost through purging, the body loses vital fluids. Vomiting purges the body of food, along with the electrolytes that are in the stomach fluids. **Electrolytes** are electrically charged minerals that include sodium, potassium, chloride, magnesium, calcium, and phosphorus, all of which are essential for the function of individual cells in the human body. The cells use electrolytes to maintain voltages across cell membranes and to carry electrical impulses to other cells. Loss of electrolytes can result in irregular

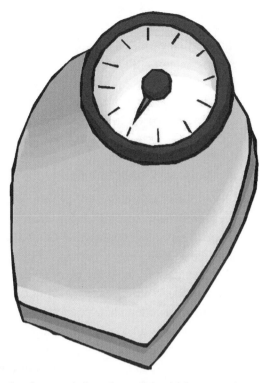

heart rhythms (leading to cardiac arrest), abnormal function of the kidneys and intestines, and muscle weakness and paralysis.

The human body is 60 to 70 percent water, so weight changes caused by dehydration may be quite dramatic. A woman with bulimia may be monitoring her weight quite closely, due to fear of weight gain. She may see her weight vary by two to seven pounds overnight after an episode of bingeing and purging. She might take a large dose of laxatives and, due to all the fluid loss, see her weight drop several pounds. When she begins drinking fluids and rehydrating, her weight rapidly increases. This leads her to believe she has gained actual body fat. So, in her mind, she feels the need to purge once again. This results in a vicious cycle of repeated episodes of dehydration, electrolyte depletion, and rehydration. The consequences of this behavior are kidney problems, edema, heart failure, and death.

In addition to the loss of fluids and electrolytes, purging causes other physical damage. Stomach acid can erode the teeth. Purging can tear the esophagus and cause bleeding. During a binge, the stomach can actually rupture because of the large volumes of food and fluids. The bowel can lose its ability to function due to damage caused by laxatives. The parotid glands, salivary glands situated below and in front of the ears, can become swollen and painful due to constant stimulation.

These physical consequences represent only the tip of the iceberg regarding the many possible conditions that can result from eating disorders. The irony is that too many times a person's goal to look more attractive ends in that person's premature aging. Patients in their forties who have a history of eating disorders from the time they were teenagers often appear much older than their counterparts who eat normally. Sadly, those with eating disorders also have much more serious health problems.

Emotional Complications

A high percentage of people who seek treatment for an eating disorder report a history of depression. Often, the eating disorder starts because of the hope that achieving a certain weight will make these patients feel better. Unfortunately, as the brain becomes deprived of the essential nutrients it needs, the depression escalates. Escalating depression may increase the symptoms of the eating disorders; hence, another vicious cycle develops.

> A high percentage of people who seek treatment for an eating disorder report a history of depression.

Anxiety is also common. Patients may experience a continual sense of discomfort that they can't quite identify. Irritability, withdrawal, and odd behaviors are common, such as compulsive rituals, strange eating habits, and division of foods into "good/safe" and "bad/dangerous" categories. People with eating disorders may fear change and new situations. They may even fear growing up and accepting adult responsibilities. They may have difficulty expressing their feelings. Many feel unworthy, inadequate, "not good enough." This leads to feelings of "craziness" or a sense that things are "out-of-control." Because the illness is often secretive, many feel too embarrassed to ask for help. This results in more isolation, fear, and hopelessness.

Relational Complications

It is easier to practice an eating disorder when no one knows about it. Once family, friends, or spouses know of the eating disorder, the patient finds it more difficult to practice the behaviors. Because of this, many patients with eating disorders feel the need to lie, deceive, manipulate people, and even break the law in order to foster their eating disorders. Repeated instances of being caught in a lie, hiding food, throwing food away, or exercising secretively in the middle of the night break down the trust that is so necessary for healthy relationships. To the person with an eating disorder, the relationship with food is often more valued than the relationship with family. Even eating in a restaurant can be a stress-filled occasion. When a patient cannot figure an exact calorie count from the menu, or finds that all her choices are in the "bad/dangerous" category, or fears she cannot purge without being discovered, she may choose to avoid socializing with friends in the future—further isolating herself from others.

Once the eating disorder is out in the open, family members often become apprehensive of addressing the disorder for fear it will "upset" the patient and "then she'll eat even less." Wives with eating disorders frequently avoid sexual relations with their spouses because of body image issues. Because they "feel fat," teens will sit at the beach in blue jeans and a sweatshirt, unable to freely play in the water with their peers. All of this further strains significant relationships in a person's life, deepening the feeling of alienation.

Shoplifting and other risk-taking behaviors are not uncommon. Teens cannot purchase diet pills in some stores, so they may decide to steal them. Sometimes those with eating disorders don't have enough money to buy food for a binge, so they borrow from others, steal money from home, or shoplift. Since buying large amounts of laxatives raises suspicion, bulimics become crafty, making small purchases at several stores. Some patients with eating disorders have been barred from entering certain grocery stores, because they have been caught bingeing and purging in those stores. These behaviors demonstrate how easily a patient's integrity can crumble and how difficult it is to regain the trust of those important to them.

■ Spiritual Complications

Eating disorders and addictive illnesses affect the most important relationship of all—one's relationship with God. Guilt, shame, and behavior choices all combine to hinder a person's walk with God. Christians may find it hard to approach God when they are struggling with behaviors that they either can't seem to stop or don't want to stop. The time, energy, and money directed toward appearance and body image can sidetrack someone's focus from the true God to a "false god." Food becomes a substitute for the true spiritual nourishment that only God can give.

In Philippians 3:19, Paul warns of those whose *"destiny is destruction, their god is their stomach, and their glory is in their shame."* Many Christians staunchly affirm that they would never use alcohol or drugs.

Yet, their continual overindulgence in food leads to much more serious health problems than those of people who eat moderately and drink alcohol sparingly.

Many people with eating disorders have asked God to heal them. As with any illness, they find it hard to understand why it won't just go away. Some Christians with eating disorders believe that God will simply deliver them, and that they will never again struggle with weight gain or the urge to binge and purge. It is true that some have been delivered in this way. Many more, however, must walk the path of recovery upon which they will struggle and continue to wrestle with their problems. Through this walk, their relationship with God can grow stronger, as they see how God meets them at their point of weakness.

Working at Recovery

If you have an eating disorder and have decided it's time to do something about it, what should you do? The first step is to see a health care professional and explain your concerns. It is important to remember that your lab tests and medical evaluation may be normal—unless you first inform your medical provider about your eating behaviors. A physician is often only as good as the information you give, so be honest and tell the whole story. Don't minimize your situation.

After you have had your physical health assessed, you probably want to talk to a mental health professional, or another person in whom you can confide about the emotional issues underlying your eating disorder. Getting at the emotional issues is just as important as treating the physical consequences of these illnesses. To avoid this step is like putting a Band-Aid on a major wound. Remember that the emotional issues are what fuel the eating disorder. Treatment depends on the type of eating disorder, the severity, the duration, and other complex psychiatric issues. If an outpatient program doesn't work, you may need a more structured inpatient treatment to help break the cycle. A registered dietician is often a part of the treatment program. This professional will help develop a meal plan and hold you accountable to the program.

Perhaps you suspect a friend or family member is suffering from an eating disorder. A good first step is to sit down with this person and share your concerns. Start with your observations and let this person know that you care and want to help. This is a critically important step for many, as being able to confide in someone and disclose the "ugly secret" is exactly what sets a sufferer on the road to recovery. Others will respond with great resistance and denial. There is a good chance that the stronger and more emotionally charged the denial, the

Exhibit 9.4. Confronting a Person with Anorexia or Bulimia

When confronting someone with an eating disorder, it is important to have a plan. A confrontation can be difficult due to the person's denial regarding the eating disorder. However, even if the individual does deny the problem, you can plant a seed. At some point in the future, the person will recognize and admit the problem. The following scheme is helpful to use when considering a confrontation.

The Plan: "**CONFRONT**"

Concern: The reason you are confronting. You care about the mental, physical, spiritual, and nutritional needs of the person.

Organize: Decide WHO is involved, WHERE to confront, WHY the concern, HOW to talk, WHEN is a convenient time.

Needs: What will you need to facilitate the confrontation? Professional help and/or support groups are available.

Face: The actual confrontation. Be empathetic, but direct. Do not back down if the person initially denies the problem.

Respond: By listening carefully.

Offer: Help and suggestions. You may want to encourage the individual to contact you when he or she needs to talk to someone.

Negotiate: Another time to talk and a time span within which to seek professional help.

Time: Remember to stress that recovery takes time and patience. However, the person has a lot to gain through the recovery process and a lot to lose if the individual makes the choice to continue the existing behaviors.

Source: The National Association of Anorexia Nervosa and Associated Disorders Web site. Retrieved 2-08-03 from http://www.anad.org/confront.htm.

greater the problem. Even if you meet with resistance, continue to be tuned in and available to that person. Watch and listen. If this person is your child, you are in a position to be more assertive about getting the child to treatment.

In some cases, intervention is best. An intervention can be formal or the result of a crisis. A crisis intervention results from an emergency situation—for example, the person with the eating disorder is admitted to the emergency room—and provides immediate assistance by focusing attention on the underlying cause of the emergency and then developing treatment for the problem. In a formal intervention, a group of people comes together to confront an individual about a specific issue, such as an eating disorder. This intervention is the result of careful planning and may be guided by a counselor or other professional trained in helping the patient come to grips with the eating disorder. Many times, when the patient is confronted by those who love and care about him/her, the patient acknowledges the problem and becomes more willing to seek help.

Recovery from an eating disorder is possible. It is difficult, of course, because food must always remain a part of our lives. However, recovery allows the person with an eating disorder to reach a point of accepting food as just food, and not as something that exerts power and control over that person's well-being. Most often, recovery is a process, not a miraculous moment of deliverance. A process takes time and requires stages of development. Eating disorder treatment facilities often quote a favorite maxim: "It's not about the food." This refers to the fact that eating disorders are about so much more than food and weight. As patients begins to address the emotional issues fueling the eating disorder, they find that food and weight concerns diminish as they move into a healthy relationship with food. Patients find that they are much less preoccupied with how their bodies look or whether to eat or not. Instead, they begin to experience a more balanced and serene life. This is what recovery is about: peace with self, peace with those around us, and peace with God.

KEY CONCEPTS

anorexia nervosa
binge
bulimia nervosa
electrolytes
lanugo

Learning Activity

1. Where do you draw the line between the pursuit of healthy living and eating-disordered behavior, evidenced by such factors as weight control and exercise?

   _____

   _____

   _____

   _____

   _____

   _____

2. What can be done to move toward acceptance of one's body, instead of trying to alter it to fit into a societal mold of what is fashionable?

   _____

   _____

   _____

   _____

   _____

   _____

3. What does Scripture tell us about our bodies? How can this affect our body image and help us to appreciate the gift God has given us?

   _____

   _____

   _____

   _____

   _____

   _____

Learning Exercises

1. Take a sheet of butcher paper long enough to accommodate your height. Without lying on the paper, draw yourself as you think you would look if someone were to trace your outline. Next, lie down on the paper and ask someone to trace your outline, using a different color marker or pen. How much does the actual tracing differ from your perception of yourself? (Most people with eating disorders and body image disturbances have markedly different tracings.)

   _____

   _____

   _____

   _____

2. Look through some current magazines, specifically ones that target teenage girls, feature celebrities, or focus on fitness and sports. How many articles in these issues are based on diet or exercises to sculpt one's body? Cut out or highlight pictures of people who appear to be unusually thin. Does what these magazines portray as "normal" match what most people consider to be normal?

   _____

   _____

   _____

   _____

References

American Psychiatric Association. *Diagnostic and Statistical Manual of Mental Disorders*. 4th ed. Washington, D.C.: American Psychiatric Publishing, Inc., 2000.

American Psychiatric Association. *American Psychiatric Association Practice Guideline for Eating Disorders*. 2nd ed. Washington, D.C.: American Psychiatric Publishing Group, 2000.

Bruch, Hilde. *The Golden Cage: The Enigma of Anorexia Nervosa*. New York: Vintage Books, 1979.

Brumberg, Joan Jacobs. *Fasting Girls: The Emergence of Anorexia Nervosa As a Modern Disease*. Cambridge, MA: Harvard University Press, 1988.

O'Neill, Cherry Boone. *Starving for Attention*. New York: Dell, 1982.

Yager, Joel, ed. *Eating Disorders: Psychiatric Clinics of North America*. Vol. 19, no. 4. American Psychiatric Press, 1996.

Zerbe, Kathryn J. *The Body Betrayed: A Deeper Understanding of Women, Eating Disorders, and Treatment*. Washington, D.C.: American Psychiatric Press, 1993.

For Additional Information

The International Association of Eating Disorders Professionals Foundation (**IAEDP**) is a professional organization for therapists, dieticians, psychologists, and physicians who treat people with eating disorders. IAEDP may be contacted at: P.O. Box 1295, Pekin, IL 61555-1295.

Remuda Ranch is a Christ-centered, biblically based treatment center for women and adolescent girls suffering from anorexia, bulimia, and related disorders. For information, write Remuda Ranch, 1 Apache East, Wickenburg, AZ 85390 or call 1-800-445-1900.

Endnotes

1. Earnie Larsen and Carol L. Hegarty, *Days of Healing, Days of Joy: Daily Meditations for Adult Children* (Hazelden Information Education, 1992), quoting Samuel Butler.
2. American Psychiatric Association, *Diagnostic and Statistical Manual of Mental Disorders*, 4th ed. (Washington, D.C.: American Psychiatric Publishing, Inc., 2000).

10

WELLNESS AND ADDICTION

"Learn what you are and be such."

—Pindar

With the help of this text, you have been learning about different aspects of everyday living that can lead to a more or less healthy body and a different state of wellness. Regardless of your age, this awareness hopefully will increase your interest in changing some current behaviors. As you begin or continue to grow in wholeness, you will discover many positive end results. In addition to less psychological and physical pain, you may come to realize better management of health problems. Better yet, you may notice that

leading a healthier lifestyle will lower your incidence of various illnesses and protect you from diseases and illnesses. Although it may appear difficult to change certain lifestyle behaviors, it need not be a struggle. As you think about yourself, where you are now, and where you want to be, remember that your life is precious. Keep in mind that you can take care of yourself and make your own decisions.

The Slide from Reliance to Habit

Every day we are confronted with substances and practices, healthy or not, that can lead to abuse and adversely impact our level of wellness. For instance, eating healthy food in moderation and exercising properly will enhance wellness. We don't think of either as a source of abuse and addiction. However, when a person repeatedly seeks relief from emotional distress through repetitive hyper-exercise or excessive overeating, this individual demonstrates abuse and even addiction. Other examples are more easily recognized. Alcohol, prescriptive, recreational and designer drugs, and even over-the-counter drugs—all have the potential to produce mood changes that can lead to reliance. Over time, this reliance becomes a habit that begins the process of abuse and leads to ultimate addiction. Often, people stumble into this behavior, certainly not with the intent of letting it control them. Unfortunately, substances used, then abused, do have the capability of controlling us.

DRUG: A chemical intended to affect the structure or function of the body.

Substance Abuse and Addictive Behaviors

In this chapter, our discussion of substances with the potential for abuse includes alcohol, tobacco, caffeine, and drugs. We defines **drug** as a chemical intended to affect the structure or function of the body. The categories of drugs we cover include

- prescription medicines,
- over-the-counter medicines, such as aspirin,
- legal substances, such as caffeine, tobacco, and alcohol, and
- illegal substances, such as marijuana, cocaine, and heroin.

We will focus particularly on **psychoactive drugs,** those that alter one's thoughts, feelings, sensations, and/or nervous system. We also will look briefly at addictive behaviors referred to as "process addictions," such as exercise or gambling, both of which have the potential for causing dependence. We turn first to alcohol. Because the usage of alcohol is so prevalent in our

> # PSYCHOACTIVE DRUG:
> A drug that alters one's thoughts, feelings, sensations, and/or nervous system.

society (approximately 70 percent of all Americans consume alcohol regularly), and because it accounts for numerous problems in our society, we will look carefully at this heavily abused substance.

Alcohol: The Socially Acceptable Drug

Not only is alcohol the most prevalent drug on college campuses, it is the most commonly used and abused drug in the country and possibly the world. Alcohol abuse is a major national health problem, with the same ranking as heart disease and cancer. Its widespread, excessive use in America and elsewhere has many causes. In the United States, alcohol is readily accessible to those who are of legal age. Massive marketing and promotion increase alcohol's visibility and make it available in a wide array of stores. Alcohol is used for many purposes, including religious rituals, celebrations, social gatherings, and as a mealtime drink.

Even though alcohol is socially accepted by most people, it is now regarded as a drug—something we tend to forget due to its great visibility and availability. We also forget that even when consumed in small amounts or occasionally, alcohol has a high potential to abuse and harm the body. Alcohol abuse is defined as usage to a degree that causes physical damage, impairs functioning, or results in harm to others. The abuse of alcohol usually follows one of four patterns:

1. Regular intake of large amounts on a daily basis
2. Regular heavy drinking restricted to weekends
3. Binges of daily or heavy drinking lasting for weeks or months, with long periods of sobriety between drinking episodes
4. Heavy drinking limited to times of stress

Approximately six million Americans have such severe physical and psychological health problems from the consumption of alcohol that they can be classified as alcoholics. Alcohol, therefore, is clearly a drug that has the potential for abuse and subsequent health hazards, even when its consumption is limited. Knowing about alcohol and other drugs will not necessarily keep them from having negative consequences on your health and your life. However, with a greater understanding of

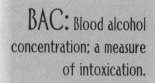

BAC: Blood alcohol concentration; a measure of intoxication.

their effects and impact, you will have the knowledge to make more informed choices when confronted with substance and chemical opportunities.

■ The Effects of Alcohol

The short-term effects of alcohol depend upon the concentration level, the amount consumed, and the time in which it has been consumed. The "proof" of alcohol is the concentration of ethyl alcohol in the liquor or drink. For example, if a drink contains 80 proof alcohol, it is 40 percent alcohol. The body can metabolize approximately half a can of beer or half of an alcoholic beverage in about an hour. The blood alcohol concentration (**BAC**) will remain low if a person drinks slightly less than this amount each hour. However, if more

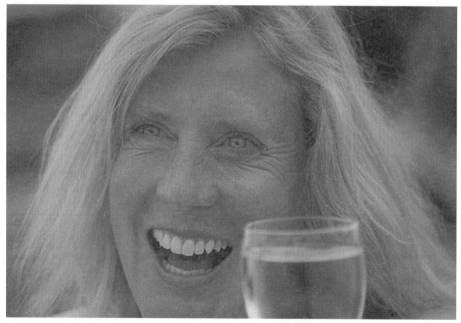

Approximately 70 percent of all Americans consume alcohol regularly.

alcohol is consumed than metabolized, the BAC will rise accordingly, and so will that person's level of intoxication.

The BAC measures levels of intoxication to determine when a person is legally drunk. States differ on that amount, but the average range is between 0.08 - 0.10. One method to estimate BAC is to assume that consumption of one standard drink per hour (one beer, one glass of wine, one mixed drink), which contains approximately one-half ounce of ethyl alcohol, gives a BAC of .02 in a male who weighs 150 lbs. If this same male drank five beers in one hour, his BAC would be .10, the level most states have designated as legally drunk. Many factors affect BAC, including gender, body size, body composition, and amount of food and liquid consumed prior to ingesting alcohol. Table 10.1 demonstrates the BAC of an average person of average weight, the behavioral effects of alcohol at specific amounts, and the approximate time for removal from body systems.

Table 10.1. The Effects of Alcohol

Number of drinks	Ounces of alcohol	BAC (g/100 ml)	Approximate time for removal	Effects
1 beer, glass of wine, or mixed drink	½	0.02	1 hour	Feeling relaxed and euphoric
2½ beers, glasses of wine, or mixed drinks	1¼	0.05	2½ hours	Decreased inhibitions; increased confidence; impaired judgment
5 beers, glasses of wine, or mixed drinks	2½	0.10	5 hours	Impaired memory and motor coordination; slurred speech; exaggerated emotions
10 beers, glasses of wine, or mixed drinks	5	0.20	10 hours	Slowed reflexes; unsteadiness in standing and walking; loss of peripheral vision
15 beers, glasses of wine, or mixed drinks	7½	0.30	15-16 hours	Stuporous; complete loss of coordination; impairment of pain and other senses
20 beers, glasses of wine, or mixed drinks	10	0.40	20 hours	May become unconscious or comatose; breathing may cease
25-30 beers, glasses of wine, or mixed drinks	15-20	0.50	26 hours	Fatal for most people

When consumed, alcohol affects virtually every system in the body, both in the short term and long term. Low doses of alcohol induce relaxation and release inhibitions. Higher doses lead to interference with motor coordination, intellectual functions, and judgment. Some other physiological effects include flushing of the skin, increased perspiration, decreased sexual performance, disturbed sleep, and what is termed a "hangover" the following day (headache, gastrointestinal upset, and muscular discomfort).

Drinking alcohol alters mood and has complex physiological effects that over time can shorten the life of alcohol abusers by ten to twelve years. Though moderate amounts of alcohol (one to two drinks a day) may protect against heart disease in some, high doses have been found to contribute to cardiovascular problems,

FETAL ALCOHOL SYNDROME:
A group of birth defects associated with the infants of women who drink during pregnancy.

such as high blood pressure. Chronic alcohol use is associated with cirrhosis of the liver, in which liver cells are destroyed and replaced by scar tissue. Other medical conditions associated with chronic alcohol abuse include diabetes, certain cancers, gout, asthma, frequent infections, nervous system diseases, and psychiatric problems.

Of particular concern is alcohol's effect on pregnant women. **Fetal alcohol syndrome** is a group of birth defects associated with the infants of women who drink during pregnancy, especially during the first three months of pregnancy. Symptoms of infants born with this syndrome include small birth size, heart defects, mental abnormalities, and atypical facial features such as small, wide-set eyes. No amount of alcohol is safe for any woman who is pregnant or in a relationship that might result in pregnancy.

Excluding pregnant women, how much alcohol is "safe"? How often can it be consumed without being dangerous? These are frequently asked questions. When considering what is safe for one person versus another, everything from personal health status to one's compulsion for drinking comes into consideration. There really are no "correct" answers to these questions. In view of the fact that you do not need to be physiologically dependent on alcohol to have a drinking problem, you need to take into account the potential for harm to yourself and others (especially when drinking and driving) when making a decision about alcohol.

■ Tobacco: It's Not Just About You

Tobacco is another legal substance (for those of age) that has a tremendous impact on health. Like alcohol, tobacco is highly addictive. The addictive component in tobacco is the psychoactive drug nicotine. Persons who are addicted to tobacco crave this drug, which causes withdrawal symptoms (headache, nausea, irritability, insomnia, and other discomforts) when it is not circulating in the blood and brain. Nicotine addiction has been described as something as powerful as an addiction to heroine, cocaine, or alcohol.

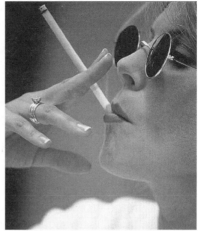

Nicotine produces a strong psychological and physiological effect that can lead to dependence.

Why and how do people become smokers or users of other forms of tobacco? Usually the habit begins in the early years when young people are attempting to model others or gain acceptance in peer groups. Soon the discovery of certain perceived benefits occurs. Some people say that smoking relaxes them. Others say it gives them a psychological lift or stimulation for intellectual tasks. Whatever the reason, this drug produces a strong psychological and physiological effect that can lead to dependence.

■ The Effects of Tobacco

The effects of nicotine and other active chemicals depend on the amount inhaled, chewed, or otherwise consumed. After the tobacco is placed in the mouth, nicotine and the other chemicals in tobacco are absorbed through the mucous membranes and then into the bloodstream. Nicotine stimulates the brain to release chemicals that alter mood. It can either excite or tranquilize the nervous system, but ultimately the pleasurable feeling turns to depression.

CARCINOGEN:
A substance or agent that produces or causes cancer.

COCARCINOGEN:
An agent that aggravates the carcinogenic effects of another substance.

Other immediate effects on the body include blood vessel constriction, increased heart rate and blood pressure, decreased urine production, increased mucous production, irritation of bronchial tubes and lungs, dulling of taste buds, and increased blood sugar. It is clearly evident that tobacco negatively affects nearly the entire body and involves several long-term complications. Most common complications include high blood pressure, emphysema, bronchitis, heart disease, and cancer of the lungs, lips, and mouth. Ultimately, life expectancy is reduced. Research continues to show that the death rate for smokers is much higher than that for nonsmokers, regardless of the cause of death. Diseases from smoking can be attributed to the many damaging chemicals in tobacco that are **carcinogens** or **cocarcinogens.** A carcinogen is a substance or agent that produces or causes

Table 10.2, Selective Hazardous Substances in Tobacco Smoke

Substance	Hazard
Arsenic	Poisonous, carcinogenic
Carbon monoxide	Reduces the oxygen-carrying capacity of blood
Hydrogen cyanide	Reduces cilia function of the lungs
Nicotine	Poisonous, addictive
Nitrogen dioxide	Irritates respiratory tract
Nitrous oxide	Reduces the number of white blood cells
Phenol, Benzoapyrene, Formaldehyde, Vinyl chloride	Cocarcinogenic

cancer. A cocarcinogen is an agent that aggravates the carcinogenic effects of another substance. Table 10.2 lists some selective hazardous substances in tobacco smoke.

Women who use tobacco during pregnancy—like women who drink during pregnancy—are more likely to have babies that suffer from low birth weight and a variety of other infant health disorders. While considering these health hazards, there is also concern for others who inhale sidestream smoke (the smoke emitted from the lighted end of cigarettes, cigars, and pipes) and secondhand smoke (smoke exhaled by smokers). Both kinds of smoke are also referred to as environmental tobacco smoke (ETS) and are known to contribute to the ill health of others. Studies show that many people subjected to ETS develop symptoms such as headaches, nasal and eye irritation, coughs, and sinus and bronchial problems. Some of the worst effects occur in children

> Women who use tobacco during pregnancy—like women who drink during pregnancy—are more likely to have babies that suffer from low birth weight and a variety of other infant health disorders.

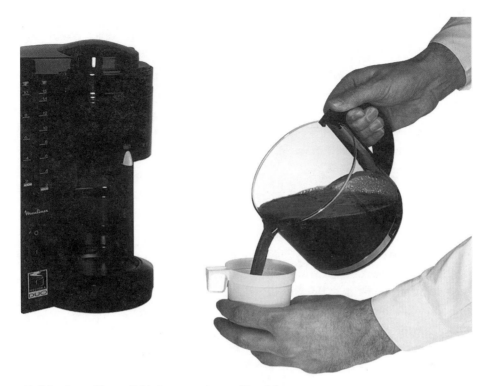

Caffeine is readily available in our society and legal for any age.

who live in the homes of smokers. It is not coincidental that these children have an increased frequency of upper and lower respiratory infections, as well as other health problems.

Realizing the many problems that tobacco can have on your health and the health of others should deter you from smoking. The strong addictive power of this drug should also make you think twice about smoking. As the cost of tobacco continues to rise and the bans on public smoking increase, now is an excellent time to make the commitment to stop or never start!

■ Caffeine: Some Unhealthy "Perks"

Caffeine is a powerful, tasteless stimulant found in coffee, tea, chocolate, certain soft drinks, and many over-the-counter medications. It is readily available in our society and legal for any age. Like alcohol and tobacco, caffeine is a drug, although we tend to place it in the categories of products that produce "energy" or "wakefulness." Caffeine is a main component in weight loss medications and menstrual pain products because it also has a powerful diuretic effect, causing urine output with water loss. Some other effects are noted below, according to dosage:

- 100 milligrams (1 cup of coffee): an increase in heart rate, blood pressure, and respiration. Most people realize a more rapid and clear flow of thought and an increased capacity for sustained performance.
- 300 milligrams (3 cups of coffee): nervousness, restlessness, tremors, and insomnia.
- 10 grams (60 cups of coffee): can produce convulsions and lead to death.

Since caffeine is a drug that has the potential for psychological dependence, chronic and excessive use may lead to long-term problems. The most common health problem associated with excess caffeine is stomach irritation, which can lead to gastrointestinal illnesses. Because it increases heart rate and blood pressure, caffeine can cause heart palpitations, which for some could be serious. Finally, with excessive consumption of coffee, some women have noted an increase of symptoms associated with premenstrual syndrome and a higher incidence of fibrocystic breast disease. For most adults who are healthy and not adversely affected by caffeine, moderate use is generally harmless. However, excessive use or overconsumption can certainly be hazardous and even toxic.

■ Other Drugs

Fewer college students and Americans in general take drugs than drink alcohol. Still, the risks of drug use are significant. The discussion in this section will focus on the various effects of drugs such as marijuana, cocaine, heroine, LSD, ecstasy, amphetamines, barbiturates, steroids, and inhalants.

■ Marijuana

Marijuana, a product of the hemp plant, is the most often used illegal drug in this country. Unlike alcohol or even cocaine, this drug contains more than 400 components. Thus, the strength of one mixture may be entirely different from another, increasing the potential danger when the content is unknown. Users mix the dried flowers and leaves (green/gray) and roll them into a cigarette or smoke them in a water pipe. Marijuana is also brewed as a tea or mixed in food.

The short-term effects of marijuana include distorted perception (sights, sounds, time, touch); trouble with thinking, learning, problem solving, and memory; increased heart rate, blood pressure, and appetite; dilated pupils, anxiety, and loss of motor coordination. Possible long-term effects include reduced sperm motility, irregularity of ovulation, and overall physical damage from impure doses. Because most users smoke marijuana, the greatest health threat to long-term users is the risk of respiratory tract and lung damage. Cancer of the tongue, jaw, mouth, and lung, in addition to impairment of the immune system, are also threats. Because users often become psychologically dependent on marijuana, it can become addictive and interfere with all aspects of one's life.

■ Cocaine

Cocaine, a product of the coca shrub found in Central and South America, is the second most commonly used illegal drug in the United States. Typically, the leaves are processed into a powder that is smoked, sniffed, or injected. Cocaine increases heart rate and blood pressure, giving the user a quick sense of euphoria that lasts from thirty to sixty minutes. Other short-term effects include increased energy, restlessness, suppressed appetite, and a sense of power. The euphoria subsides quickly and the user experiences a letdown that leads to craving another dose. Tolerance to cocaine usually develops quickly, and users find themselves wanting more pure forms to get the same "high." Overdose is not uncommon and may induce seizures or lead to respiratory and heart failure.

Users of cocaine can quickly develop not only a psychological dependence, but also a physiological dependence. Long-term effects include chronic

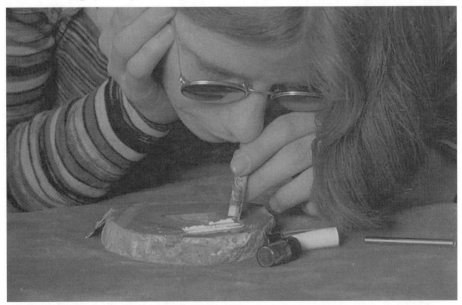

For those who snort cocaine, nasal bleeding and perforation are possible outcomes of chronic use.

confusion, toxic psychosis, and behavior that is paranoid or violent. For those who snort cocaine, nasal bleeding and perforation are possible outcomes of chronic use. When cocaine is injected, the user is at an increased risk of developing hepatitis B, HIV, and other infections from shared needles. In addition to the dangers associated with this drug, it is particularly addictive and an extremely difficult habit for the user to stop. Increasing the public's awareness of cocaine's dangers is necessary to prevent people from falling into its grip.

■ Heroin

Heroin is a highly addictive narcotic that depresses the central nervous system and causes many health problems, primarily due to uncertain dosage levels. It can be smoked, snorted, or injected. The immediate effects include euphoria, drowsiness, and the reduction of pain. The potential for physical and psychological dependence is high, and complications from usage include dizziness, nausea, and respiratory depression. Like other injected drugs, such as cocaine, there is a high risk for contracting diseases from shared needles. Withdrawal from heroin can take up to or over a week, with symptoms that range from insomnia and muscle cramps to elevated blood pressure, respiration, and temperature.

■ LSD

LSD, one of the most commonly known psychedelic drugs, has regained popularity in recent years. Also known as acid, LSD is less expensive than most other illegal and abused drugs. It is packaged in various forms such as tablets, pellets, gelatin chips, and thin paper squares. The blotter paper form (which is special paper that has been soaked in LSD) often features designs or characters, making it attractive to younger people. The effects are dose related, and usually include an increase in various body rates (heart, blood pressure, temperature), loss of appetite, sleeplessness, dry mouth, and tremors. Euphoria is often mixed with hallucinations, disorientation, paranoia, and even psychosis. Users may experience several thoughts simultaneously, exaggerated body distortion, flashbacks, panic, and fear of death. Many LSD users become depressed for one or two days following the use of LSD—referred to as a "trip"—and may resort to use again for relief of depression. Although there is no evidence that LSD leads to physical dependence, it is known to cause psychological dependence.

■ Ecstasy

Ecstasy is a synthetic drug that comes in a tablet/pill often branded with an insignia such as CK, Nike swoosh, or Playboy bunnies. It is often consumed at "rave" parties for mood enhancement and to prolong energy for dancing. Short-term effects include psychological difficulties, such as confusion, depression, sleep problems, severe anxiety, and paranoia. Other physical symptoms that can occur immediately or even weeks after consumption include muscle tension, involuntary teeth clenching, blurred vision, rapid eye movement, faintness, chills or sweating, and nausea. Recent research on Ecstasy has linked long-term damage to parts of the brain that are critical to thinking and memory.

■ Amphetamines

Amphetamines are drugs that stimulate the central nervous system. Although they come in tablet form, users may crush the drug and inhale or inject the substance. The short-term effects include increased talkativeness, aggressiveness, respiration, heart rate, and

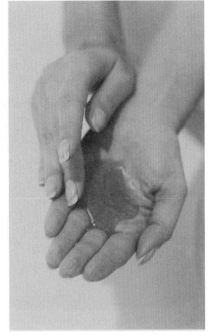

Many illegal substances can cause physical and psychological dependence.

blood pressure. Other short-term effects are decreased appetite, dilated pupils, visual and auditory hallucinations, compulsiveness, repetitive action, and nervousness. The effects of large doses can include fever and sweating, dry mouth, headache, paleness, blurred vision, dizziness, irregular heartbeat, tremors, loss of coordination, and collapse. The possible long-term effects include tolerance, dependence, violence, aggression, and malnutrition due to appetite suppression. The potential exists for physical and psychological dependence, and even death from overdosage.

■ Barbiturates

Barbiturates are prescription sedatives that depress the central nervous system. Of the several multicolored tablets and capsule medications manufactured, the most abused are Nembutal, Seconal, Amytal and Phenobarbital. These sedatives are used most often to treat the unpleasant effects of illicit stimulants, to reduce anxiety, and to obtain an euphoric high. Like amphetamines, they may be swallowed or crushed, and then inhaled or injected. Barbiturates mimic the effects of alcohol, causing mild euphoria, loss of inhibition, relief of anxiety, and sleepiness. Other short-term effects include

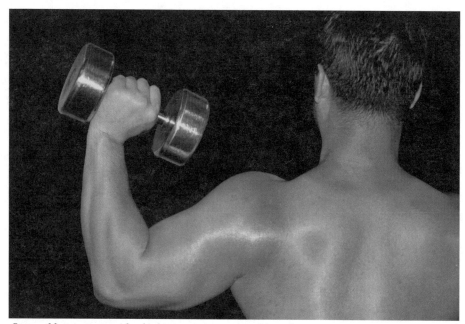

Some athletes use steroids, thinking to gain a competitive advantage.

slurred speech, shallow breathing, sluggishness, fatigue, disorientation, lack of coordination, and dilated pupils. In higher doses, barbiturates cause impairment of memory, judgment, and coordination. They also lead to irritability, paranoia, and suicidal thoughts. Tolerance to these drugs develops quickly, and as larger doses are used, the danger of an overdose increases. With an overdose or in conjunction with other drugs like alcohol, death is due to depression of the respiratory center in the brain.

■ Anabolic Steroids

Anabolic steroids are a group of powerful compounds closely related to the male sex hormone testosterone. These drugs are used legitimately for medical purposes, such as to treat certain anemias, severe burns, and some forms of breast cancer. Illegally, they are used by various athletes who want a competitive advantage and/or to improve their physical appearance. Most steroids used illegally come from the black market, so quality and purity are virtually unknown. Steroids come in tablets or liquid form, and are taken orally or injected. Athletes and other abusers typically take them in cycles of weeks or months, rather than continuously.

More than seventy side effects are possible from the abuse of steroids. These range in severity from acne and aggressive behavior to liver damage and cancer. Reports indicate that the use of anabolic steroids produces increases in lean muscle mass, strength, and ability to train longer and harder. Many health hazards associated with short-term effects are reversible. The major effects of anabolic steroid use include liver tumors, jaundice, fluid retention, and high blood pressure. Additional side effects for men include shrinking of the testicles, reduced sperm count, infertility, baldness, and development of breasts. For women, additional side effects include growth of facial hair, changes in or cessation of the menstrual cycle, and deepened voice.

In addition to these physical side effects, steroid users often begin a vicious cycle of dependence. Due to the cyclical method of usage, users frequently experience "shrinking," during which previous enhancements diminish. At this time, panic may set in and the user may begin taking the drugs in even larger amounts. When steroid use is stopped, the user often goes into a deep depression due to a perceived loss of euphoria, power, and invincibility. Some long-term effects may not be evident for several years. If steroids are taken during adolescence, growth may be retarded through premature skeletal development. Of worse consequence is the increased risk for strokes and heart attacks due to vascular damage from steroid abuse.

■ Inhalants

Hundreds of ordinary household products on the market today are inhaled or sniffed by children and adults in order to produce various kinds of intoxicating effects. The inhalants most commonly used for recreational purposes fall into these categories:

- commercial chemicals, such as model airplane glue, nail polish remover, correction fluid, paint thinner, and gasoline
- aerosols, such as hair spray, cooking spray, spray paint, and fabric protector
- anesthetics, such as amyl nitrate, nitrous oxide ("laughing gas"), diethyl ether, and chloroform

These products are sniffed, snorted, bagged (fumes inhaled from a plastic bag), or "huffed" (inhalant-soaked rag, sock, or roll of toilet paper in the mouth) to achieve a high. Inhalants are also sniffed directly from the container. When inhaled through the nose or mouth into the lungs in sufficient concentrations, inhalants cause intoxicating effects. Intoxication can last only a few minutes or several hours if inhaled repeatedly.

> # PROCESS ADDICTION:
> Any activity or interaction upon which a person becomes dependent.

Initially, users may feel slightly stimulated. With successive inhalations, they may feel less inhibited and less in control. Finally, a user can lose consciousness. Other effects include headache, muscle weakness, abdominal pain, severe mood swings, violent behavior, numbness and tingling of the hands and feet, nausea, hearing loss, limb spasms, fatigue, and lack of coordination. Sniffing highly concentrated amounts of the chemicals in solvents or aerosols can directly induce heart failure and death. Death also can result from suffocation. This happens when oxygen is displaced first in the lungs and then in the central nervous system so that breathing ceases. Inhalation from an attached bag or in a closed area greatly increases the chances of suffocation. Other irreversible effects may include permanent hearing loss and damage to the central nervous system or brain.

Process Addictions

To this point you have read about mood-altering substances and their addictive potential. Included in addictive behaviors are **process addictions.** We define these addictions as any series of activities or interactions upon which a person becomes dependent. Examples of process addictions include exercise, food, work, money, love, and sex.

■ The "Rush" of Exercise

Many Americans include exercise as part of a healthy lifestyle. The physical and psychological benefits are many, as you read in chapter 3 and other sections of this book. However, as individuals find themselves making such gains, they sometimes get too absorbed in exercise. Research has shown that aerobic exercise like running causes the brain to release endorphins. This causes a sense of euphoria which, when combined with the stress released from activity, increases the desire for even more exercise. In this sense, exercise can become a habit that has the potential to become an addictive behavioral pattern.

◾ Filling the Emptiness with Food

The chapter on nutrition explains that the main purpose of food is to fuel our bodies. However, we also eat for pleasure. Family togetherness, social gatherings, dating, and celebrations frequently revolve around eating food. Because it is a pleasurable event, eating food can become addictive. For example, think about certain foods associated with special times or remember the kinds of food you associate with being nurtured by an adult. These very foods may be ones you are drawn to in spite of your level of hunger. Even if full or satiated, some people are compelled to keep eating due to their preoccupation with food. Many compulsive eaters begin eating and simply cannot stop—much like others who are addicted to alcohol or drugs. Chapter 9 discusses several eating disorders in detail.

As with substance abuse, these people experience similar symptoms of withdrawal, like mood swings and depression in the absence of food. Other people addicted to food substitute it for something lacking in their lives, such as intimacy. Another reason for addiction to some foods, especially sugary foods, is that they stimulate the release of endorphins. This is the same chemical that when released by the brain elevates mood during aerobic exercise. Whatever the reason, we now know that a compulsion for eating can develop into an addiction.

◾ Driven to Work

You have probably heard the term workaholism coined in reference to those who are "driven" to work more than others. The same could be said about students who are driven to study excessively and to achieve academic excellence. For both types of individuals, the need is to get ahead and be at the top. Often, the need is also to avoid other interests, friends, and family. Part of the issue seems to be related to a lack of self-esteem. This form of addiction leaves little room for the pursuit of relaxation, social activities, or other recreational pastimes. In that regard, not only does the individual suffer from self-imposed isolation, but others also suffer from the workaholic's frequent absences.

◾ The Financial Trap

Addictions related to money can take several directions, including spending, borrowing, and/or gambling. A common theme in the lives of compulsive spenders, borrowers, and gamblers is the need for excitement, euphoria, and relief from

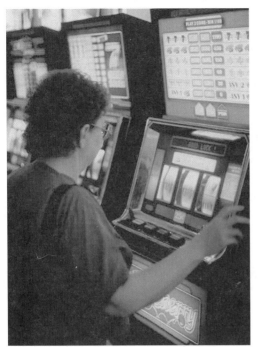

An addiction to gambling can lead to financial ruin for the addict and for the addict's family.

powerlessness and anxiety. Gratification is often instant, but when it dwindles, these persons return for more of the same. Some compulsive spenders, borrowers, and gamblers come from homes in which parents also were addicted to these behaviors or to other substances. Additional reasons include low self-esteem and a sense of helplessness. This process addiction can lead to rapid financial ruin, not only for the person addicted, but also for the addict's family.

■ Love and Sex Addictions

Love addiction results from a romantic obsession with one person or a series of relationships. Like so many of the aforementioned process addictions, an addiction to love seems to be related to a lack of self-esteem. Often those addicted to love rely upon partners to fulfill their emotional needs, with identification of self-worth derived through their partners. Love addicts frequently ignore their own needs and desires, as they are incapable of separating their own feelings from those of their partners. Frequently, the love addict will select someone whose affection is difficult to obtain, with subsequent pursuit costing great time and effort. This can lead to many conflicts in the life of a love addict, including an unhealthy relationship.

Sexual addiction is generally considered by experts to differ from love addiction. In recent years, sexual addiction has been studied from a biological perspective. Phenylethylamine, a chemical in the brain, is responsible for the euphoria and excitement that accompanies falling in love. Therefore, it is felt that sex addicts may be addicted to the physical and psychological arousal that results from a repeated release of this chemical. However, the sex addict does not view this compulsive behavior as pleasurable or expressive of love. Rather, the sex addict sees it as an act of control that may evolve into a cycle of abuse. Studies of sex addicts have found that many were abused or neglected as children, and that they suffer from a lack of self-esteem. This may be partly to blame for the wide range of possibly sexually addictive behaviors evident in today's society.

What Prompts Substance Abuse and Addictive Behaviors?

One factor common to most people who abuse substances or who suffer from process addictions is a lack of self-esteem. People who have not developed confidence or faith in themselves are more susceptible to substance abuse and addictive behaviors than those with a strong sense of self-esteem. However, many other factors can contribute to these tendencies. In this section we will examine psychosocial factors, such as family and peer relationships, life stresses, social and cultural customs, and the media. We also will look at biological factors and how they are related to substance abuse and addiction.

■ The Psychosocial Connection

Good family relationships help family members develop self-esteem, self-respect, respect for one another, and respect for those outside the family. In families that lack love, care, and support, family members may look outside the family for social attachments. They may make some of these social attachments with persons who use and/or encourage substance abuse. They also may make social attachments directly to objects of possible abuse, such as alcohol and/or drugs.

Perhaps one of the greatest invitations for substance abuse and addiction in early life is association with the wrong peer groups. Vulnerability is high in adolescence, and as this age group struggles to develop identity, the influence of other people of similar age can positively or negatively impact their decisions and actions. Young people sometimes make bad choices more quickly and frequently when they are with others who behave similarly. In addition, peer pressure to cope in an unhealthy way—such as drinking alcohol—often is more powerful when young people are attempting to cope with stress.

Just as young people experience life stresses, so do adults. These stresses may be infrequent major events, such as marriage, divorce, death, or job loss. They also can be ongoing events like chronic illness, a strained relationship, a stressful job, or difficult home situation. Whatever the stress, how the individual copes with it may be detrimental to health if it triggers substance abuse or addictive behavior.

> Perhaps one of the greatest invitations for substance abuse and addiction in early life is association with the wrong peer groups.

Social and cultural customs may encourage the use of substances like alcohol or tobacco during ceremonies, rituals, or parties. Where such use is acceptable, the incidence of abuse and even addiction is higher. For example, a person born into a family that provides and supports the use of alcohol (e.g., wine with meals) or tobacco will be influenced more toward the use and possible abuse of such substances. The same could be said for persons who decide to join a group, club, or organization that similarly promotes smoking and/or drinking. In situations in which others encourage the use of illegal substances, the most vulnerable people are those who have difficulty making decisions for themselves. They are unable to sort through their feelings about substance use and often choose to do as others do, regardless of the health hazards.

> When people learn who they are and become less vulnerable, they are less influenced by what others "out there" are telling them to do.

Another very strong psychosocial influence comes simply from what we see and hear as we go about our daily activities. More and more the public is flooded with messages from the media promoting certain products that can lead to substance abuse and addiction. Magazine ads, billboards, commercials, and electronic messages all send powerful images of the pleasure associated with such products. The television, film, and music industries often portray illegal substances in a glamorous light. Included in this promotional blitz are process addictions such as excessive exercising, overeating, shopping, and even gambling. Whether the suggestions are subtle or strong, the messages are nearly constant. We are saturated with mixed messages, such as smoking and sex appeal, or eating and exuberant happiness. This can lead to a "quick fix" before we are able to consciously evaluate our decision. When people learn who they are and become less vulnerable, they are less influenced by what others "out there" are telling them to do.

■ The Biological Connection

In addition to identifying psychosocial factors, research has proven that substance abuse and addiction have biological roots, grounded in biochemical, metabolic, or genetic disorders. In particular, addiction has been described as a disease of brain function. Research findings have concluded that addicts often have deficiencies in brain hormones and/or neurotransmitters that cause them to react differently than nonaddicts do to the same substance, encounter, or experience.

Scientists continue to investigate the genetic link of substance abuse and addictive behavior within families and even certain ethnic groups or cultures. Children of parents who abuse substances are at greater risk for similar abuse, or even abuse of different substances due to genetic predisposition. Certainly the influence is greater for these children when parents and others within their environment use and abuse substances openly.

We now realize the inaccuracy of society's message that includes the notion that substance abusers and addicts are weak-minded. In actuality and for over fifty years, addiction has been described and defined as a disease. For substance abusers and persons with addictive behaviors, the capacity to make choices has been taken away by genetic deficiencies, environmental influences, and/or the very real pain of stopping the drug or addiction.

The Impact of Substance Abuse and Addiction

■ A Rippling Effect

Substance abuse and addictive behaviors create serious problems, not only for the abuser/addict, but also for family members, friends, and others. These problems may include angry and frustrated family members, reprimands at work, reassignment or loss of jobs, strained or severed friendships and other personal relationships, loss of personal/family money from substance purchases or legal penalties, and even the death of the abuser/addict or someone else when the abuser/addict is under the influence of a substance. If the abuser/addict is convicted of driving under the influence of a substance, financial penalties are not the only negative outcome. Vehicle forfeiture almost always is indicated for a specific time period, making travel contingent upon public transportation systems or the charity of others. In addition, hefty increases are applied to the offender's insurance coverage, another strain on the family budget. The abuser/addict's actions have a rippling effect far beyond that individual's perception.

■ Emotional Turmoil

> **CODEPENDENCY:**
> A relationship in which a person is controlled or manipulated by an abuser/addict.

In addition to frustration and anger, the families of substance abusers/addicts also may feel shame and guilt. Family members often feel that they are to blame for the substance abuse and/or addictive behaviors. For example, the parents of an adolescent who abuses drugs may blame themselves, citing anything from excess work to other pressures that may have prevented closer supervision. In other situations, family members may blame one another for the problem and even push the person blamed into taking responsibility for the abuser/addict's behavior.

Some families of abusers/addicts suffer from codependency. **Codependency** is a relationship in which a person is controlled or manipulated by an abuser/addict.

ENABLING: Allowing another to persist in abusive/addictive behavior by making excuses or helping the abuser/addict to avoid responsibility.

Not only is the addictive behavior allowed to continue, but the codependent person may even deny that it exists. Denial or rationalization can lead to **enabling,** the process of allowing the abuser/addict to continue the destructive behavior by either excusing the abuser/addict's actions or protecting that person from the consequences of the destructive behavior. Examples of enabling include making excuses for the abuser/addict's absence from work, school, or other obligations. Intentional or not, this form of protection fosters the destructive behavior and keeps affected individuals from assuming responsibility for their actions.

When relationships are strained by any of the voluminous problems caused by substance abuse and addictive behaviors, difficulties may lead to the ruin of a marriage or committed relationship. When children are involved, the destruction of this unit can result in the destruction of an entire family. Often, the substance abuser or addict loses custody of children due to problems cited during court proceedings. This means that for the majority of affected families, parents no longer are involved together in the daily activities of raising their children. This can cause children to withdraw or exhibit other emotional difficulties during a time when they most need family support.

A Tragic Legacy

Regardless of relationship status or stability, children who experience parental role modeling inclusive of substance abuse and addictive behaviors are at greater risk for developing similar behaviors as they mature. The chances for this development are further increased when children come in frequent contact with others similarly affected, such as older siblings, extended family, and neighbors. Children tend to replicate what they see others doing within and around their homes. In addition, children in this type of home environment usually have more free time to watch television. The programs they watch also may influence use of harmful substances. Children are incapable of making decisions for themselves and therefore rely upon others to show or tell them how to act. With poor parental guidance and other negative influences, these children are certainly in a position to experience a more tragic life than other children the same age.

Solving the Problem of Substance Abuse and Addictive Behavior

Several strategies have been developed over the years to offer solutions for substance abuse and addictive behaviors. These strategies focus on intervention, treatment, relapse, and prevention, and are based on the study and experience of individuals who have gone through various programs. Just as there are many factors that can lead to substance abuse and addictive behaviors, there are also different methods for approaching a solution to these problems. Positive outcomes depend largely upon the person, the substance and behavior, and such factors as environment and personal motivation.

■ The First Step

Most individuals who suffer from substance abuse and addictive behaviors deny that they have a problem. They may be aware that their actions are unsafe and unhealthy, but frequently they will not acknowledge the potential for ruin or the impact their behavior has on their lives and the lives of others. When the abusers/addicts realize and accept that they have a problem, they have taken the first step toward effective treatment.

The realization may come from hearing how someone's life has been negatively affected by the abuser/addict's behavior. The abuser/addict may see him/herself in someone else who has been identified as having a problem. A "signal" may flare as the abuser/addict reads literature about the warning signs of substance abuse and addictive behavior. (See Exhibit 10.1 for the warning signs of substance abuse or addictive behaviors.) Or a health screening may confirm the existence of a problem. Regardless of how realization and acceptance come about, at this point intervention is necessary.

■ Intervention

Interventions can be informal, formal, or crisis interventions. Informal interventions may occur over months and even years. These involve family, friends, and colleagues who offer concern and support regarding the abuser/addict's problem.

A formal intervention is a planned, face-to-face confrontation between the abuser/addict and other significant people in the abuser/addict's life. It generally involves several weeks of planning and preparation and is guided by a counselor who leads family and friends through the process.

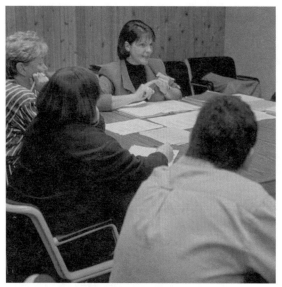

A formal intervention is guided by a counselor who leads family and friends through the process.

A crisis intervention is more immediate, intense, and powerful. It occurs as the result of a physical crisis; e.g., an abuser/addict is admitted to the emergency room for acute hepatitis, an auto accident while under the influence of a substance, or because of a suicide attempt. The crisis intervention provides immediate emergency assistance by focusing attention on the underlying cause of the physical emergency and then developing treatment for the problem—without delay.

The ultimate goal of any intervention is to diminish and ultimately eliminate the abuser/addict's denial—denial which may have been going on for months or years. Intervention helps to identify the problem and the abuser/addict's part in it. Whether informally or formally, those involved in the intervention must proceed with care and concern, avoiding moral judgments. In considering intervention, look at the following "Do's" and "Don'ts" before trying to help someone:

■ Intervention "Do's"

- Provide facts and data relevant to the substance or addictive behavior.
- Be supportive and caring. Listen with open ears and an open mind.
- Suggest counseling and other forms of help.
- Emphasize the advantages of recovery over the continued substance abuse and behavior.

■ Intervention "Don'ts"

- Nag, plead, beg, manipulate, or threaten. This will end in a power struggle with you as the loser.
- Criticize or shame the abuser/addict. This will cause the abuser/addict to withdraw.

- Pry or give advice, unless requested. This often will sabotage your efforts to help.

■ Intervention Reminders

- Recovery is the responsibility of the affected person, not you.
- Don't overestimate what you can accomplish. Providing support and encouragement may be all you can offer. People will make only the changes they truly want to make.
- Maintain your own health and happiness. You are a good and caring person trying to help another human being!

Exhibit 10.1. The Warning Signs of Substance Abuse or Addictive Behavior

1. Relying on alcohol, other substances, or addictive behaviors to build self-esteem and confidence.
2. Drinking alcohol or taking other substances before going to work or to a social event.
3. Drinking, using substances, or continuing addictive behaviors to avoid academic, work, and/or personal problems.
4. Missing classes, work, or other obligations due to substance abuse or addictive behaviors.
5. Driving while under the influence of alcohol or other substances, or getting a DWI charge.
6. Experiencing a memory loss from drinking or using other substances.
7. Borrowing money to purchase alcohol or addictive substances.
8. Associating with friends who share your substance abuse or addictive behavior.
9. Disassociating from certain friends after developing a substance abuse or addictive behavior.
10. Drinking more or taking more substances than other friends, or doing so alone.
11. Hiding the amount of substances used or time spent in addictive behaviors.
12. Consuming alcohol or other substances until they are completely gone.
13. Getting irritated by others who suggest you may be using too much alcohol or other substances, or overindulging in a certain activity.
14. Getting annoyed with classes or lectures on substance abuse and addictive behaviors.
15. Realizing that your use of certain substances or addictive behaviors has caused difficulties with your social life, family life, or friendships.

Note: Refer to the Learning Activity at the end of this chapter for additional signs of substance dependency.

■ Treatment

The treatment field of substance abuse and addictive behaviors contains an enormous diversity of treatment philosophies and techniques. Treatments offered by different disciplines range from medicine to psychiatry, psychology, social work, and pastoral counseling. In addition to outpatient treatment options, inpatient programs are available for everything from substance abuse to addictive behaviors such as gambling. Though more costly, inpatient programs seem to have a higher success rate. This is especially true for individuals with various and complicated addictions, minimal family and social support, and/or a medical history of unsuccessful previous attempts or relapse. In addition to cost, other factors to consider when selecting a program include location, facility environment, staff, and other clients involved in treatment. Most program basics include an abstinence-based philosophy, education component, individual counseling, group therapy, recreational therapy, and family therapy.

■ Relapse

Whether a person obtains inpatient or outpatient help, the chances of relapse are lowered when the individual continues some type of self-help support group similar to Alcoholics Anonymous. Groups exist for all types of addictions from substance abuse to overeating and gambling. These programs provide the support necessary to live one day at a time, putting the past behind, and cherishing each day with enthusiasm.

In spite of multiple programs and therapies that one might complete, the fact remains that substance and behavior addicts are prone to regress. Recovery, like addiction, involves a long period of adaptation. During that time, the body attempts to heal and restore balance. Unfortunately, withdrawal, which can last months and even years after the individual has ceased the substance or behavior, can overpower the individual. Research has provided clear and strong evidence of long-term effects from neurological addiction. While physical reasons often prompt a relapse, other reasons exist as well. Some of these reasons include

- an inability to recognize or control certain personality traits, such as compulsiveness;
- a narrow view of recovery, such as the belief that treatment is minimal and quick;
- a tendency to substitute one addiction for another; and/or

- the incapability of avoiding environmental factors that previously encouraged and motivated the substance abuse and addictive behaviors.

Relapse should never be interpreted as a symptom of weakness or an inability to live life without certain substances or behaviors. All chronic illnesses that have some behavioral component, such as cardiovascular disease and diabetes, have the potential for relapse. In other words, the patient does not always follow the treatment plan. Understanding why relapses occur can help to prevent them. Professionals agree that relapse is best prevented when recovery is viewed as a lifelong adventure and treatment programs are geared specifically to each person.

■ Prevention

Throughout this chapter and others, the aspect of prevention has been a common theme. Taking part in preventive measures is far better than the lifelong necessity for treatment of substance abuse and addictive behaviors. Realizing that you may have the predisposition for substance abuse or addictive behaviors often comes from looking inward at yourself and/or outward at your family, friends, and environment. Sometimes this realization comes after involvement in a college course, or simply through a health screening or self-risk test. Special academic courses or programs on a college campus offer help to prevent substance abuse and addictive behaviors. These programs usually include the following information and assistance:

- Recognizing and accepting responsibility for the role of substance abuse and addictive behaviors in one's life
- Learning how to minimize emotional and psychological susceptibility to abuse and dependency
- Taking actions that foster responsibility when confronted with certain substances and situations that can lead to addictive behaviors

Some of these concepts are reflected below in three methods for preventing a downfall associated with substance abuse and addictive behaviors:

1. **Take Responsibility.** When potentially harmful substances or situations become available or even encouraged, remember that in the end you are responsible for what you put in your body or how you act. Likewise, you are responsible for the

consequences of your choices. If you discover that you are particularly susceptible to a harmful substance or addictive behavior, cultivate a course of action, including behavior patterns that are a deterrent to the substance or activity.

2. **Minimize Emotional and Psychological Susceptibility**. Masking emotional and psychological pain with potentially harmful substances or behaviors does not correct the source of pain. If you are experiencing chronic emotional discomfort, such as conflict, loneliness, or values clarification, develop skills to handle these challenges. Counseling and developing healthy ways to feel good are positive ways to help yourself. Turning to substances or addictive behaviors is a negative course of action.

3. **Develop Alternative Actions**. Have an alternative action plan when you are confronted with situations in which addictive substances or activities are present. Ideas include an "alternative bar" where nonalcoholic drinks are served, taking your own nonalcoholic drink where beer or other alcohol is being served, volunteering to be the designated driver, or taking a limited amount of money or no money when you are with others who are gambling or on a shopping spree.

If you now realize that you have a problem with substance abuse or an addictive behavior, or if you want to make a concentrated effort to prevent this from happening, take advantage of the many resources that can give you perspective and support. If you recognize the symptoms of substance abuse or an addictive behavior in a friend or family member, know that you can help. Go back to the section on intervention and reread the "Do's" and "Don'ts" before you attempt to help another in need of intervention. Additionally, whether for yourself or for someone else, ask the following questions:

1. Why do you think you are having a problem with the substance or addictive behavior?
2. What do you think you can do about it?
3. What are you going to do about it?
4. What kinds of support do you need in order to discontinue or curtail the substance or behavior?

Developing Control

At the beginning of this chapter, we explained that every day we are confronted with substances and practices, healthy or not, that can lead to abuse and that can adversely impact our level of wellness. We also saw how easy it is to fall into the cycle of substance abuse and addictive behavior. Someone may first look for mood alteration, then drift into reliance, from reliance to habit, and from habit to abuse or addiction. Often, people stumble into abuse or addiction, not intending to let it control them.

How contrary this is to the teachings of Christ. He has told us that through God's strength we can develop control. With this realization, we understand that God and not some substance or behavior is in control of our lives. God is always seeking to teach us the way of faith. Through faith comes strength. This strength will help us resist the temptation to give in to substances and activities that have the potential to damage our bodies.

Never fail to remember that the Bible tells us we should care about our bodies. The body is the temple of the Holy Spirit. Our bodies, minds, and spirits are in a constant state of change until we return to God. Therefore, keep seeking the truth and answers to questions about wholistic wellness. Our capacity for maximal wellness is far greater than we probably believe!

In the final analysis of substance abuse and addictive behavior, we return to the Bible to remind us that our Lord has never promised a life free of problems. However, He has promised to stay by our sides and help us through adversity. True contentment comes from dependence on our Lord to guide us throughout life. We cannot really be content until we relinquish dependence on all other things except Him. We remember this when reading Psalm 55:22 (NIV):

KEY CONCEPTS

BAC
carcinogen
cocarcinogen
codependency
drug
enabling
fetal alcohol syndrome
process addiction
psychoactive drug

> *"Cast your cares on the Lord and he will sustain you;*
> *he will never let the righteous fall."*

Learning Activity

Signs of Substance Dependency

If you are wondering whether you are becoming dependent on a substance, answer the following questions. The more times you answer yes, the more likely it is that you are developing a physical or psychological dependence on the substance. If you answer yes to more than two or three of these questions, you should seek professional help.

YES   NO

_____   _____   1. Do you ingest the substance on a regular basis?

_____   _____   2. Have you been ingesting the substance for a long time?

_____   _____   3. Do you always take the substance in certain situations or when you are with certain people?

_____   _____   4. Do you find it difficult to stop using the substance? Do you feel powerless to quit?

_____   _____   5. Have you tried repeatedly to cut down or control your use of the substance?

_____   _____   6. Do you need larger amounts of the substance in order to get the same high?

_____   _____   7. Do you feel specific symptoms if you cut back or stop using the substance?

_____   _____   8. Do you frequently take another substance to relieve withdrawal symptoms?

_____   _____   9. Do you take the substance to feel "normal"?

YES   NO

_____ _____ 10. Do you go to extreme lengths or put yourself in dangerous situations to get the substance?

_____ _____ 11. Do you hide your substance use from others?

_____ _____ 12. Do you think about the substance when you're not high, figuring out ways to get it?

_____ _____ 13. If you stop using the substance, do you feel bad until you can ingest it again?

_____ _____ 14. Does the substance interfere with your ability to study, work, or socialize?

_____ _____ 15. Do you skip important occupational, social, or recreational activities in order to obtain or use the substance?

_____ _____ 16. Do you continue to use the substance despite a physical or mental disorder, or despite a significant problem that you know is worsened by the substance use?

_____ _____ 17. Have you developed a mental or physical condition or disorder because of prolonged substance use?

Helpful Information
Available at These Web Sites:

Healthy People 2010: objectives, tobacco use, substance abuse
    http://www.health.gov/healthypeople
Mayo Clinic: http://www.mayoclinic.com
Mayo Health Oasis: http://www.mayohealth.org
National Institute on Alcohol and Alcoholism: http://www.niaaa.nih.gov
The National Association for Children of Alcoholics:
    http://www.health.org/nacoa
The National Council on Alcohol and Drug Dependence:
    http://www.ncadd.org
The National Clearinghouse for Alcohol and Drug Information:
    http://www.health.org
The American Society of Addiction Medicine: http://www.asam.org
Mothers Against Drunk Driving: http://www.madd.org
Students Against Drunk Driving: http://www.saddonline.com
Alcoholics Anonymous: http://www.alcoholics-anonymous.org

Helpful Information is also available at the following toll-free numbers:

800 – COCAINE	Around-the-clock information and referral service
800 – NCA – CALL	National Council on Alcoholism and Drug Dependency Information Line, providing information and referrals to families and individuals seeking help with an alcohol or other drug problem
800 – 662 – HELP	National Institute on Drug Abuse information and referral line, providing written materials on drug use and treatment referrals

References

American Cancer Society. *Cancer Facts and Figures – 1993*. New York: American Cancer Society, 1993.

American Heart Association. *Heart and Stroke Facts*. Dallas: American Heart Association, 1993.

American Heart Association, American Cancer Association, and American Lung Association. *Smoke-Free Class of 2000 Facts*. Dallas: American Heart Association, 1995.

Anderson, David. *Breaking the Tradition on College Campuses: Reducing Drug and Alcohol Misuse*. Fairfax, VA: George Mason University, 1994.

Centers for Disease Control and Prevention. "Perspectives in Disease Prevention and Health Promotion—Smoking-Attributable Mortality and Years of Potential Life Lost—United States, 1984." *Morbidity and Mortality Weekly Report* (MMWR) 46, no. 20 (23 May 1997): 444-51.

Eriksen, M. P., C. A. LeMaistre, and G. R. Newell. "The Health Hazards of Passive Smoking." *Annual Review of Public Health* 9 (1988): 47-70.

Ketcham, Katherine, and William F. Asbury. *Beyond the Influence: Understanding and Defeating Alcoholism*. New York: Bantam Books, 2000.

Liska, Ken. *Drugs and the Human Body: With Implications for Society*. 3rd ed. New York: Macmillan, 1990.

Marlatt, G. Alan, and Judith R. Gordon. *Relapse Prevention: Maintenance Strategies in the Treatment of Addictive Behaviors*. New York: Guilford Press, 1985.

Noble, John, ed., et al. *Textbook of Primary Care Medicine*. 2nd ed. St. Louis: Mosby, 1996.

Ray, Oakley S., and Charles Ksir. *Drugs, Society, and Human Behavior*. 4th ed. St. Louis: Mosby, 1987.

Schuckit, Marc A. *Educating Yourself About Alcohol and Drugs: A People's Primer*. New York: Plenum, 1995.

Substance Abuse and Mental Health Services Administration. *Summary of Findings from the 1998 National Household Survey on Drug Abuse*. Rockville, MD: U.S. Department of Health and Human Services, SAMHSA, Office of Applied Studies, 1999.

U.S. Department of Health and Human Services. *Healthy People 2010: Understanding and Improving Health*. Washington, D.C.: U.S. Department of Health and Human Services, Government Printing Office, 2000.

Worick, W. Wayne, and Warren E. Schaller. *Alcohol, Tobacco, and Drugs*. Englewood Cliffs, N.J.: Prentice-Hall, 1977.

Yoder, Barbara. *The Recovery Resource Book*. New York: Simon and Schuster, 1990.

11

WELLNESS AND DISEASE PREVENTION

"Half the spiritual difficulties that men and women suffer
arise from a morbid state of health."

—Henry Ward Beecher

The absence of disease does not ensure that a person is well or healthy; however, the presence of disease certainly undermines a state of wellness. Seventy percent of diseases that cause early disability and/or death are preventable with good lifestyle choices.[1] That is an amazing statistic: 70 percent! This chapter will examine the most prevalent diseases affecting society today and focus on methods of preventing disease from robbing us of long, healthy lives.

Identifying and Preventing Infectious Diseases

Infectious diseases kill more people worldwide than any other kind of disease.[2]

Ironically, some infectious diseases that we thought had been eradicated have struck again—tuberculosis is one example. Food-borne infectious diseases also have been on the rise, as well as many newly discovered disease-causing bacteria and viruses. Infectious disease is a issue of importance to all of us. An infectious disease is a disease that is communicable. Most at risk for infectious diseases are underdeveloped, poverty-stricken countries, whose populations continue to die from such diseases as malaria, cholera, AIDS, and tuberculosis. Improved sanitation, better immunizations, healthier nutrition, and better personal hygiene are all valuable in reducing infectious diseases.

■ Mode of Attack

Most infectious diseases are carried by microorganisms. Microorganisms live everywhere in the environment—in water, soil, and even in our bodies. Not all microorganisms in or on our bodies are harmful; in fact, many perform very helpful functions. For example, some microorganisms normally found in the intestines produce a substance that kills infection-causing bacteria. Another interesting fact is that some bacteria normally found in one bodily system can produce disease in another bodily system. *Escherichia coli* is normally present in the intestine, but would cause an infection if it turned up in the urinary tract.

■ Mode of Defense

The human body's immune system is a phenomenal thing. The skin is our first line of attack against infection. It acts as a barrier to most harmful microorganisms. The mucous membranes in the nose, mouth, throat, and

LEUKOCYTE: A white blood cell.

eyes—as well as the lining of other major organs—secrete substances that wash away potential disease-producing germs. If a harmful microorganism does enter the bloodstream, special cells called **leukocytes** or white blood cells increase in number and fight off the invading germs.[3] Healthy diets, adequate sleep, regular exercise, and low levels of stress are all important in maintaining a healthy immune system.

Immunizations help the immune system recognize and attack disease-producing germs. Thousands of people die yearly as the result of the flu and other diseases that might have been prevented by an immunization. Health care providers are continually researching diseases and immunizations, making recommendations for those most at risk (age and health factors). Since these recommendations can change as new disease strains appear, it is best to consult your family doctor or Public Health Department for the most up-to-date information on immunizations that may be appropriate for you or a family member.

In the next section, we will examine the symptoms and effects of some of the most common infectious diseases. We also will offer prevention strategies in dealing with these diseases.

■ Gastroenteritis and Food Poisoning

Gastroenteritis and food poisoning have very similar symptoms: nausea, vomiting, abdominal cramping, diarrhea, and sometimes fever. However, these two diseases are caused by very different things. Gastroenteritis is caused by a viral infection in the digestive system. Food poisoning is usually caused by bacteria in food that has not been stored properly.

There is little you can do to prevent gastroenteritis, except to avoid others who have it. However, you can avoid food poisoning by taking precautions such as these:[4]

1. Do not eat raw eggs or uncooked sauces made with eggs.
2. Defrost meats in the refrigerator, not on the countertop.
3. Do not use a wooden cutting board.
4. Wash hands, countertops, and cutting boards frequently.
5. Cook hamburger until it is well done. Cook chicken until the juices are clear.
6. Discard any cans or jars of food with bulging lids or leaks.
7. Follow home canning and freezing instructions carefully.
8. Keep hot foods hot and cold foods cold.
9. Confirm that your refrigerator's temperature is between 34 and 40 degrees.
10. Do not eat meats, salads, or other foods that have been out of the refrigerator for more than two hours.

■ Colds and Flu

Viruses that attack the respiratory tract cause colds and flu. Colds last about seven days and are evidenced by a runny nose, cough, sore throat, congestion, and a general sense of "not feeling well." Colds usually do not result in serious illness. Treatment includes fluids, rest, and over-the-counter cold medications.

Influenza or the flu is also caused by a virus, but not the same virus that causes a cold. The flu can be much more serious than a cold. The symptoms of the flu are body aches, fever, and loss of appetite. Weakened by the flu, the patient may develop pneumonia. To prevent colds and the flu, follow these guidelines:[5]

1. Keep your resistance up by getting sufficient sleep, eating nutritious meals, and getting adequate exercise.
2. Avoid being near people who have a cold or flu.
3. Keep your hands away from your eyes, nose, and mouth.
4. Wash your hands often.
5. Humidify your home, especially your bedroom.
6. Get a flu shot each year in the fall before the cold and flu season begins. This is especially important if you are over sixty-five years of age or if you are at high risk of exposure.

■ Hepatitis

Hepatitis is an inflammation or infection of the liver. There are at least five different viruses that can cause hepatitis.[6] Hepatitis A and hepatitis E are spread mainly by fecal-oral transmission. This transmission occurs when food or water is contaminated with fecal material. It also occurs when people do not wash their hands after going to the bathroom, and then handle food that others will eat. Symptoms are diarrhea, stomach pain, and **jaundice** (yellowing of the eyes and/or skin). This type of hepatitis usually is not life threatening.

JAUNDICE: Yellowing of the eyes and/or skin; one of the side effects of hepatitis.

Hepatitis B, C, and D can be very serious, causing chronic liver infections that may lead to liver cancer or liver failure. Many people die every year from hepatitis-related liver cancer. Hepatitis B lives in the blood and other body fluids. It can be spread by blood contamination, sexual contact, and by shared needles. A pregnant woman who is hepatitis B-positive can pass it on to her baby. Hepatitis C was once spread through blood transfusions, but now is transmitted primarily among drug users who share needles. Symptoms of these diseases are nausea, headache, sore muscles, fatigue, and perhaps jaundice. Some people experience right-sided abdominal pain. In advanced cases, symptoms include cirrhosis and chronic liver dysfunction. To avoid hepatitis, follow these guidelines:

1. Wash hands thoroughly after using the restroom.
2. Everyone, especially young children and those at exposure risk, should receive the hepatitis B vaccine.
3. People at risk for hepatitis A—those traveling to South America, Asia, or Africa—should receive the hepatitis A vaccine.
4. Do not share needles.
5. Have monogamous sexual relationships.

■ Sexually Transmitted Diseases

Sexually transmitted diseases (STDs) are prolific in both their variety and in the number of people they infect. Sexually transmitted diseases infect more people than any other disease except the common cold.[7] These infectious diseases are passed from person to person during sexual contact. A majority of those infected are under twenty-five years of ago. Two-thirds of gonorrhea and chlamydia cases occur in persons under twenty-four years of age. Our society pays a high social, economic, and spiritual price for this epidemic of STDs. Let's look at some of these diseases individually.

■ Chlamydia

Chlamydia is the most common sexually transmitted disease in America and the Western world. It is caused by the microorganism *Chlamydia trachomatis*, which infects mucous membranes in the genital tract, mouth, anus, rectum, conjunctiva of the eye, and sometimes the lungs. It frequently occurs simultaneously with gonorrhea. Newborns are at risk if their mothers are infected at the time of delivery.

> Sexually transmitted diseases infect more people than any other disease except the common cold.

Chlamydia has mild to no symptoms in the early stages of the disease. Thus, people often do not realize they have this STD and may pass it on unknowingly. Symptoms can occur one to three weeks after exposure. For women, these symptoms include vaginal discharge, irregular menstrual bleeding, pain when urinating, and lower abdominal pain.

In men, there may be pain when urinating and a discharge from the penis.

Chlamydia is easily treated with antibiotics. However, undetected and untreated chlamydia can create major health problems, including pelvic inflammatory disease, which may lead to ectopic pregnancy and/or infertility. It is estimated that about 10,000 woman become infertile each year as the result of chlamydia.

■ Gonorrhea

Gonorrhea is caused by the bacterium *Neisseria gonorrhea.* This bacterium generally infects the mucous membranes of the genital tract, reproductive organs, mouth, throat, eyes, and anus. It is usually transmitted through genital, oral, or anal sexual contact. Newborns may contract it when passing through the infected birth canal of their mothers. Most states require a prophylactic eye medication to be given to newborns to prevent blindness caused by gonorrhea. Contrary to popular myths, gonorrhea cannot be transmitted via toilet seats, doorknobs, or bath towels.

Although very different types of bacteria cause chlamydia and gonorrhea, their symptoms are similar. Symptoms of gonorrhea appear two days to two weeks after exposure and may include painful or frequent urination, vaginal discharge, irregular menstrual bleeding, or a thick discharge from the penis. Many people who are infected have no symptoms. In nearly half the cases of gonorrhea, chlamydia is also present.

Gonorrhea may cause infertility. It can lead to prostate infection in men, and also may spread to the joints and cause arthritis. It is best treated with a regimen of antibiotics. However, new strains of the disease are evolving which are antibiotic resistant. It is important that both sex partners are treated so they do not reinfect one another.

■ Syphilis

Syphilis is caused by the bacterium *Treponema pallidum.* It is spread through sexual contact or by sharing blood-contaminated needles. It also may be given to a fetus from an infected mother as early as the ninth week of pregnancy.

CHANCRE: A primary sore or ulcer at the site of entry of a pathogen; the initial lesion of syphilis.

The first symptom of syphilis to appear is a painless open sore called a **chancre.** This usually appears on the genital area, mouth, or rectal area, and will occur three weeks to three months after exposure. If the infection is not treated, the sore will heal and the disease will then enter its second phase. This phase is characterized by a skin rash, patchy hair loss, fever, swollen lymph nodes, and flu-like symptoms. If the disease remains untreated, these symptoms may disappear, but the syphilis organism continues to multiply, can invade and damage vital organs, and result in premature death. Syphilis can be treated with antibiotics at any stage of the disease.

■ HIV Infection and AIDS

Human immunodeficiency virus (HIV) causes illness by destroying cells in the immune system. When the body's immune system is weakened, the HIV-infected person is then susceptible to many other bacterial, viral, and fungal infections. AIDS is the last and most serious phase of the HIV infection. AIDS usually occurs twelve to thirteen years after exposure to HIV and results in the body's inability to fight infection or disease.

HIV is spread through the blood, semen, and vaginal fluids of infected persons. Sexual transmission is a common method of exposure. All blood donations are now screened for HIV, so this route of transmission is minimal. The sharing of dirty needles is a source of exposure. In fact, the majority of new cases of AIDS are among injection drug users who share needles and those who have sex with them. Babies born to infected women or breast-fed by infected women are also at risk. HIV is not spread by casual contact. Being hugged, touched, or lightly kissed by someone who is HIV-positive will not transfer the virus.

When exposed to HIV, the body produces large amounts of antibodies to HIV. An HIV test is positive if these antibodies are identified. Within a few weeks to six months, the infected individual will experience flu-like symptoms, but soon will recover from the symptoms. Even symptom-free, the infected person can still pass the disease on to another person.

There is no vaccine for HIV at this time, and there is no way to rid the body of the HIV virus. Thus, treatment is aimed at managing the opportunistic infections that arise from the weakened immune system, and suppressing the HIV infection as long as possible to avoid earlier occurrence of AIDS. The combination drug treatment necessary is about 10,000 dollars per year. Many infected persons are economically disadvantaged and cannot afford the treatment. The only effective way to control the spread of HIV is to prevent the spread of the virus. This can be done by reducing exposure to infected persons, using condoms during sex with infected persons or persons with unknown HIV status, avoiding casual sex, and avoiding the practice of sharing needles.

Preventing STDs and HIV

The Christian wellness perspective includes the belief that God intended for sex to be shared only between a man and woman who are married to one another. Monogamous relationships

> The Christian wellness perspective includes the belief that God intended for sex to be shared only between a man and woman who are married to one another.

between a husband and wife or sexual abstinence are the only sure ways to eliminate the risk of HIV and other sexually transmitted diseases. Other less effective prevention strategies include these:

1. Avoid sexual contact while you or your partner are being treated for a STD.
2. Take time to find out if your partner has been exposed to or infected with a STD, or participates in any high-risk behavior.
3. Avoid unprotected sex with anyone who has symptoms or who has been exposed to STDs or HIV. Remember that a person may be able to spread the infection even if no symptoms are present.
4. Use latex condoms and spermicide every time you have sex (vaginal, anal, or oral) until you are certain you and your partner are disease free and in a monogamous relationship.
5. Never share needles, syringes, or other personal items that could be contaminated with blood.
6. If your job puts you at risk for coming into contact with contaminated blood, use precautions and contact a health professional immediately if you suspect exposure.

Identifying and Preventing Noninfectious Diseases

Heart Disease

Next we will look at noninfectious diseases, beginning with the leading cause of death in the United States: cardiovascular disease. The irony of cardiovascular disease is that while it is a major health problem for Americans, it is also one of the most *preventable* lifestyle-related illnesses.

■ How the Healthy Heart Works

The heart is a muscle about the size of a fist. It squeezes or contracts and then relaxes in order to pump oxygen-rich blood throughout the body. The heart muscle itself needs oxygen-rich blood to stay alive. It receives

ATRIA: The heart's two upper chambers; the atria receive blood.

this blood from blood vessels called **coronary arteries.** The left main coronary artery splits into two branches, which supply blood to the front, left side, and back of the heart muscle. The right coronary artery supplies blood to the bottom, right side, and back of the heart.

The inside of the heart is divided into right and left sides. Each side has an upper chamber called the atrium and a lower chamber called the ventricle. The two upper chambers or **atria** receive blood from the lungs and body. When the atria contract, blood is pumped into the lower chambers or **ventricles.** As the

---

Figure 11.1, Inside the Heart

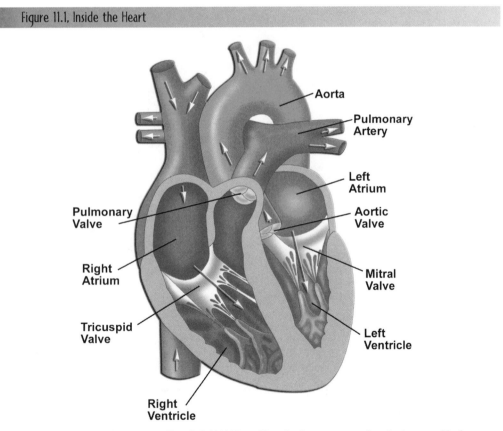

Source: "Anatomy of the Human Heart." © 2003 Texas Heart Institute www.texasheartinstitute.org. Used by permission.

VENTRICLES:

The heart's two lower chambers; the ventricles pump blood to the body and lungs.

lower chambers contract, blood is pumped into the lungs and body. The right side of the heart pumps blood to the lungs, where it receives oxygen. This oxygen-rich blood returns to the heart, and the left side of the heart pumps the oxygen-rich blood through the body. When the body has used the oxygen, the blood returns to the heart and the cycle begins again.

There are four valves inside the heart: the pulmonary, tricuspid, aortic, and mitral valves. When the heart beats, the valves keep the blood moving forward through the heart in a one-way direction. The heart also has a special electrical system that creates and sends electrical signals. Groups of special cells in the right atrium, called nodes, send the heart's electrical impulses. The signal travels along pathways called bundle branches. The SA (sinoatrial) node sets the pace of the heartbeat and starts each heartbeat by releasing a signal telling the atria to squeeze. The AV (atrioventricular) node receives the signal from the SA node. The AV node is the gateway between the atria and the ventricles, channeling the signal into the ventricles. The bundle branches carry the signal through the ventricle walls causing the ventricles to squeeze.[8]

This brief description of how the healthy heart works cannot do justice to the amazing complexity of this vital organ. In the next section, we will examine what happens when the heart functions at less than maximum efficiency or is damaged.

■ Coronary Artery Disease

When the openings inside the coronary arteries narrow or become blocked, the resulting disease is called coronary artery disease (CAD). Healthy coronary arteries with no blockage enable

CORONARY ARTERIES:

Blood vessels that supply the heart muscle with blood.

blood to flow easily to the heart. CAD signals that too much fatty material called **plaque** has built up inside the walls of the coronary arteries. The flow of oxygen-rich blood to the heart muscle is then reduced. If not corrected, plaque buildup can cut off the flow of blood to part of the heart muscle and result in a heart attack.

CAD begins when an artery wall is damaged. This usually occurs because of high blood cholesterol, high blood pressure, or diabetes. Other causes can be smoking, obesity, and lack of physical activity. Once the artery wall is damaged, the plaque begins to build up, reducing the blood flow to the heart. Early in this process there are no signs or symptoms.[9]

■ The Cholesterol Connection

High blood cholesterol is one contributing factor to plaque buildup. What exactly is high cholesterol? Blood cholesterol is a fatty substance that travels through the bloodstream. Your body's cells need cholesterol to function properly. However, excess cholesterol in the blood causes **arteriosclerosis** or narrowing of the arteries. This is the starting point for most heart and circulation problems. Cholesterol travels through the bloodstream attached to a protein called a lipoprotein. Two lipoproteins are the main carriers of cholesterol: low-density lipoprotein (LDL) and high-density lipoprotein (HDL).

PLAQUE: A deposit of fatty material within the artery walls.

Low-density lipoprotein is less healthy and is often called bad cholesterol. It carries cholesterol from the liver to other parts of the body. This is the cholesterol that can build up on the artery walls and cause heart disease. High-density lipoprotein is healthy and is referred to as good cholesterol. It helps clear bad cholesterol from the body by picking it up in the bloodstream and taking it back to the liver. There it is processed into waste products for later elimination. Increasing HDL cholesterol may reduce the risk of heart disease.

Cholesterol levels may be checked by a simple blood test. The results can tell how much total cholesterol is in the blood, as well as the amount of HDL and LDL. A normal total cholesterol level should be 200 or below. A desirable level of HDL is above 35 in men and 45 in women. A level of LDL below 130 in either gender is considered normal. It is also important to assess the ratio of HDL to the total cholesterol level. If the ratio of total cholesterol divided by the HDL level is around 4.5, the risk of cardiac disease is said to be average.

ARTERIOSCLEROSIS: Narrowing of the arteries caused by excess cholesterol in the blood.

A ratio above 4.5 increases the risk of heart disease; a ratio below 4.5 decreases it. Triglycerides are other fatty substances in the blood that can lead to plaque buildup. A blood level of less than 200 would be considered a good triglyceride level.[10] See Chart 11.1 for healthy levels.

Chart 11.1, Normal Adult Cholesterol Values For Laboratory Tests

Serum Cholesterol
<200 mg/dl or 5.2 mmol/L (SI units)

Serum Triglyceride
Male   40-160 mg/dl or 0.45-1.81 mmol/L
Female   35-135 mg/dl or 0.40-1.52 mmol/L

High Density Lipoprotein (HDL)
Male   >35 mg/dl or >0.75 mmol/L
Female   >45 mg/dl or >0.91 mmol/L

Low Density Lipoproteins (LDL)
Male and Female 130-180 mg/dl or <3.7 mmol/L

Cholesterol to HDL	4.5 average
Male 5.0	above 4.5 - increased risk
Female 4.4	below 4.5 - decreased risk

Adapted from S. Wilson and J. Giddens, *Health Assessment for Nursing Practice* (St. Louis: Mosby, 2001). Used by permission.

The following are recommendations for lowering blood cholesterol:

1. Eat less fat. Your total fat intake should be 30 percent or less of your total calories.

2. Watch your intake of saturated fat especially. This type of fat does the most harm. It is found mainly in foods that come from animals: meat, chicken skin, cheese, whole milk, and butter. Any fat that solidifies at room temperature is saturated fat.

3. Eat more fiber: oats, dried beans, brown rice, vegetables, and fruit.

4. Increase physical activity. Being active raises HDL levels, lowers LDL levels, and improves the ratio of HDL to total cholesterol.

5. Lose weight. Losing even five to ten pounds can raise HDL levels and lower LDL and triglyceride levels.

■ The Danger of High Blood Pressure

High blood pressure is another factor in developing CAD. Blood pressure is the pressure exerted by the blood against the walls of the blood vessels, especially the arteries. A blood pressure reading consists of two numbers; e.g., 120/80. The first or top number in the reading is called the systolic pressure, which measures the force the blood exerts on the artery wall as the heart contracts. The second or bottom number in the reading is the diastolic pressure, which is the force the blood exerts on the artery walls between heartbeats or when the heart is at rest. A person is said to have high blood pressure if the systolic is consistently above 140 and the diastolic is above 90. A rule of thumb is that if your blood pressure is 140/90 on three different occasions, you are considered to have high blood pressure.

Chart 11.2, Classification and Management of Blood Pressure for Adults*

BP Classification	SBP mmHg	DBP mmHg	Lifestyle Modification	Initial Drug Therapy	
				Without Compelling Indications	With Compelling Indications
Normal	<120	and <80	Encourage		
Prehypertension	120-139	or 80-89	Yes	No antihypertensive drug indicated.	Drug(s) for compelling indications.‡
Stage 1 Hypertension	140-159	or 90-99	Yes	Thiazide-type diuretics for most. May consider ACEI, ARB, BB, CCB, or combination	Drug(s) for the compelling indications.‡ Other antihypertensive drugs (diuretics, ACEI, ARB, BB, CCB) as needed.
Stage 2 Hypertension	≥160	or ≥100	Yes	Two-drug combination for most† (usually thiazide-type diuretic and ACEI or ARB or BB or CCB).	

DBP, diastolic blood pressure; SBP, systolic blood pressure.
Drug abbreviations: ACEI, angiotensin converting enzyme inhibitor; ARB, angiotensin receptor blocker; BB, beta-blocker; CCB, calcium channel blocker.

*   Treatment determined by highest BP category
†   Initial combined therapy should be used cautiously in those at risk for orthostatic hypotension.
‡   Treat patients with chronic kidney disease or diabetes to BP goal of <130/80 mmHg.

Source: *Seventh Report of the Joint National Committee on Prevention, Detection, Evaluation, and Treatment of High Blood Pressure*. U.S. Department of Health and Human Services, National Institutes of Health, National Heart, Lung, and Blood Institute, National High Blood Pressure Education Program. NIH Publication No. 03-5233, May 2003.

High blood pressure usually has no signs or symptoms. Therefore, it is extremely important to have your blood pressure routinely checked. Factors that put someone at risk for developing high blood pressure include: a family history of high blood pressure, being overweight, being of African American descent, an inactive lifestyle, drinking too much alcohol, smoking, too much salt in the diet, not enough potassium, calcium, or magnesium in the diet, and taking certain medications such as birth control pills, steroids, decongestants, and anti-inflammatory drugs. To lower blood pressure, follow these guidelines:

1. Maintain a healthy weight. Losing even ten pounds can lower your blood pressure.
2. Exercise regularly. Thirty to forty-five minutes of brisk walking three to four times a week will help to lower blood pressure.
3. Drink alcohol in moderation.
4. Use salt moderately.
5. Make sure you get enough potassium, calcium, and magnesium in your diet. Eating fruits (bananas and oranges), vegetables, legumes, and low-fat dairy products will ensure that you get enough of these minerals.
6. Reduce the saturated fat in your diet.
7. Do not smoke.

■ Angina and Heart Attack

Plaque buildup can cause a clot to form. The blood clot may plug the narrow opening in the plaque-filled artery walls. When blood is prevented from reaching part of the heart muscle, the heart is damaged and stops working. This is called a heart attack, also referred to as a **myocardial infarction** or MI. A heart attack

MYOCARDIAL INFARCTION:
Another term for heart attack. Also called MI.

can cause permanent heart muscle damage.

Angina is a warning that your heart muscle is not getting enough oxygen-rich blood. It is preceded by ischemia, which is tissue anemia due to an obstruction of arterial blood. Angina is chest

ANGINA: Chest pain and other symptoms that signal the heart is not getting enough oxygen-rich blood.

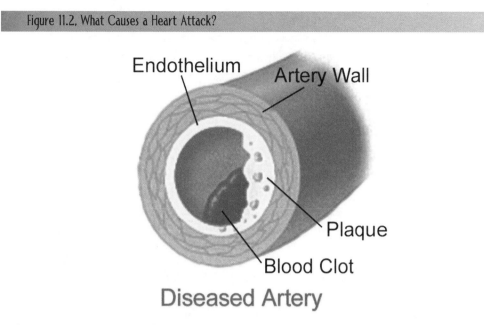

Endothelium   Artery Wall

Plaque

Blood Clot

Diseased Artery

Source: "Heart Attack." © 2003 Texas Heart Institute www.texasheartinstitute.org. Used by permission.

pain, but also can feel like mild indigestion or a burning in the stomach. It may occur in other parts of the upper body. Angina usually lasts just a few minutes and almost always goes away with medication and rest. It happens most often during physical activity, but can occur if you are upset or even after you have eaten a large meal. Unlike a heart attack, angina does not cause permanent damage to the heart muscle. If angina occurs with more frequency, lasts for longer periods of time, or causes more discomfort than normal, seek medical help, as any of these symptoms could indicate that your CAD is getting worse. Medication, lifestyle changes, and certain medical procedures can help to control angina.

The symptoms of a heart attack vary from person to person and not all symptoms occur in every person. The most common symptoms are uncomfortable pressure, fullness, squeezing or pain in the center of the chest that lasts more than ten minutes, or that goes away and comes back. Other symptoms include pain that spreads to the shoulders, neck, or arms, along with lightheadedness, fainting, sweating, nausea, and shortness of breath. Less common warning signs of heart attack are atypical chest pain, stomach or abdominal pain, nausea or dizziness (without chest pain), unexplained anxiety, weakness or fatigue, shortness of breath (without chest pain), palpitations, cold sweat, and paleness.

The pain of heart attack usually will not go away with rest. It is often described as feeling like someone is sitting on your chest. Many people mistake heart attack symptoms for other problems, such as indigestion, heartburn, or a pulled muscle. It is important to recognize the signals the body sends during the early stages of a heart attack and to seek emergency medical care. If a person receives medical care early enough, it is possible for medications to be given to prevent heart muscle damage caused by the heart attack.

■ Risk Factors for CAD

The American Heart Association has identified several risk factors for CAD, which can lead to heart attack.[11] The more risk factors you have, the greater the probability that you will develop heart disease. These risk factors are divided into two types: those outside your control and those within your control.

Risk factors outside your control are things you cannot alter or change. They include:

1. **Increasing age**. About four out of every five people who die from heart disease are over sixty-five years of age. At older ages, women who have heart attacks are twice as likely as men to die from the attack within a few weeks.
2. **Heredity**. If you have a parent with heart disease, your chances are greater of developing the disease. Since African Americans have a higher risk of high blood pressure, they also have a higher risk of heart disease.
3. **Gender**. Early in life men have a greater chance of developing heart disease than women. However, the death rate for women who die of heart disease increases after menopause.

The major risk factors for heart disease that are within your ability to stop, change, or modify are:

1. **Smoking**. A smoker's risk of heart attack is twice that of a nonsmoker. Cigarette smoking is the biggest risk factor for sudden cardiac death. Smokers who have a heart attack are more likely to die and die suddenly (within the hour) than nonsmokers. Evidence now shows that chronic exposure to secondhand smoke increases the risk of heart disease. Smoking is a woman's single biggest risk for a heart attack.

2. **High blood cholesterol**. The risk of heart disease rises as blood cholesterol levels increase. Refer back to the discussion on cholesterol and review ways to lower blood cholesterol.

3. **High blood pressure**. High blood pressure makes the heart work harder to circulate the blood. This causes the heart to enlarge and weaken over time. When high blood pressure exists along with obesity, smoking, high blood cholesterol, or diabetes, the chances of heart attack or stroke increase several times.

4. **Physical Inactivity**. Lack of physical activity is a risk factor for CAD. Regular exercise plays a significant role in preventing heart and blood vessel disease. Even modest levels of low intensity exercise are helpful if done regularly and over the long term. Exercise helps to control blood cholesterol, diabetes, and obesity, and may even lower blood pressure.

5. **Obesity**. People who are overweight are more likely to develop heart disease and stroke even if they have no other risk factors. Extra weight puts more strain on the heart. Weight influences blood pressure, blood cholesterol, triglyceride levels, and also makes it more likely that diabetes will develop. Losing ten to twenty pounds can help lower your risk of heart disease.

6. **Diabetes**. We will discuss this disease in more detail later in this chapter. However, it is important to realize that persons who are diabetic have a seriously increased risk of developing cardiovascular disease. Even when blood glucose levels are under control, diabetes increases the risk of heart disease and stroke. More than 80 percent of people with diabetes die of some kind of heart or blood vessel disease. It is very important for persons with diabetes to monitor and control any other risk factors they may have.

7. **Stress**. Some scientists who have studied the relationship between stress and heart disease believe that there is a correlation. For example, when people are under a lot of stress, they may tend to eat more or smoke more. Managing stress is important in order to lower the risk of heart disease.

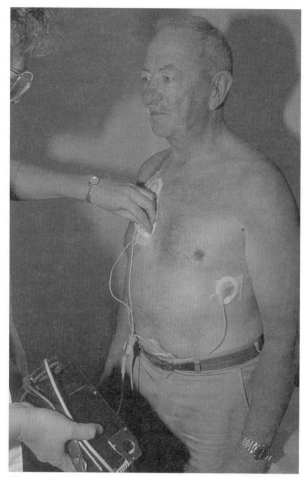

The more risk factors a person has, the greater the probability of developing heart disease.

■ Stroke

A stroke occurs when a blood vessel supplying blood to the brain bursts or becomes blocked by a blood clot.[12] In a very short period of time, the nerve cells in that area of the brain are damaged and die. When this happens, the part of the body controlled by those nerve cells cannot function properly.

The outcomes of a stroke vary from moderate to severe and may be temporary or permanent. A stroke can affect the ability to move any part of the body—even causing paralysis in some patients. It also may affect speech, vision, the thought process, or behavior. A stroke may result in coma or death. The effects of a stroke depend on which brain cells are damaged, how much of the brain is affected, and how quickly blood supply is restored to the affected area.

■ TIA: Early Warning

A transient ischemic attack (TIA) may occur before a person has a stroke. These are often called mini-strokes because their symptoms are similar to those of a stroke. Unlike stroke symptoms, TIA symptoms disappear within minutes (ten to twenty minutes). A TIA can occur months before a stroke. However, it needs to be treated as an emergency because it is a warning sign that a stroke is impending. The symptoms of stroke include these:

1. Severe dizziness, loss of balance, or loss of coordination
2. Any new weakness, numbness, or paralysis in your face, arm, or leg—especially on only one side of your body
3. Blurred or decreased vision that will not improve with blinking
4. Newly developed difficulty speaking
5. Inability to understand simple statements
6. Sudden and intense headache unlike any you have had before

If a symptom occurs and then goes away after a few minutes, call the doctor immediately. It may be a TIA or an impending sign of a stroke. If medical care is provided quickly enough, fewer brain cells may be damaged. Medication can be given to reduce the effects of the stroke, but this medication must be given within a very short time frame of the initial symptoms. Time is of the essence!

■ Preventing Strokes

The prevention guidelines for stroke are the same as for heart disease. Look over this quick review:

1. Maintain normal blood pressure.
2. Maintain normal blood cholesterol.
3. Do not smoke.
4. Maintain a normal body weight.
5. Stay physically active.
6. Manage symptoms of diabetes.
7. Drink alcohol in moderation, if at all.[13]
8. Manage stress. Keep a reasonable schedule, get enough sleep, and create time for relaxation and play.

■ Diabetes

Diabetes is a disorder of metabolism.[14] When diabetes is present, the human body does not properly process food for growth and energy. In the normal human body, most of the food eaten is broken down into glucose in the stomach. After food is digested, glucose—the body's main source of fuel and energy—enters the bloodstream, where it becomes available to cells. It is at this point that the blood glucose level or blood sugar level rises, a normal result of the process.

For glucose to get into the cells, insulin must be present. Insulin is a hormone produced by the pancreas, which is a large gland behind the stomach. In the normal human body, after food is digested, the pancreas automatically produces the right amount of insulin to move glucose from the blood into the cells. The cells then metabolize or burn the glucose to give the body energy.

In people with diabetes, however, the pancreas produces little or no insulin, or the cells do not respond properly to what insulin is produced. Glucose builds up in the blood, overflows into the urine, and passes out of the body. The body loses its main source of fuel and energy, even though the blood contains large amounts of glucose. Over long periods of time, high blood sugars may damage blood vessels and nerves, increasing the risk for problems associated with the eyes, heart, kidneys, legs, and feet.

High blood glucose can lead to both short-term and long-term health problems. Diabetes is the fourth leading cause of death by disease and is the leading cause of new cases of kidney disease, blindness, amputation, and impotence. Heart disease and stroke are two to six times more common in people with diabetes.

Diabetes is classified into two types. Type 1 diabetes (also called juvenile or insulin-dependent diabetes) occurs when the pancreas makes little or no insulin. This kind of diabetes usually develops in childhood or adolescence, but can develop at any age. People with type 1 diabetes must give themselves insulin shots every day in order to survive.

Type 2 diabetes (also called adult-onset or non-insulin-dependent diabetes) occurs when the pancreas cannot make enough insulin to meet the needs of the body or when the body does not use insulin properly. This type of diabetes often occurs in adults who are over forty years of age and overweight. In fact 80 percent of people with type 2 diabetes are considered to be overweight. Many people with type 2 diabetes are able to control their blood sugar with a healthy diet, regular exercise, and weight control. Some need oral medication or insulin shots. These are the risk factors associated with diabetes:

1. Being overweight (20 percent more than your ideal weight)
2. Being forty years of age or older
3. Having a family history of type 2 diabetes
4. Having an inactive lifestyle
5. Being of African American descent, as well as Hispanic, Pacific Island, or Native American descent
6. Having a history of gestational diabetes (diabetes during pregnancy)

Table 11.1. Estimated Risk of Developing Diabetes

Estimated Risk of Developing Diabetes		
Relationship to Person with Diabetes	**Approximate Chance of Developing Diabetes**	
	Type 1	Type 2
No diabetes in family	1%	11%
Identical twin with diabetes	25–50%	58–75%
One parent with diabetes	1–6%	7–14%
Sibling with diabetes	10%	45%
Anyone Can Get Diabetes—But Your Risk Is Greater Than Normal If You . . .		
• Are 40 years or older • Are overweight		

Source: LifeScan Risk Chart retrieved 2-11-03 from www.allenlee.com.

Because the symptoms of diabetes can be vague or may mimic another illness, a doctor should do a blood test to accurately diagnose diabetes. The most common symptoms are dry mouth and increased thirst, frequent urination (especially at night), increased appetite, unexplained weight loss, frequent skin infections and slowly healing wounds, recurrent vaginal infections, blurry vision, tingling or numbness in the hands or feet, and feelings of weakness, fatigue, and/or dizziness.

At present there is no way to prevent type 1 diabetes. The risk for developing type 2 diabetes runs in families. However, even with a family history of diabetes, you may be able to delay or prevent its onset by maintaining a healthy weight and exercising regularly. About sixteen million Americans have diabetes, but only eight million are treating it.

Gestational diabetes is diabetes that is first diagnosed during a pregnancy. Women who have had no prior history of glucose intolerance but demonstrate hyperglycemia (high blood sugar) during pregnancy have gestational diabetes. Usually this is diagnosed in the fourth to sixth months of pregnancy when the baby's nutrient demands are high, the mother's calorie intake is higher, and the mother's insulin resistance increases.

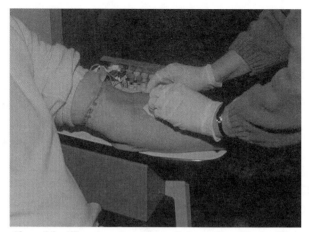

About 16 million Americans have diabetes, but only 8 million are treating it.

Most women can manage gestational diabetes with modifications to their diets. Some may need insulin injections immediately. This condition usually reverses itself completely following the delivery of the baby. However, many women who have gestational diabetes will develop type 2 diabetes later in life. The following factors put women at risk for gestational diabetes:

1. Previous birth of a large newborn (nine pounds or more)
2. Family history of diabetes
3. Weight above 200 pounds
4. Previous newborn with a congenital defect
5. High blood pressure
6. Loss of baby through stillbirth or miscarriage, cause unknown
7. History of one or more pregnancies

■ Osteoporosis

During the normal human life, bones go through continuous bone-building cycles in which old bone is broken down and new bone is formed. Osteoporosis, a condition in which more bone is lost than replaced, is caused by an imbalance in this cycle. Some thinning and weakening of the bones happens to everyone as part of the aging process. Bone mass usually peaks between the ages of twenty-five and thirty-five; most women begin to lose bone after age thirty-five. One-third of a woman's bone loss can occur in the first five years after menopause. As bones become weaker and thinner, they become more susceptible to fractures or breaks. Bones in the hip, wrist, and spine are especially at risk. Fractures can result in pain, height loss, a humped back, disability, loss of independence, and even death if complications set in.[15]

Bone loss is usually a painless process until a fracture occurs. Thus, many women are often unaware that they have osteoporosis until they have a sudden and painful fracture. Bone density tests are available to help determine a woman's risk for osteoporosis. Bone density tests are simple, safe, painless, and take only a few minutes to perform. The most commonly tested bones are the hip, spine, wrist, heel, and finger. Low bone density at any site indicates that there is an increased risk for fracture there. Bone density tests also can be used to monitor the rate of bone loss and a person's response to therapy.

All women over the age of sixty-five should have a bone density test, as well as postmenopausal women under the age of sixty-five who have other risk factors for developing osteoporosis. Test scores are called T-scores and determine bone density in comparison with that of a population of young women. A T-score above -1 indicates normal bone mass. A score of -1 to -2 indicates low bone mass, which means the bone mass is 10 to 20 percent below normal and at a double risk of fracture. A score below -2 indicates a diagnosis of osteoporosis, with a quadrupled risk of fracture.

Relatively few women with osteoporosis even know they have it; thus, they have not been diagnosed and are not receiving treatment. Doctors have identified factors that put a woman at risk for osteoporosis:

1. Being of Caucasian or Asian descent
2. Having a family history of osteoporosis
3. Being thin or petite
4. Taking certain medications, such as steroids or too much thyroid hormone
5. Smoking
6. Drinking several caffeinated or alcoholic beverages a day
7. Too little calcium or vitamin D
8. Lack of physical exercise

Even if these risk factors do not apply to you, you may still have or develop osteoporosis. You can take a proactive approach to protect yourself against this disease. You cannot slow the passing of time or change the effects of aging on your body. However, it is never too late to act on the things over which you do have control. Osteoporosis is a potentially devastating disease that is preventable and treatable.

First, get regular exercise. Regular exercise helps to prevent bone loss. Exercises that strengthen muscles and improve flexibility help prevent falls. You do not have to exercise vigorously to obtain benefits. What is important is that the exercise is consistent and weight bearing. Before starting any exercise program, it is a good idea to talk to your doctor.

Second, make sure your diet has enough calcium and vitamin D. One of the most important ways to reduce your risk for developing osteoporosis is to have a strong skeleton in the first place. By making sure that children have enough calcium in their diets, we ensure that their bones will be strong. However, maintaining a good calcium intake is important at any age. A daily calcium intake of 1,000 mg is sufficient for most adults, although if you are postmenopausal, you may need to increase your daily intake to 1,500 mg.

Another lifestyle change that can prevent or slow down the development of osteoporosis is the cessation of smoking. If you are not motivated to stop smoking for the sake of your lungs, heart, and circulation—then osteoporosis may be another good reason to stop. Limit drinks with caffeine. Caffeine in coffee and soft drinks increases calcium loss from the body. A small amount of alcohol may not harm you, but if you drink alcohol regularly, you may increase your risk of osteoporosis. Medications, including some steroids such as hydrocortisone or prednisone, can increase bone loss. Talk to your doctor about reviewing your medications—especially for bone-related side effects.

■ Cancer

Cancer is a broad term for a group of more than 100 different diseases. Cancer in its various forms occurs when abnormal cells divide and form more abnormal cells without control or order. All organs of the body are made up of cells. In a healthy body, cells divide to produce more cells only when new ones are needed. If cells divide when new ones are *not* needed, however, they form a mass of excess tissue called a tumor. Tumors can be benign (not cancerous) or malignant (cancerous).

METASTASIS: The spread of cancer cells to other areas of the body by way of the lymph system or bloodstream.

The cells in malignant tumors can invade and damage tissues and nearby organs. The cancer cells also can break away from a malignant tumor and travel through the bloodstream or lymphatic system to form new tumors in other parts of the body. This spread of the cancer is called **metastasis.**

Generally, cancer's symptoms are easily identified. The acronym CAUTION can help you remember the most common warning signs of cancer.[16]

> **C**hange in bowel or bladder habits
> **A** sore that does not heal
> **U**nusual bleeding or discharge
> **T**hickening or lump in the breast or any other part of the body
> **I**ndigestion or difficulty swallowing
> **O**bvious change in a wart or mole
> **N**agging cough or hoarseness

These symptoms do not always signify cancer, of course. They can indicate the presence of a less serious illness. However, if you are experiencing any of these symptoms, see your doctor. It is also important to remember that pain is not a symptom of early cancer; if you wait until you are feeling pain, the cancer may be advanced. Only a doctor can make an accurate diagnosis. A biopsy is the only sure way to diagnose cancer. This is a minor surgical procedure in which a sample of tissue is removed. The tissue is then examined under a microscope to identify cancer cells.

Can cancer be prevented? The answer is yes in many cases. Avoiding the harmful rays of the sun, not using tobacco products, and choosing foods with less fat and more fiber are just a few lifestyle choices that can help to prevent cancer. In addition, regular checkups and self-exams can catch cancer at an early stage when treatment is most likely to be effective. In the next section, we will look at four of today's leading forms of cancer.

■ Lung Cancer

Lung cancer is the leading cause of cancer death among men and women.[17] Smoking cigarettes is the number-one cause of lung cancer, causing 80 to 90 percent of all cases. Thus, it is almost an entirely preventable disease. Lung cancer is often not diagnosed until it is very well developed and has already spread to other parts of the body. The five-year survival rate for people diagnosed with lung cancer is only 10 to 15 percent—not very good odds. Another issue to consider is the issue of secondhand smoke. Research is indicating that exposure to secondhand smoke also puts one at risk for lung cancer.

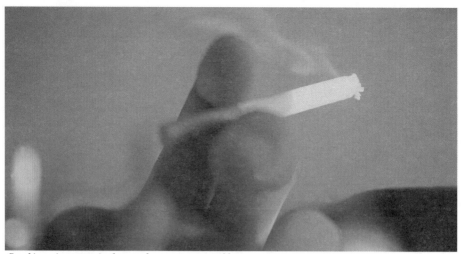

Smoking cigarettes is the number-one cause of lung cancer.

■ Skin Cancer

Skin cancer is the most commonly diagnosed type of cancer. However, most skin cancers can be cured if detected and treated early. Skin cancer is preventable! Most skin cancers are caused by exposure to the sun. Ninety percent of skin cancers occur on the face, neck, and arms where sun exposure is the greatest. Most damaging sun exposure occurs by age twenty, so children and adolescents must be protected from damage by the UV (ultraviolet) rays of the sun. Tanning beds can cause the same damage as the sun, if the skin is burned or blistered.

There are three forms of skin cancer. *Basal cell carcinoma* usually appears as a small, fleshy bump on the head, neck, or hands. These lesions seldom occur in African Americans, but are frequently found in fair-skinned persons. People who have this cancer often have light-colored eyes, hair, and complexions. This cancer is very slow growing. Although it seldom metastasizes, it can extend below the skin to the bone and cause considerable local damage.

Squamous cell carcinoma might appear as a bump or as a red, scaly patch. This is the second most common skin cancer found in fair-skinned persons. It is often found on the rim of the ear, the face, lips, and mouth. This type of skin cancer does metastasize and can develop into large masses. When found early and treated properly, the cure rate for both basal cell and squamous cell cancers is 95 percent.

Malignant melanoma is the most deadly skin cancer. Every year an estimated 7,300 Americans will die from melanoma. Melanoma may appear suddenly or it may begin in or near a mole or other dark spot on the skin. It is important to know the location and appearance of the moles on your body, so any changes can be quickly recognized and treated. Melanoma tends to spread;

thus, early treatment is essential. If treated early, melanoma can be cured.

Call your doctor if you notice any of the following changes in a mole. The A-B-C-D format should help you remember these important warning signs:[18]

> **A.** **A**symmetrical shape: one half does not match the other half.
> **B.** **B**order irregularity: the edges are notched, ragged, or blurred.
> **C.** **C**olor is not uniform: watch for shades of red and black, or a red, white, and blue mottled look.
> **D.** **D**iameter: the mole is larger than a pencil eraser.

Other signs to be aware of are any changes in the appearance of the mole, itching, tenderness, pain, scaliness, oozing, bleeding, or spreading of pigment into surrounding skin.

To repeat, most skin cancers can be prevented. Repeated sun exposure and severe sunburns are major factors in the development of skin cancer. Sun exposure accumulates day after day and occurs whenever you are outdoors— gardening, swimming, boating, hiking, or just walking to and from your car. Sunlight reflects off water, sand, concrete, snow, and reaches below the water's surface. To prevent or restrict sun exposure, follow these tips:

> 1. Limit sun exposure between 10 a.m. and 4 p.m. when ultraviolet rays are the most intense.
> 2. Wear a shirt and pants to protect as much skin as possible.
> 3. Choose and use a sunscreen with a sun protection factor (SPF) of 15 or higher. Reapply often, especially when coming out of the water.
> 4. Wear a hat. Choose a hat that shades the face, neck, and ears.
> 5. Wear sunglasses to protect your eyes from UV rays.
> 6. Remember that sunlamps and tanning beds can be as harmful to your skin as the sun.
> 7. Check with your pharmacist. Some prescription drugs can greatly increase your skin's sensitivity to UV rays.
> 8. Avoid sunburn during childhood and adolescence. This is very important in reducing the risk of skin cancer later in life.
> 9. Sunscreen is not recommended for children less than six months of age. Keep infants in the shade and protected by clothing.

■ Breast Cancer

Breast cancer is the leading cause of cancer deaths in women who are forty to fifty-five years of age.[19] Breast cancer often can be cured if it is detected and treated early. Early detection involves three different methods: mammography, clinical breast exam, and breast self-exam.

Mammograms are breast X-rays that can reveal breast tumors too small to be felt by self-exam or clinical exam. Studies have shown that in women over age fifty, mammograms reduce breast cancer deaths by one-third. Doctors usually recommend mammograms every one to two years for women ages forty to fifty, and every year for women over fifty.

In a clinical breast exam, a doctor or nurse examines the breasts and gently feels them for lumps or other unusual changes. A clinical breast exam is recommended every one to two years after the age of forty, or whenever a woman has symptoms indicating a problem with her breast or breasts.

The monthly self-exam is an important way for women to learn what is "normal" for their breasts. Thus, they will be able to better identify lumps, cysts, and other breast problems. A good time to do a monthly breast self-exam is a few days after the monthly period has ended, when the breasts are less sore and swollen. If a woman finds anything unusual—a lump that is different or harder than the rest of the breast tissue, for example—she should immediately consult her doctor or nurse.

The risk factors for breast cancer are few. They include age (the risk goes up considerably after age fifty) and a family history of breast cancer, particularly if a mother or sister had breast cancer before menopause.

Call a doctor if you notice these signs or symptoms of breast cancer:

1. A lump of any kind that hasn't been there before

2. A bloody or greenish discharge from the nipple

3. A watery or milky discharge that occurs without pressing on the breast

4. A breast that changes shape; the appearance of a dimple or pucker, especially when the arm is raised

5. A change in the color or feel of the skin

6. A change in the areola (dark area around the nipple)

7. A new pain in one breast that is not due to injury (particularly for postmenopausal women)

8. Any signs of infection in the breast: swollen, tender lymph nodes under the arms, redness, heat, or tenderness in the breast, pus draining from the breast

Prevention and early detection of breast cancer are key factors in reducing deaths associated with this disease. Prevention and early detection guidelines include these:

1. Have a mammogram every year after age fifty.
2. Have a clinical breast exam every one to two years after age forty.
3. Perform monthly breast self-exams.
4. Eat a low-fat diet. Fat in the diet is linked to an increased risk for breast cancer.
5. Limit alcohol intake. Even moderate drinking increases the risk of breast disease.
6. Eat foods that contain vitamins A and C (dark green and orange vegetables and fruits), and cruciferous vegetables (broccoli, cabbage, kale). There is some research that suggests diets high in these foods reduce the risk of breast cancer.

■ Colon Cancer

Deaths from colon cancer are exceeded in the United States only by lung cancer; about 60,000 persons will die annually from colon cancer. It affects men and women equally. However, like most other cancers, if it is detected early, a cure is possible. Colon cancer is most often found in people over age fifty. Another risk factor is a family history of the disease. Certain inherited genes are known to increase a person's risk for colon cancer.

The main screening tests for colon cancer are occult blood test and flexible sigmoidoscopy. In the occult blood test, stool samples are studied for the presence of blood, which could indicate that cancer is present. In the sigmoidoscopy, a flexible, lighted instrument is inserted into the rectum, allowing the physician to examine the lining of the lower colon. If abnormalities are found, further testing is required. Neither of these tests provides completely accurate results. A positive result will necessitate follow-up testing.

Prevention and early detection of colon cancer includes the following:[20]

1. Eat a well-balanced, low-fat diet. Pay special attention to adequate amounts of fiber.
2. Call the doctor if you observe blood in the stool.
3. After age fifty, ask your doctor if you should have a sigmoidoscopy or a colonoscopy.
4. Report any change in bowel function.

There are many more types of cancer that affect many parts of the body. We have addressed only four in this chapter. While a diagnosis of cancer is serious, the good news is that most cancers are preventable or curable with early diagnosis. Current research is continuing to find better diagnostic and treatment modalities for cancer. Your most important line of defense is still *prevention*.

Disease and the Wellness Connection

As we saw earlier in this text, wellness is composed of six primary components: physical, emotional, spiritual, social, intellectual, and occupational. What is the relationship of these wellness components to the prevention or cure of disease? Medical science has been researching this question for years. Recent data demonstrate a positive relationship between emotional, spiritual, and vocational wellness.[21]

For example, your brain can create endorphins, gamma globulin, and interferon. Endorphins are natural painkillers, gamma globulin builds up the immune system, and interferon combats infections.[22] The quantity or quality of the substances the brain produces, however, depends somewhat on the individual's emotional state at the time, as well as that person's attitude toward an illness.

Persons who create positive expectations for health and healing usually have better health outcomes.

> Persons who create positive expectations for health and healing usually have better health outcomes.

The earlier chapters on stress explain how stress creates reactions in the body that can negatively influence health. Among these physical reactions to stress are increased pulse rate, increased blood pressure, and pupil dilation to name a few. These reactions have short-term benefits, of course, as a way to prepare the body to fend off attack or escape danger. However, if these reactions are the result of constant stress, negative physical consequences become evident: headache, backache, lower resistance to infection, upset stomach, exhaustion, and irritability.

Vocational wellness relates to a safe work setting.[23] This means working in an environment where injuries are not a risk, where sanitation is good, where work-related risks are identified and managed, and where stress is managed. Let's look at a hypothetical truck driver with these risk factors:

- Back injury from sitting for long periods of time with inadequate back support

- Accidents from driving while he is sleep deprived
- High blood pressure from lack of exercise and frequent snacking on unhealthy food
- Stress from pushing hard to meet deadlines

If this truck driver's work environment is changed to meet vocational wellness guidelines, he will have:

- Adequate back support
- Adequate time to deliver his goods, including rest stops to exercise and sleep, as well as time to eat well-balanced meals

It is obvious that the truck driver needs to bear some responsibility for his health. Even given enough time does not ensure that he will make the healthiest choices regarding food and exercise.

The relationship between nutrition, exercise, and the prevention of disease has been very well established. Poor nutrition and lack of exercise are the common culprits of many preventable diseases. Nutrition and exercise have direct cause-and-effect relationships to heart disease, infection, and some cancers, just to name a few.

Spiritual wellness has a direct relationship to illness and the prevention of illness.[24] A spiritually well person usually has a healthier lifestyle. A spiritually well person seeks God's direction for day-to-day living and for making difficult decisions. Faith, prayer, and spiritual beliefs give people hope when they are not well, thus improving their chances for positive outcomes.

The role of disease prevention is deeply intertwined with the other areas of wellness discussed in this textbook: nutritional, physical, emotional, spiritual, family and social, career and educational, as well as the related areas of healthy aging and stress reduction. Disease prevention means active participation in managing your health concerns—taking charge of your life and doing what needs to be done to prevent physical illness. As people begin to comprehend that wellness is not simply the absence of disease or just the traditional medical treatment of an already-existing disease, they will better understand that disease prevention is pivotal to maintaining a state of wellness.

KEY CONCEPTS

angina
arteriosclerosis
atria
chancre
coronary arteries
jaundice
leukocyte
metastasis
myocardial infarction
plaque
ventricles

Learning Activity

1. Do a risk assessment for stroke and heart attack.

2. Evaluate your risk for STDs and AIDS.

3. List your personal risk factors for developing cancer. Develop a plan to modify your lifestyle to reduce these risk factors.

4. Keep a log for a week and record your cholesterol intake. Develop a plan to reduce your cholesterol intake by 20 percent.

5. Develop an overall disease prevention plan for yourself. Prioritize lifestyle changes you want to make and work on them one at a time. Reevaluate your plan in six months.

Endnotes

1. The Centers for Disease Control and Prevention, *National Center for Chronic Disease. Prevention and Health Promotion* (November 2, 2002). Retrieved December 25, 2002 from http://www.cdc.gov/aging/health_issues.htm#health.

2. "Investing in Health for Economic Development," *The World Health Organization Report on Infectious Disease.* Retrieved from the World Wide Web on December 27, 2002 at http://www.who.int/infectious-disease-report/2002/investinghealth.html.

3. J. Spicher, *Hematology and Lymphatics* (CO: University of Colorado at Colorado Springs, n.d.). Retrieved from the World Wide Web on December 27, 2002 at http://web.uccs.edu/jspiche2/N674/Hematology%20Lymphatics%20outline.pdf.

4. Shands Healthcare Site (FL: University of Florida, n.d.). Retrieved from the World Wide Web on December 27, 2002 at http://www.shands.org/healthy/guide/diet/poison.htm.

5. National Center for Infectious Disease, "Influenza: The Disease." Retrieved from the World Wide Web on December 27, 2002 at http://www.cdc.gov/ncidod/diseases/flu/fluinfo.htm.

6. The United States Department of Health and Human Services. The Food and Drug Administration. "The Five Faces of Hepatitis." Available from http://www.fda/gov/fdac/graphics/1999graphics/hepa.pdf.

7. National Institute of Allergy and Infectious Disease. National Institutes of Health. "An Introduction to Sexually Transmitted Diseases (1999)." Available from http://www.niaid.nih.gov/factsheets/stdinfo.htm.

8. The Conduction System of the Heart. Southern Illinois University School of Medicine, 2000. Available at http://www.siumed.edu/peds/teaching/cardiology/conduct.htm.

9. Ron Winslow, "Coronary Culprit: Heart-Disease Sleuths Identify Prime Suspect: Inflammation of Artery—The Body's Efforts to Repair Irritated Lining of Vessel Can Backfire Disastrously—Plaques Burst Like Popcorn," *Wall Street Journal*, Eastern Edition (October 7, 1999): A1. Can be read online at http://www.gordonresearch.com/coronary_culprit.html.

10. The Heart Center Online at http://www.heartcenteronline.com.

11. The American Heart Association at http://www.americanheart.org.

12. The American Stroke Association at http://www.strokeassociation.org.

13. Liz Applegate, *Runner's World* 37, no. 3 (March 2002): 86. There is some confusion over the idea of drinking alcohol in moderation. Some research concludes that drinking alcohol in moderation could have some cardiac health-related benefits. Moderation is defined as no more than one drink a day for females and no more than two drinks a day for males. However, this moderation policy does not mean you *should* drink alcohol. The use of alcohol in any amount is related to several types of disease. So, if you do not drink now, do not start. If you do drink, drink in moderation.

14. The American Diabetes Association at http://www.diabetes.org.

15. The National Osteoporosis Foundation at http://www.nof.org/.

16. Scott and White Center for Cancer Prevention and Care at http://www.sw.org/cancer/seven_signs.htm.
17. The American Cancer Society at http://www.cancer.org.
18. Ibid.
19. Ibid.
20. Ibid.
21. Joan Borysenko, *A Woman's Book of Life: The Biology, Psychology, and Spirituality of the Feminine Life Cycle* (New York: Riverhead/Penguin Putnam, 1998).
22. Immune Deficiency Foundation. *Patient/Family Handbook: For the Primary Immune Deficiency Diseases* (1993). Retrieved December 25, 2002 from http://www.primaryimmune.org/library/handbook/page89.html.
23. The Wellness Center. Chicago: Loyola University. Retrieved from the World Wide Web on December 27, 2002 at http://www.luc.edu/wellness/welldef/html#vocational.
24. The Nemours Foundation's Center for Children's Health Media. Kids Health for Parents (2002). Retrieved December 25, 2002 from http://kidshealth.org/parent/positive/family/spirituality_p3.html.

12

WELLNESS AND THE REALITY OF AGING AND DEATH

"Where, O death, is your victory?
Where, O death, is your sting?"

—1 Corinthians 15:55 NIV

A wellness perspective implies a positive outlook. So, how can we find anything positive about aging and death? These are the grim inevitabilities of life—no one is exempt. From newborn to octogenarian, we age moment by moment and we all eventually face death. There's an ironic twist to the reality of aging in contemporary society. Life expectancy has continued to increase over the past several decades. However, older adults also suffer poorer physical health and greater activity limitations than any other age group in our country. Thus, the length of our lives is increasing, but the quality of our lives is decreasing.

OBJECTIVES

- Identify what influences the human aging process.

- Discuss the myths and facts of aging.

- Identify the steps and outlooks of aging well.

- Explore perspectives of those dealing with death/grieving.

- Recognize and discuss issues relevant to death.

- Establish a personal spiritual foundation to counter the inevitability of death.

Aging: What's Your Outlook?

Most people don't like to think a lot about aging and death. But a wellness perspective requires that we act rather than react to issues affecting our overall well-being. Ask these questions:

- How are you "preparing" to age?
- What positive thoughts and activities are you pursuing in the areas of body, mind, and spirit as you enter the different stages of your life?
- Have you thought about "what's next" when your heart beats for the last time? Are you at peace about where you will be when you take your last breath?
- What is your personal perception of death? Do you see it as the end of life or as a transition to a new and better life?

It's important to ponder these questions and seek the answers that will lead to personal peace. Every one of our thoughts and actions influences our overall well-being. Are we focusing on positive steps and outlooks as we age, or have we accepted a "what's-the-use" attitude? As we have seen throughout this book, a negative outlook can present a major barrier to positive thoughts and actions—thoughts and actions that not only could add *quantity* (years) to our lives, but could also influence the *quality* of our lives.

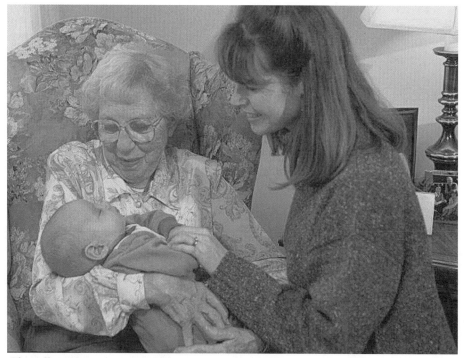

The wellness perspective sees every day as a blessing.

The wellness perspective sees every day as a blessing, but with each day comes a personal wellness responsibility to focus on positive physical, emotional, and spiritual goals to support that blessing. It is never too late in life to experience positive benefits from positive actions. Aging is an ongoing process. It is a wellness responsibility to make that process a positive one through action choices—actions over which we have control.

■ Aging and the Stages of Life

How we perceive aging depends in part on what stage of life we're going through. For young people, aging can't happen fast enough! Have you ever heard the following?

- I can't wait until I turn sixteen and get my driver's license!
- I look forward to being eighteen and voting in the next election.
- I want to be older and be considered an "adult."

As we approach middle age, however, we begin to view aging from a completely different perspective. A sense of human mortality suddenly looms on the horizon and we're not quite so excited about reaching that next birthday! Contrast the previous statements with these from a middle-age perspective:

- This is the twelfth celebration of my twenty-ninth birthday.
- I'm telling you, life is all downhill after forty!

Once past middle age, people in the later stages of life often feel a peaceful sense of acceptance about the aging process. You'll frequently hear comments like these:

- I have led a full life and I am satisfied with what I have accomplished.
- I would not trade these years for any of my earlier years.

Critical to an individual's ability to progress from basically "fighting" the aging process to accepting it is the perception of one's physical, emotional, and/or spiritual well-being at any particular stage. This perspective of peacefully accepting the aging process is much more prevalent in individuals who have aged "well" and who have a sense of purpose in their later years.

Acceptance and peace are not as prevalent for older individuals who, for any number of reasons, have not aged well and do not have a sense of quality in their present stage of life. A negative cycle can occur in the aging process when people have a negative outlook regarding their current or past situations. This negative outlook creates barriers to positive thoughts and actions, which then erodes individual well-being and invites greater risk into the aging process.

■ The Stages of Psychosocial Development

Psychologist Erik Erikson presented a model of psychosocial development built around eight stages in the life cycle. He saw each stage as involving certain "tasks" to be mastered, including basic social skills and the ability to adapt to one's changing environment. The first five stages encompass the time from infancy to adolescence. The last three stages are young adulthood, middle or mature adulthood, and late adulthood.

- Young adulthood is expected to be a time of developing relationships and a sense of personal intimacy.

- Middle adulthood focuses on generativity, a concern for the next generation. The purpose of middle adulthood is to contribute, guide, teach, and provide positive models to members of that future generation.

- Erikson's late adulthood stage focuses on what he terms "ego integrity," defined as a need to be aware of the meaning and limitations of one's life.[1]

In their book, *The Graying of America*, authors Donald and Barry Kausler cite research indicating that a sense of generativity is just as prevalent in the older adult stage as it is in the middle adulthood stage. The authors see **generativity** as concern for the next generation and a desire to help guide that generation. Maintaining this sense of purpose and mentoring younger people is related to higher degrees of life satisfaction in older adults.[2] This is an important consideration when coming into contact with older adults. The older adults will benefit from sharing their experiences and mentoring the younger generation. The younger generation will also benefit, gaining insight and direction from those who have walked before them.

GENERATIVITY: Concern for the next generation of humanity and a desire to guide that generation; framing one's goals in life to benefit family, work, and community, ensuring society's continuation.

■ Aging Well

We've heard the terms "aging well" or "successful aging," but what sets apart someone who has "aged successfully" from someone who has not "aged well"?

A longitudinal study at Duke University stated that normal aging is usually accompanied by a decline in both mental and physical functioning. The report also stated that what they classified as a "substantial" minority of individuals were exceptions to this

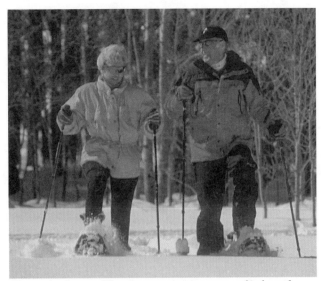

Those who "age well" strive to maintain a sense of independence.

common decline, indicating that mental and physical decline may not be directly related to the aging process. This suggests there may be factors other than aging that influence a decline or lack of decline in mental and physical functioning.[3]

In *Successful Aging*, authors John W. Rowe and Robert L. Kahn define the term "successful aging" as it relates to three key areas of life. They suggest that successful aging involves these abilities:[4]

1. Maintain a low risk of disease and disease-related disabilities.

   - taking steps to reduce the presence of disease risk factors

   - developing an awareness of the signs and symptoms of disease

   - taking necessary steps when noticing these signs, such as changing related lifestyle habits

   - developing an awareness of new medical alternatives to deal with threatening conditions

2. Maintain high mental and physical functioning.

   - striving to maintain a sense of independence

   - overcoming unrealistic fears of losing this independence (only 10 percent of individuals over sixty-five have Alzheimer's disease and only about 5 percent of adults over sixty-five are confined to nursing homes)

- staying mentally active, challenging the mind (most mental capacity losses come very late in life; many older adults are not significantly affected by even minor losses of mental ability)

- maintaining physical activity (declining physical ability is termed both inevitable and preventable; more often it is preventable)

3. Maintain an active engagement with life.

- taking part in "happy" activities

- maintaining close relationships with others (social networking has been related to longevity)

- seeking meaningful and purposeful activities (activities seen as being productive in some way)

> Successful aging includes maintaining and developing one's spiritual foundation (church, church groups, prayer).

Each of these areas should harmonize in supporting the goal of successful aging. While Rowe and Kahn focus primarily on the physical and emotional dimensions of well-being as people age, we would include the importance of fostering a Christian worldview. Spiritual well-being is a key aspect of overall well-being. Successful aging includes maintaining and developing one's spiritual foundation (church, church groups, prayer). A strong spiritual foundation offers a sense of peace, not only about the aging process itself, but also about the final stage of life—making the transition from a temporal life to an eternal life.

Cultivating a positive outlook on aging means realizing we have personal choices to make and actions to take if we are going to "age successfully." Once we have the right mind-set, it then becomes our personal wellness responsibility to make positive personal choices in these areas, as well as to be supportive of others attempting to make positive changes in their lives.

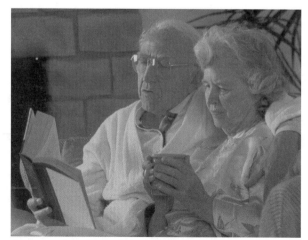

A strong spiritual foundation offers a sense of peace.

■ The Myths of Aging

In contrast to those who age successfully, there are those who succumb to misconceptions about the aging process. Myths and "old wives' tales" persist on the subject of aging and its supposed "debilitations." Rowe and Kahn highlight some of the more glaring myths, along with evidence to refute these myths:[5]

Myth: To be old is to be sick.

Fact: Older Americans are generally healthy. The percentage of older adults (over sixty-five years of age) reported with disabilities, high blood pressure, high cholesterol levels, and dental problems has declined significantly over the past thirty years.

Myth: The elderly cannot broaden or sharpen their minds.

Fact: Research has shown that the aged brain is capable of making new connections, absorbing new data, acquiring new skills, and improving short-term memory with practice. The speed of learning does slow with age.

Myth: By the time you reach old age, it is too late to attempt to reduce health risks and take positive steps toward better health.

Fact: Research has demonstrated that it is almost never too late to take healthy steps to improve health, including exercise, good nutrition, and eliminating health risks like smoking.

Myth: As we advance in age, heredity totally accounts for the rate of decline in the body's functions.

Fact: There is a meaningful connection between aging and genetics, but the role of genetics has been overstated. Family habits and environment are important influences on disease prevention, as are maintaining high physical and mental functioning and actively engaging in strong interpersonal relationships.

Myth: The elderly are not interested in sex or able to participate in sexual activity.

Fact: Sexual activity does decrease with age, beginning around the age of fifty. But there are significant individual differences in this aspect of life. Research indicates that at age sixty-eight, approximately 70 percent of males are sexually active on a regular basis. For older women, sexual activity is mainly dependent on the availability of an appropriate partner. A basic human need for affection and physical contact persists throughout all stages of life.

Myth: Elderly people are unproductive.

Fact: Over two-thirds of older men and women either work for pay or work as volunteers. Others provide informal assistance to community, church, and/or neighborhood concerns and causes. Often older workers are not given the same consideration for paid employment opportunities as younger workers are.

To these myths, Kausler and Kausler add the myth that people over age sixty-five are incapacitated and are incapable of functioning on their own. In fact, 90 percent of those over sixty-five years of age function on their own and are capable of carrying out the activities of daily living.[6]

Table 12.1. Statistics on Aging

Largest percentages of populations	Projected greatest increases in population	Life expectancy at birth in 2000
Ages 65 and Older in 2000:	65 and older, 2000 - 2030	for various countries (in years):
Italy: 18.1 percent	Singapore: 372 percent	Japan: 80.7
Greece: 17.3	Malaysia: 277	Australia: 79.8
Sweden: 17.3	Colombia: 258	Canada: 79.4
Japan: 17.0	Costa Rica: 250	Italy: 79.0
Spain: 16.9	Philippines: 240	France: 78.8
Belgium: 16.8	Indonesia: 240	Israel: 78.6
Bulgaria: 16.5	Mexico: 227	United Kingdom: 77.7
Germany: 16.2	South Korea: 216	Germany: 77.4
France: 16.0	Egypt: 210	United States: 77.1
United Kingdom: 15.7	Bangladesh: 207	Mexico: 71.5
United States: 12.6	United States: 102	Russia: 67.2
		Egypt: 63.3
		Brazil: 62.9
		Pakistan: 61.1
		Kenya: 48.0
		Zimbabwe: 37.8

Source: Genaro C. Armas (AP), "An Aging World Population Challenges Nations," *The Indianapolis Star,* 12 December 2001, A11, citing the U.S. Census Bureau, National Institute on Aging.

Table 12.2, Population Changes in the United States

Age Groups with the largest population change from 1990 – 2000

45 – 54	49.4 percent increase
85 – up	37.6
55 – 59	27.9
75 – 84	22.9

Growth Rate of 85 and older population in the United States

1980	2.24 million
1990	3.08 million
2000	4.24 million

Source: Adapted from "An Aging World: 2001," November 2001. Issued by the U.S. Department of Health and Human Services, National Institute of Health, National Institute on Aging, in conjunction with the U.S. Department of Commerce, Economics and Statistics Administration, Bureau of the Census.

■ Quality v. Quantity of Life

Since 1900, the overall life expectancy of individuals in the United States has dramatically increased. A primary reason for this marked increase is a reduction in infant death rates, along with improvements in medical science and treatment methods. The older population has also increased its overall life expectancy. In 1900, individuals who reached the age of seventy-five could expect to live an additional eight years. In 2000 those at age seventy-five could expect an additional twelve years of life.[7]

Life expectancy seems to be influenced by many variables, including gender, race, occupation, geographical location within the United States, and geographical location globally. Statistics support that those living in underdeveloped, third-world countries generally have a lower life expectancy than those who live in industrialized, technologically advanced countries.

GERONTOLOGY: The study of aging and the problems associated with aging.

When we speak of life expectancy, the major emphasis is often given to the number of years an individual may expect to live — the *quantity* of years. Naturally, that is a positive goal and an expected outcome of the wellness lifestyle. However, as we saw in the introduction of this chapter,

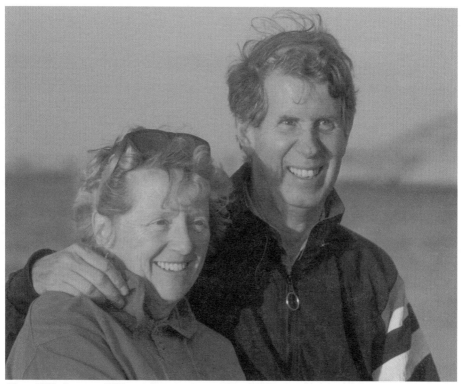

Since 1900, the overall life expectancy of people in the United States has dramatically increased.

the *quality* of life at any given stage is just as important as the number of days we live. This is as true for those in the later stages of life as for those in the early stages of life. In seeking to determine the quality of your life, ask these questions:

- Did you have a good day today?
- Are you looking forward to tomorrow?

The answers to these questions will speak volumes about the perceived quality of your life. What factors contribute to a "Yes" answer by older adults? This is one of the concerns of gerontologists. **Gerontology** is the study of aging and the problems associated with aging. Gerontologists and others who study aging have determined that the presence or absence of certain factors is directly related to quality of life in older adults.

■ Religion

A key point of this text is the importance of a spiritual foundation to overall well-being. Faith can powerfully affect our attitudes and direct our actions in life. A strong faith is instrumental in overcoming the sense of helplessness that many older people feel. Helplessness fosters a "what's-the-use" outlook on life, which leads to apathy toward taking positive physical, emotional, or spiritual actions.

Fortunately, religion is important to most people in the later stages of life. Between 60 and 95 percent of the elderly population pray daily and are likely to use prayer as a means of coping with stress. Elderly individuals who are involved in religious activities report a more positive outlook on life and greater personal satisfaction than do those who are not involved in religious activities.

Why, then, does church attendance decline in the elderly population? Sadly, this has nothing to do with a decrease in their level of faith. Instead, it is commonly related to factors that limit mobility, such as poor health, bad weather, and a lack of transportation.[8]

■ Social Support

A sense of connectedness with other people is important to the well-being of all individuals, particularly to that of older adults. Rowe and Kahn report four major findings concerning connectedness as it relates to older adults:[9]

1. Isolation is a risk factor for poor health. On the average, older adults who participate in social relationships (phone calls, visits, church activities, community groups) are healthier than people who lack these contacts. The frequency of these contacts and the contributions made are strong predictors of well-being.
2. Support can come in many forms—emotional, physical, and spiritual.
3. Support can actually reduce some of the health-related effects of aging.
4. The type of support is not carved in stone. The effectiveness of support depends on the person, the situation, and/or the individual needs involved.

Long past midnight, hours before dawn
I jump up from my bed, pull my longjohns on.
Peeking out the window, the snow has started to fall.
Slipping on my overalls, I race quickly down the hall.
Rushing to the closet, grasping my old wrap,
I throw it over my shoulder, give the button a snap.
Working all ten fingers, through the holes of much worn mitts,
I stick my feet into the boots that thankfully still fit.
Faster than is possible, I head straight for the door.
Behind me I am dragging a sled from years before.
The wind is loud and howling, snow is blowing all around.
Already what has fallen has covered the ground.
Tramping through the deepness, only my footprints to see,
I head straight for the meadow, the hill is waiting for me.
A few more steps, I reach my goal, as always in the past
I'll be the first to sled this hill, and I'll be the very last.
Breathing in the cool air, I witness the year's first snow.
Perhaps this is my favorite spot, in all the sights I know.
Holding tight in a world of silence, I shove off with my feet.
Wind is picking up my hair, snow hits against my teeth.
Traveling faster and faster, I struggle not to tip.
Stretching out my snow-damp legs, I lean from hip to hip.
What a big delight, this morn has given thee.
As all years before have done, when it's just this hill and me.
Now if I do my best to hurry, I can take another run.
The sun will soon be rising, the day will have begun.
But before that can happen, I must be back in bed.
For whatever would the children think . . .
. . . if they knew Grandma used their sled!

—Betty J. Reid

Source: Used by permission of Betty J. Reid. "The Hill" first appeared in *Chicken Soup for the Unsinkable Soul*, eds. Jack Canfield and Mark Victor Hansen (Deerfield Beach, FL: Health Communications, Inc., 1999), 302-03. Cited 17 April 2000 from cs-html-weekday-reply@SoupServer.com.

Related to social connectedness is what Kausler and Kausler call the "activity theory." This theory proposes that older adults continue as much as possible the activities of middle age, finding alternatives to those they cannot continue because of decreased abilities. These activities fall into three classifications and are rated in the order of their reported level of life satisfaction:[10]

1. Informal Activity: Activities with family, friends, and neighbors
2. Formal Activity: Participating in voluntary organizations
3. Solitary Activity: Leisure pursuits and the responsibility of maintaining a household

■ Disease Prevention

Taking steps to prevent disease or reduce the risk factors for disease can positively affect the quality and quantity of life. Three factors generally helpful in reducing the risk of chronic diseases are: (1) having a high lung function, (2) being of normal weight, and (3) participating in either moderate or strenuous exercise.

> As activity declines, the elderly can experience a feeling of weakness, which then leads to less activity and increased reports of weakness.

For obvious reasons, exercise can assist in increasing lung function and reducing weight. Exercise in the correct form and the correct amount can increase individual strength, flexibility, and stamina in elderly adults. It is not far-fetched to say that in the older population a prescription for exercise is just as important as a prescription for medication.[11]

Other barriers to successful aging include obesity, high blood pressure, high

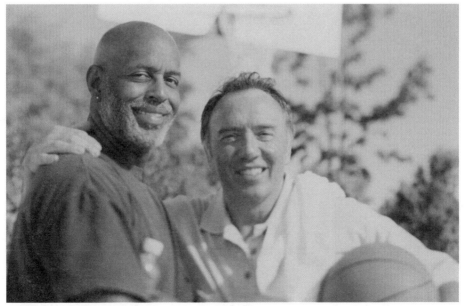

Exercise can increase strength, flexibility, and stamina.

levels of cholesterol, and a lack of mental alertness.[12] Exercise and moderate physical activity again can positively influence these risk factors. Exercise helps to counter a frequently seen negative spiral that affects both the quality and quantity of life in older adults. As activity declines, the elderly can experience a feeling of weakness, which then leads to less activity and increased reports of weakness. This negative spiral invites a sedentary lifestyle that feeds on dependency, loneliness, and isolation.

Another potentially threatening situation arises from overmedication. Approximately 25 percent of older adults take three or more prescription medicines. The dangers of overmedication include serious side effects and drug interaction. Physicians should carefully and regularly monitor the medications of their elderly patients, assessing any lifestyle changes related to the effectiveness of these drugs.[13]

■ Retirement Planning the Wellness Way

The decision to retire can be one of the most stressful decisions an older person will make. Whether the decision is voluntary or involuntary will in large part determine the retiree's attitude and outlook toward retirement. Contingent on how well one adjusts to retirement is the financial planning that precedes the decision to retire. Will the retiree be able to enjoy a satisfactory lifestyle in retirement? Preplanning or *acting* to take steps before retirement instead of *reacting* to the sudden reality of retirement will help facilitate a successful transition.

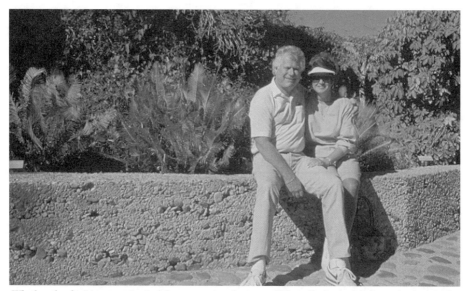

Whether the decision to retire is voluntary or involuntary will largely determine the retiree's attitude and outlook toward retirement.

Wellness retirement planning looks at retirement as it relates to physical, emotional, and spiritual well-being. Ask these questions:

- What steps are you currently taking to ensure good physical health for your future retirement years?
- What steps are you currently taking to ensure a positive attitude and outlook in your future years?
- What steps are you currently taking to develop a stronger spiritual foundation for your future?

These steps may be instrumental in helping to plan for retirement *the wellness way*. The most comprehensive financial plan will be of little value if you arrive at the retirement stage of life in a negative wellness condition—or if you fail even to reach retirement.

■ "I Wish I Would've" . . . Measuring Life Satisfaction

How do you measure satisfaction in life? For those in the later stages, satisfaction can be measured by (1) their positive experiences, (2) the people they have impacted or who have influenced them, and (3) the belief that they have made a positive contribution to society. It is never too late to start developing goals in all of these areas. Taking steps now will help you avoid an "I-wish-I-would've" attitude later.

What better way to prepare for your own later years than by interacting with the elderly today? Begin making time to get to know older people. As we saw earlier in this chapter, not only will you benefit from their experience and wisdom, but you also will help them feel a sense of purpose as they mentor you. Because of prevailing myths and misunderstandings, this population is often the most forgotten population in our society. Time with these individuals is often sacrificed to "other" priorities in life. Reevaluate these priorities and consider spending time with some elderly individuals around you. As you get to know these individuals, you may hear some of the same stories or encounter other communication or physical issues. Nevertheless, spending time with elderly family members, church members, and/or community members may provide some of the most rewarding times you will ever experience. Doing for others in need can provide positive benefits and increased well-being for all of those involved in that contact.

Death: The Final Frontier?

■ Accept or Fight?

Nobody likes to talk about death and dying. It's something we tend to avoid in normal conversation. However, a wellness perspective requires us to look closely at death issues as they impact physical, emotional, and spiritual well-being.

Earlier in this chapter, we looked at aging and Erik Erikson's eight stages of life, particularly the last three (adult) stages. In *Human Relations: A Game Plan for Improving Personal Adjustment*, author and psychologist Loren Ford expands the life-stage theory and proposes the inclusion of death in the life cycle.[14] This somewhat reflects the thinking of the past, when death was accepted as an inevitable and "normal" aspect of life. Today, however, there seems to be more of a focus on "fighting" death. **Cryonics** is one extreme example of this focus. Cryonics is the science of freezing a dead, diseased human body with the intent of reanimating the corpse at a future time, when a cure for the disease has been found.

> **CRYONICS:** The science of freezing a dead, diseased human body with the intent of reanimating the corpse at a future time, when a cure for the fatal disease has been found.

As you consider whether to accept or fight death, it might be helpful to ponder these questions from a Christian worldview:

- Is death the end of earthly life, or merely a transition to an eternal life?
- Do you know how to access that eternal life?
- Do you feel secure about your place in eternity?
- What is the nature of your relationship with Jesus Christ?

Please thoughtfully and prayerfully evaluate your responses to these questions, seeking a level of spiritual peace and comfort. If these questions cause you to feel uncomfortable, consider this discomfort a sign that you need to act immediately to deal with your death issues. Don't stop until your comfort level is aligned with the general principles of wellness—emotionally, physically, and spiritually. This includes assuming responsibility for your death issues and taking appropriate action steps instead of leaving these issues to chance.

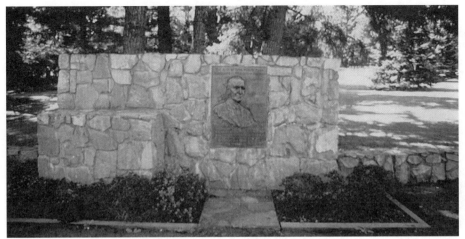

Is death the end of earthly life, or merely a transition to an eternal life?

■ The Stages of Death

You may have had the opportunity to spend time with a terminally ill person, perhaps a family member. If so, you probably noticed an emotional progression as this person came to grips with impending death. *On Death and Dying* by Elisabeth Kubler-Ross details five stages as a terminally ill patient approaches death:[15]

1. Anger—A nearly universal response as the reality of the situation becomes apparent. Can often result in the outlook that "Life is not fair."
2. Denial—Disbelief that this is actually happening, specifically that "this is happening to *me*."
3. Depression—Reality sets in. Much stronger than ordinary sadness, depression can overwhelm a terminally ill person, clouding judgment and contributing to even further deterioration of health.
4. Bargaining—A desperate technique to try to change the situation. Promising, usually to God, to take positive actions in the future or to refrain from future negative actions.
5. Acceptance—After passing through all of the other stages— perhaps more than once—finally accepting the reality and inevitability of the situation.

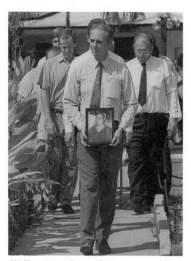

Wellness involves taking responsibility for your death issues.

As you may have noted in your own experience with a terminally ill person, these stages can appear in no particular sequence, varying from person to person. People may even return several times to one or more stages during the course of their illness.

■ What About Hope?

An important consideration when you are involved with a terminally ill individual is how long you or the individual should hold out hope for recovery. When do you move into acceptance and "letting go"? This is not an easy decision. Without hope, a person's sense of purpose and desire to live can be extinguished. Stories abound of gravely ill people far outliving the predicted "timetable" of their impending deaths—because they had hope, purpose, and a positive attitude.

In dealing with the issue of hope, consider first and foremost the reasonable wishes of the terminally ill individual. Seek out and heed the advice of the medical personnel involved. Consult with them when you find information or have suggestions that you think might be helpful to the situation. Pray for wisdom and guidance as you work to make decisions in this area. A unified effort to progress from *support through hope* to *peaceful support through letting go* should be the focus of all those involved in the care and support of the terminally ill person.

■ The Stages of Grief

No matter how well prepared you are for the death of a loved one, no matter how secure you feel about your "definition" of death, you still must deal with a deep void once that person has died. Just as the terminally ill person experiences stages in coming to grips with approaching death, so too does the grieving survivor. These stages include:

- Denial—Disbelief that a family member or friend is terminally ill, that death is near, or that death has occurred.

- Anger—This is similar to the anger of the terminally ill individual, along with the feeling that "Life is not fair." Questions such as "Why this person?" and "Why now?" often become evident during this stage.

- Depression—Different from the normal sadness expected over the loss of a close friend or family, depression lasts for an extended period of time and may signal the need for professional assistance.

- Acceptance—Accepting that the loss is real and that a loved one has made the transition from a physical existence to a spiritual existence.

It is important to remember that grieving can occur before the death of the loved one. This pre-death grief can involve some of the same emotions present during the normal post-death grieving process. Pre-death grief also may include:

- Resentment—The result of the additional responsibilities, worries, and/or separation the illness causes.

- Guilt—Feeling responsible for the illness or for not having done enough to respond to the illness.[16]

In coping with any kind of grief, a strong spiritual foundation is especially helpful in making the transition to peaceful acceptance. This spiritual support is mirrored in such comforting Scriptures as Psalm 34:18a: *"The Lord is close to those whose hearts are breaking."*

■ "A Time to Every Purpose"

The stages of grief present opportunities for the survivor to address issues underlying the loss of a loved one. In that sense, grief serves specific purposes. Loren Ford explains that grieving or mourning helps the survivor to:

- Accept the reality of the loss. Realizing that the loved one will not be returning is an intensely emotional process.

- Work through the pain of grief. Even if the survivor's faith is strong and based on the assurance that the loved one is in a better place, the survivor still must deal with the void that person leaves in this physical world.

- Adjust to a new environment that will not include the deceased. This adjustment can involve coming to grips with new roles and responsibilities previously filled by the deceased. The survivor may need to seek support in dealing with decisions and direction.

- Emotionally relocate the deceased individual and move on with life. This does not mean giving up thoughts and memories of the deceased, but finding an appropriate place for the deceased in the survivor's emotional life. The turning point occurs when the survivor accepts that while the physical person is gone, the spiritual person lives on.[17]

The grieving process varies from person to person. However, we are including a general time frame below, along with the emotions characteristic of each stage.

- The first two or three days:

  A time of strong grief and possibly shock and/or denial. The survivor may feel numb or overwhelmed by having to deal with funeral arrangements and other complex decisions at a time of vulnerability.

- The first two or three weeks:

  During this time, survivors commonly experience loss of appetite, difficulty focusing, inability to sleep, and a tendency to cry.

- The first three or four months:

  In this time frame, many support people return to their own lives, leaving the survivor to handle things alone. Survivors often feel vulnerable, even abandoned. Support during this time is especially meaningful. Some survivors require eight months to a year before the intensity of their loss diminishes.

- The first two or three years:

  The survivor may find holidays and special anniversary dates difficult to handle. The one-year mark seems to be an important turning point regarding healing and the ability to move on with life. However, it is not uncommon for survivors to have emotional reactions during special times of the year.[18]

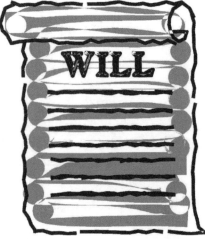

■ Proactive Planning

Making plans relevant to one's passing is not a normal topic of family conversation. Because of our general reluctance to discuss death and death issues, too many times we make no "proactive" plans at all. Instead, many families confronted with the death of a loved one respond in a "reactive" way, after the fact. This is an especially emotional and stressful time to be making the complex decisions necessary— funeral arrangements and otherwise. As evident in the time table above, it is during the early days after a death that the survivors have the most difficulty focusing on the decisions they have to make. Proactive planning—discussing important topics related to death and making decisions ahead of time—can save stress on the part of the survivors and can better ensure that the family follows the desires of the deceased. Proactive planning as it relates to death involves four areas.

> Proactive planning—discussing important topics related to death and making decisions ahead of time—can save stress on the part of the survivors and can better ensure that the family follows the desires of the deceased.

■ Traditional Will

A will provides the legal authority for the distribution of material assets and the care of any remaining dependent family members. Even if others are aware of a family's wishes and needs, without legal documentation these wishes and needs cannot be recognized. This means that many of the decisions for distributing assets or even relocating family members will come under the authority of the court systems. The unwillingness to plan in advance for these contingencies potentially deprives the family of what the deceased may have intended them to have. Equally disturbing is the mind-set that only the elderly need wills. This is another barrier to positive actions related to the preparation of a family will.

> **LIVING WILL:** A legal document giving directives for medical decisions should the person become incapable of making such decisions.

■ Living Will and Power of Attorney

Either a **living will** or a **power of attorney** will designate a person as a decision-maker for medical decisions when the ill or injured individual is not capable of making those decisions. The specific document required and the scope of that document can vary from state to state, so it is important for you and your family to investigate and become familiar with your state's regulations. Designating a decision-maker in advance and "putting in writing" your choices

> **POWER OF ATTORNEY:** A legal document that designates someone other than the grantor to make decisions should the grantor become incapacitated.

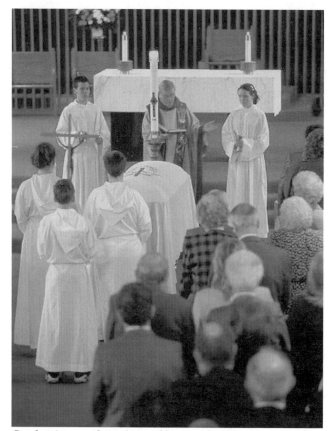

Preplanning your funeral can add to your family's peace of mind.

about treatment options will spare your family great stress during an already stressful time.

■ Organ donation

Thousands of people around the country are awaiting organ transplant surgery, a surgery that may add to the quantity and quality of their lives. Unfortunately, while these individuals wait, many potential organ donors are lost because they either did not make a decision regarding this option or they failed to make their decision known to others. This is, of course, a personal choice, but one that should be discussed in advance. To authorize the use of your organs for organ transplants, make your personal wishes known and be assured that you have been clearly understood. It may not matter that you carry an organ donation card or have indicated on your driver's license that you wish to be an organ donor—in most states, the family makes the final decision regarding organ donation. If you have not clearly communicated to them your decision in this matter, they may overrule your wishes.

■ Funeral Preplanning

Making decisions in advance and preplanning your funeral allow you to customize your funeral or memorial service—both for your own peace of mind and for that of your family. Funeral preplanning, like the previous three topics, is not an easy subject to discuss. By focusing on the positive aspects, however, you can make your wishes known, set limits and express preferences, share family members' feelings, and take comfort in their concern and input. Preplanning will help to lighten the load your family will face at your death, eliminating at least some of the stress during a very stressful time. Knowing that they have had a part in the funeral preplanning also will offer the family some release from difficult emotions, something that brings balance and peace of mind.

As you make decisions in these areas, be sure that family members are aware of your plans and decisions, that they accept your decisions, and that they know where to find supporting documentation when necessary.

■ Home Hospice: The Personal Touch

Excerpt 12.2, Hospice Statistics

Only 17 percent of terminally ill people die at home. But a Yale University School of Medicine study suggests that if people were given a choice, that number would be 2.5 times higher.

Of those who die somewhere other than home, two-thirds of people now die in hospitals and the rest in nursing homes, a practice that may ignore the wishes of terminally ill patients.

A study of 246 recently hospitalized patients showed that while 48 percent would prefer to die in a hospital, 43 percent preferred home care. Those who chose home care generally said they wanted to be near their families, while those who preferred hospital care said they didn't know if they could get adequate end-of-life care at home and they did not want to be a burden to their families.

Source: Based on Terri R. Fried, Carol van Doorn, et al., "Older Persons' Preference for Site of Terminal Care," *Annals of Internal Medicine* 131 (20 July 1999): 109-12.

Many individuals die in hospitals or other medical facilities away from their homes. These institutional settings may inhibit consistent visitation from family members and other people important to the patient. Terminally ill people often express the desire to die in the personal setting of their homes, with family and friends nearby. Institutions may provide modern technology and medicine that can extend the *quantity* (days) of life, but they often sacrifice the patient's dignity and *quality* of life in the process.

Home hospice services can provide a way to keep the dying at home in a more comfortable environment and closer to family members. Hospice service provides **palliative care,** an emphasis of which is to maintain the quality and

> **PALLIATIVE CARE:** Seeks to address all the symptoms of illness, with the aim of promoting comfort, dignity, and the best possible quality of life for patients and their families.

dignity of the client's remaining life. Services are centered on daily living needs, medications to reduce pain, support contacts for spiritual and social needs, and support and educational services for family members. Home hospice care may be an important option to consider if or when you or a family member face a terminal illness. Be sure to gather

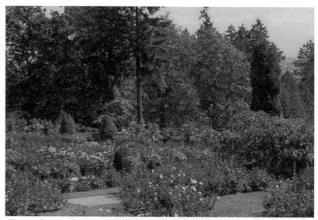

Every day in this worldly life is a gift from God, but our days on earth are numbered.

information on the home hospice organizations in your area as you proactively plan for the future.

■ In Advance

In looking at the major areas of preplanning as it relates to death issues, you came across the phrase "in advance" several times. If you put all of this into a spiritual context, you quickly realize that when it comes to physical death, no one on earth knows what "in advance" might mean. Every day in this worldly life is a gift from God, but our days on earth are numbered.

Be sure of your spiritual foundations and your answers to the questions at the beginning of this section on death and dying. If you have any doubts or misgivings, resolve them now. Do not leave this matter to chance or relegate it to something you will do "when you get around to it." As you deal with passing from this world—yourself or someone close to you—remember that God's Word offers the strongest building blocks to your spiritual foundation, giving you peace and understanding whenever you approach the subject of death.

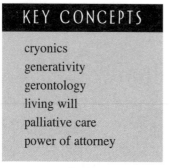

KEY CONCEPTS

cryonics
generativity
gerontology
living will
palliative care
power of attorney

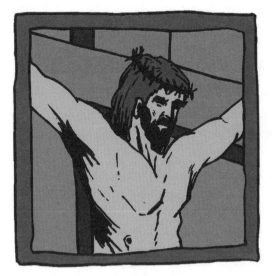

"So that anyone who believes in me will have eternal life."
John 3:15

"Because of his kindness you have been saved through trusting Christ."
Ephesians 2:8

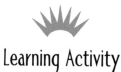

Learning Activity

1. A focus important in the middle and later adult stages of life is a concern for future generations and a desire to teach and guide them.

   a. Considering that perspective, what can you do to guide or teach people with whom you come into contact in either your professional or personal environments?

   _____

   _____

   _____

   _____

   b. Considering the elderly population around you, what elderly individuals (family, church members, neighbors) could you commit to spending time with, helping them to meet a need in their lives?

   _____

   _____

   _____

   _____

   c. Considering your own aging process, what outlooks and action steps can you initiate now to help build a positive personal foundation of wellness?

   Physical actions:

   _____

   _____

   _____

   _____

Emotional outlooks:

_____

_____

_____

_____

Spiritual foundations:

_____

_____

_____

_____

2. With which family members do you need to discuss the topics of wills, living wills, organ donation, and/or funeral preplanning?

_____

_____

_____

_____

3. What questions do you personally need to answer in order to have peace of mind concerning the issues of death and dying (either your own death or the death of a loved one)?

_____

_____

_____

_____

4. Who might be able to help you explore and develop answers to any of the above questions?

_____

_____

_____

_____

Additional Activities and Resources

1. How have any "myths of aging" influenced your relationships or contacts with elderly individuals? How have these myths influenced your responses to them or your decisions about them? How have any of these myths influenced decisions related to your own aging process?

   _____

   _____

   _____

   _____

2. What are some of your primary fears or concerns about death (either your own death or the death of someone close to you)? What steps can you take to help deal with these fears?

   _____

   _____

   _____

   _____

3. Review the following resources in order to gain more information about aging and death:

   www.aoa.dhhs.gov

   www.griefnet.org

Endnotes

1. Barbara C. Matchette and Sarah Anders, "Socialization," in *Sociology: A Christian Approach for Changing the World*, ed. Cynthia B. Tweedell (Marion, IN: Triangle Publishing, 2002), 70-71.
2. Donald H. Kausler and Barry C. Kausler, *The Graying of America: An Encyclopedia of Aging, Health, Mind, and Behavior* (Urbana, IL: University of Illinois Press, 1969), 144.
3. Ibid., 108-09.
4. John W. Rowe and Robert L. Kahn, *Successful Aging* (New York: Dell, 1998), 41-48.
5. Ibid., 13-38.
6. Kausler and Kausler, *The Graying of America*, 205.
7. Ibid., 174.
8. Ibid., 257-58.
9. Rowe and Kahn, *Successful Aging*, 163-66.
10. Kausler and Kausler, *The Graying of America*, 11.
11. Ibid., 124.
12. Rowe and Kahn, *Successful Aging*, 61-63.
13. Kausler and Kausler, *The Graying of America*, 219.
14. Loren Ford, *Human Relations: A Game Plan for Improving Personal Adjustment*, 2nd ed. (Upper Saddle River, NJ: Prentice Hall, 2001), 253.
15. Elisabeth Kubler-Ross, *On Death and Dying* (New York: Macmillan, 1969), 38-137.
16. Ibid., 157-61.
17. Ford, *Human Relations*, 254.
18. Ibid.

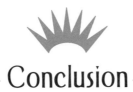

Conclusion

WELLNESS: PUTTING IT ALL TOGETHER

"Be very careful, then, how you live—not as unwise but as wise,
making the most of every opportunity . . ."

—Ephesians 5:15-16

Congratulations! You have made it to the final chapter of this book. You now should have a very clear understanding of wellness as a multifaceted concept. Furthermore, you should recognize that while wellness in large part is individual and personal, certain indicators signal good or poor states of wellness. The elements of wellness are interrelated and must be approached in totality and not solely on an item-by-item basis. However, you *can* assess each wellness element and determine your level of wellness.

Throughout this text we have given you ample opportunities to perform several wellness assessment tests. The results of these tests are very personal and may or may not be considered positive. However, a healthy way to approach the assessments is to consider all of the results to be positive. Even if the assessments indicate a poor state of wellness in one or more areas, view these results as a positive motivator to improve in those particular areas. If the assessments indicate a good state of wellness, view that as a positive reinforcement of what you already are doing.

Promoting Change through Goals

This brings us to an important wellness issue—change. We have stressed throughout this text that change is an ever-present reality in our lives. How we approach and accept/reject these changes determines our ongoing state of wellness. After reading this text, it should be evident that wellness doesn't "just happen." It requires effort and careful attention. We cannot achieve or maintain wellness without paying close attention to each of the components of wholistic wellness. That brings us back to change. As a result of reading this text, completing course requirements, and performing the assessment tests, what areas of your life need change? What areas of your personal wholistic wellness are in need of attention? What are you going to do now: Accept the challenge of change or reject it?

■ Setting Goals

When you consider change, the first thing you usually ask is this: "What needs to change?" Once you have determined what to change, you then need to decide how to get from "where you are" to "where you want to be." The "where you want to be" is a goal.

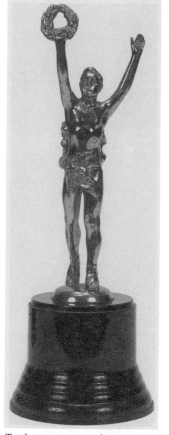

To change, you must have a goal.

To successfully change, you must have a goal. Without a goal, progress is at best the result of chance. Without a clearly defined goal, it is nearly impossible to develop an effective personal wellness plan. A study of wellness means very little if you do not develop personal goals for change. This text not only has allowed you to assess several different areas of wellness, but it also has taught you how to change. You have learned what steps are necessary to improve your personal wellness. You even have been given some sample wellness goals as a way to help you determine your own goals. However, it is important to remember that personal wholistic wellness is ongoing and not simply a matter of attaining a goal. It would be foolish to think that once you have made a friend, secured a new job, lost ten pounds, and read the Bible that you would suddenly arrive at social, occupational, physical, and spiritual wellness.

When you set goals, realize that *attaining* the goal is not the primary purpose of wellness. Actually, *pursuing* and *maintaining* the goal offers a better picture of ongoing wholistic wellness.

> When you set goals, realize that *attaining* the goal is not the primary purpose of wellness.

Nonetheless, you continually need to change/adapt/fine-tune aspects of your personal wellness. How do you effect change? How do you set goals? Because wholistic wellness is so personal, many people already have goals in mind. If you don't currently have goals, consider your results on some of the assessment tests. The results should give you some ideas for specific goals. The key is to take the goals you have in mind and transform them into a change in behavior that will result in meeting your goals.

■ Four Criteria

For change to be effective, a goal must meet four criteria:

1. It must be measurable.
2. It must be specific.
3. It must be realistic.
4. It must be dependent on you.

First of all, is the goal measurable? If it isn't measurable, you could work

Wellness doesn't "just happen." It requires effort and careful attention.

the rest of your life trying to reach the unreachable. Common wellness goals that are *not* measurable include these:

> 1. "I want to be more spiritual."
> 2. "I want to get in better shape."
> 3. "I don't want to be an emotional train wreck."

While these "goals" are good, they are not measurable. How do you define "more" or "better"? To have measurable goals, be specific. Let's modify the above examples to make them more specific and measurable:

> 1. "I want to attend church three times per month and Bible study once a week."
> 2. "I want to be able to walk a mile in ten minutes."
> 3. "I want to learn and practice three new emotional coping mechanisms."

Do you see the difference? Think in measurable and specific terms. Of course, this will involve more effort and may involve more goal setting. That is okay. It is far more likely you will improve each of the components of wellness if you set several goals instead of just saying, "I want to be in a better state of wellness." The more goals you have, the more likely you are to improve specific components of wellness. If your only goal is to improve wholistic wellness, you will never reach it, because it is not a measurable or specific goal. Remember that wellness depends on the ability to change. Goals should promote changes that will lead to success.

There are two other criteria for effective goal setting. Goals must be realistic and should not be dependent upon the actions of others. A bad physical wellness goal would be to say, "I want to beat Sally in a 500 m swim." The outcome of that goal is beyond your total control—it is at least in part dependent upon Sally. A better goal would be to say, "I want to develop my aerobic fitness and swimming skill to the point that I can swim 500 m in 'x' amount of time." The goal is no longer dependent upon someone else.

Goals also must be realistic. You cannot have an occupational goal of being hired by Friday and promoted by the end of next month. That simply is not realistic.

While outrageous goals may sound impressive, they actually become a deterrent to improvement the longer you go without realizing the goal. To summarize, goals should be specific, measurable, realistic, and dependent on you alone.

■ Classifying Goals

In selecting goals, it is important to categorize them into two types: long-term goals and short-term goals. **Long-term goals** are what you consider the outcome or the final product of your actions. Examples of long-term goals include these:

> 1. Achieving a specific weight or BMI fitness rating
> 2. Reading all the books of the Bible
> 3. Regularly volunteering for community service
> 4. Being able to walk three miles without stopping

These are exciting goals to develop and enjoyable to visualize. They are also often the easiest to develop. Consider establishing two or three long-term goals for each area of personal wholistic wellness.

The second type of goal is the short-term goal. Because it leads to a long-term goal, it also is called a process goal. **Short-term goals** are the consistent steps you will take daily or weekly to reach the desired long-term goals. These short-term steps are essential for the successful accomplishment of long-term goals, but they are not as exciting and glamorous to discuss and visualize. These are the goals that require you to take action and actually put effort into developing new habits and outlooks. They require you to make time for additional activities in your life. Although the outcomes of these short-term actions are positive, you may find it difficult to keep at these steps week in and week out.

LONG-TERM GOAL: The outcome or final result of a wellness action.

Short-term goals and steps are often forgotten or may never develop into a habit. It is important to achieve short-term goals in small, progressive steps instead of attempting too much at one time. Short-term goals can be viewed as steps of progress toward the long-

SHORT-TERM GOALS: The consistent steps required to reach a long-term goal; also called process goals.

term goal. Many long-term goals cannot be reached without several incremental goals along the way.

Your goal may be to graduate from college with a bachelor's degree. However, before you ever can reach that goal, you will need to pass the classes in which you are currently enrolled. Before you can pass your current courses, you have to pass the exams and complete the course work. These are examples of short-term goals. Short-term goals are important, but they don't carry the weight of long-term goals—that is, unless you don't achieve the short-term goals!

■ The Role Motivation Plays

EXTERNAL MOTIVATION:
An outside force—another person, a circumstance, a company policy—that moves you toward a goal.

As you set your goals, think about whether your motivation is internal or external. **Internal motivation** for a goal comes from within. These are goals that are not dependent or greatly influenced by outside forces. Goals that are driven by internal motivation are often more powerful and fulfilling. **External motivation** comes from some other source. Study the examples below to see how two people with the same goal are motivated differently:

1. Phyllis regularly sets educational and occupational personal wellness goals. She notices that her company is offering a three-week course on personal computing. Phyllis eagerly signs up and takes the course. She enjoys herself, learns a great deal, and successfully completes the course requirements.
2. Gerald's supervisor notifies him that everyone in his department is required to take a three-week course on personal computing. While Gerald is not opposed to the idea, he had never considered it before.

Which of the two was internally motivated? Phyllis, of course, who had internal motivation for her educational improvement. Gerald may have embraced the training and even may have learned a great deal. However, his initial motivation was strictly external.

Both types of motivation can be effective, although sometimes it becomes easy to disregard external motivation as burdensome. When the going gets tough, those with external motivation may question why they are permitting themselves to experience

INTERNAL MOTIVATION:
Your own desire to achieve a goal; something that is not influenced by or dependent on outside forces.

such discomfort. The person with internal motivation is usually a little more persistent when faced with adversity. That is not to say that internal motivation is faultless. If you haven't shared your goals or your motivation with others, then it is often easy to "bail out" when the going gets tough. When thinking about your goals and what motivates them, it is a good idea to utilize a good mix of internal and external motivators.

Developing a Personal Wellness Action Plan

As we have seen throughout this text, goals don't "just happen" by chance. They are the result of conscious change. Change involves effort and action. Harnessing change to accomplish goals requires a plan of action. Your plan must be thorough and must cover all the bases. While success is not guaranteed just because you have a plan, it is almost certain that without a plan you won't experience success.

Now that you have developed goals for each component of wholistic wellness, it is time to develop an effective plan to accomplish those goals. Your plan should:

1. Focus on the benefits.
2. Create specific action steps.
3. Follow timelines.
4. Measure progress.
5. Anticipate barriers.
6. Develop support resources.

If you address each of these areas and execute your plan, you should attain your goals within a reasonable length of time.

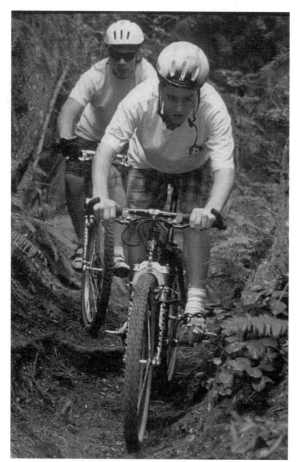

If you haven't shared your goals or your motivation with others, then it is often easy to "bail out" when the going gets tough.

■ Focus on the Benefits

The benefits of reaching a goal can be a strong motivating factor in striving for that goal. These can be very powerful incentives. Consider these two benefits:

1. "Once I get my degree, I'll be qualified for a new job with better pay."
2. "If I achieve better aerobic fitness, I will be able to play longer with my grandchildren."

This is the stuff dreams are made of. Benefits are what get you moving and help you follow your action plan. Be sure to recognize and dwell on realistic benefits. Think about what logical and likely benefits you will enjoy once you reach your goals. Create a list of these benefits for each of the areas of wholistic wellness. Reference this list when you need a powerful shot of motivation. Your list should be in writing. Sometimes it is especially helpful to place it where you can see it on a daily basis. This daily reminder not only will help you to stay motivated as you work toward your goal, but will stimulate your anticipation of the benefits that go along with achieving your goal.

■ Create Specific Action Steps

The specific action steps are where the rubber meets the road. In other words, this is the part of the plan that will either carry you to your goal or run you off the track. When developing action steps, ask these questions:

> 1. What are you going to do?
> 2. How are you going to do it?
> 3. How often will you do it?

Utilize what you have learned from this text and develop specific action steps that will lead you toward your goal. Remember, this is an area that requires realism. If you are completely out of shape and overweight, don't plan to run ten miles for your first day of exercise. That is not rational or reasonable. Be progressive in your action steps. Begin at an appropriate level and give yourself time to develop and improve.

What do action steps look like? For physical wellness, an action plan may include these steps:

- Start with a physical from the family doctor to determine your ability to embark on a fitness program.
- Complete the physical assessment tests in this textbook.
- Develop a weekly plan for physical activity.
- Monitor your progress toward your goal.

For intellectual wellness, the action plan may include these steps:

- Enroll in and attend a class.
- Complete your degree.
- Develop a reading list (and read the books).
- Join a book discussion group.

For spiritual wellness, you may wish to include these steps:

- Plan to visit and/or join a new church.

- Join a small group Bible study.
- Develop a reading list.
- Complete a volunteer service project.

Your action plan should include specific steps to follow daily. Personal wellness requires regular attention, and that is best achieved when addressed daily. Create a written personal plan of action for each area of wholistic wellness.

■ Follow Timelines

Some of us set unreasonable timelines for personal wellness improvement. Others ignore or overlook timelines. All too often, the only things we actually set down in writing are the start dates and end dates. To

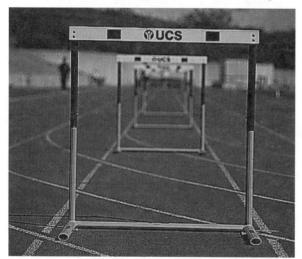

Your action plan should include specific daily steps.

illustrate this point, consider the person who says that by next Christmas he wants to lose twenty-five pounds, and he intends to start exercising on Monday. While he has certainly determined a start date and an end date for this goal, he has not established any short-term goals to assure steady progress toward the goal. Timelines require not only a start date and an end date, but incremental dates as well. These incremental dates can be one method of establishing short-term goals.

Timelines may differ according to the area of wellness on which you are focusing, but all effective timelines will include incremental steps, such as built-in dates. Short-term goals must be specific and should help to motivate you as you continue toward the primary goal. When planning a cross-country vacation, you plan to stop and "refuel," as well as "rest for the night." At other times, you will "really press forward." These points on a cross-country journey are like points on a timeline. As you approach and complete incremental steps, you can visualize your progress and determine if you are

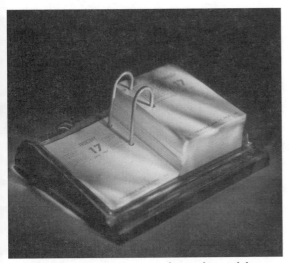

Timelines require not only a start date and an end date, but incremental dates as well.

still on target. Anticipate progress and improvement in your timeline and then plan accordingly. The more incremental steps you build in to your plan, the more likely you are to be continually reminded of your primary goal.

Would you be surprised to learn that your timelines should be specific? Probably not. As you can see by now, being specific is critical in every step of the goal process—from forming long-term and short-term goals, to identifying benefits, to planning timelines. Develop a reasonable and specific timeline for your personal wellness plan of action and be sure to include each component of wholistic wellness.

■ Measure Progress

After you are several weeks into your personal wellness action plan, how will you measure progress? Your timelines and short-term goals can be beneficial in measuring progress, but what actual methods will you use? Certainly the timeline is a good tool for determining *when* you should measure your progress. You will also know that if you haven't been following your plan, you probably won't be experiencing much progress. If several weeks have passed during which you haven't followed your specific action steps, any progress is going to be minimal at best.

The best way to measure progress is to retest yourself; that is, reassess each of your

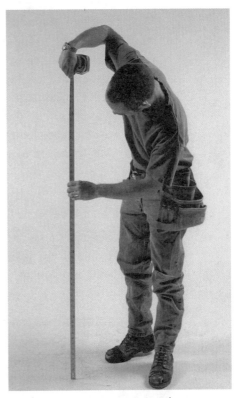

The best way to measure progress is to reassess each wellness component using the original assessment tool.

components of wellness using the same assessment tool you originally used. You also can measure your progress by your performance on an assessment test, the hours you devote to your action plan, the books you read, the courses you complete, the meetings you attend, etc. Reaching the halfway point of your goal is an especially meaningful source of motivation. However, the best way to achieve that kind of motivation is to have incremental points by which to measure your progress.

To accurately measure progress, follow these guidelines:

1. Be certain to measure the same thing each time.

   To get an accurate picture of progress, compare "apples to apples." Don't measure one attribute of physical wellness at the onset of your program and expect to get accurate feedback by measuring a different attribute partway through your action plan.

2. Use the same test.

   Maybe you took some form of wellness assessment at the onset of your program. The best testing instrument to measure progress is the same one you initially used. However, the improvements you experience may invalidate the initial test, necessitating a new kind of assessment test. Utilize the new test to measure progress. Improvement will be most evident when you have a series of "scores" to compare; e.g., "This is what my wellness rating was at the beginning of my program. Here's how much I improved when I was tested six months later. When I reach my goal, I expect this rating."

3. If possible, use the same test administrator.

   Some assessment tests or tools require someone skilled in administering them. If you are relying on a form of assessment in which someone else conducts the assessment, always utilize the same test administrator.

Some assessment scores can be skewed by the way the test is administered. If you use the same assessment tool, measure the same item, and utilize the same test administrator, you can accurately compare results over an extended period of time. Consider your goals, action steps, and timelines, and determine how you will measure your progress. Plug these measurement methods into your action plan and timeline.

■ Anticipate Barriers

It would seem that barriers are the last things you might want to think about when you are setting goals and developing action plans. However, if you are aware of what barriers you might eventually face, you will be much better prepared to handle them. Every area of wellness can be hindered by a variety of barriers. Some barriers are so significant that they can hinder improvement in every area of wellness.

Barriers come in a variety of shapes, sizes, and degrees of difficulty. Think creatively and develop a list of barriers you could possibly face. Think of barriers as a positive aspect of the process rather than as a negative aspect. This positive outlook comes from cultivating a perspective of awareness. If you are aware of possible barriers to your desired

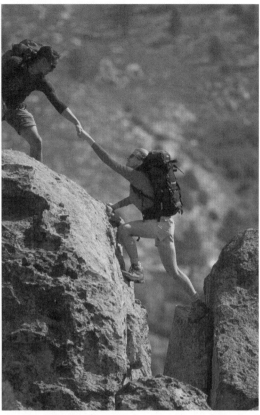

If you are aware of possible barriers to your desired goals, you can develop actions and recruit support to help overcome these barriers.

goals, you can develop actions and recruit support to help overcome these barriers. The apostle James reminds us:

"Consider it pure joy, my brothers, whenever you face trials of many kinds, because you know that the testing of your faith develops perseverance. Perseverance must finish its work so that you may be mature and complete, not lacking anything." James 1:2-4 NIV

When we face barriers or trials in any area of wellness, we know that we are facing a test, that the test will help us develop perseverance, and that perseverance will lead to maturity.

Write a list of anticipated barriers for each component of wholistic wellness. Examples might include age, weight, ability, time, equipment,

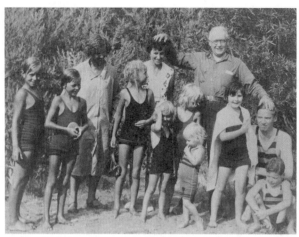

Many times, the most effective support resources are people—people who know you, love you, and believe in you.

finances, skill, intelligence, and self-image. After you have been working your personal wellness plan for some time, reevaluate your list of barriers. It is possible that you will encounter barriers that you didn't envision. Add these new barriers to your list. When you have completed your list of barriers, sit down and develop a plan to help overcome each of the barriers. Remember that these barriers are standing in the way of the benefits you hope to achieve and about which you have been dreaming for quite some time. Be tenacious—attack the barriers in such a manner as to build your confidence. You will be stronger for the experience and even more determined to reach your long-term goals. When you have a plan for overcoming barriers, you are less likely to be significantly hindered as obstacles pop up. In developing your plan, consider resources that might help to overcome the barriers. Include the resources in your plan.

■ Develop Support Resources

Support resources are critical to helping you overcome barriers and develop an effective personal wellness plan. Support resources can come in a variety of forms—from textbooks and training manuals to family and friends.

When developing your personal wellness plan, consider virtually any source of information about your subject of interest to be an invaluable resource. Surround yourself with textbooks, training manuals, periodicals, and guidebooks. Digesting this information will better prepare you for what you hope to accomplish. You also will become more and more excited about the possibilities of your goals. As you see improvement in each area of wellness, your resources will provide constant feedback on how you might adjust your goals. Many times periodicals can provide you with the latest information on how to attain your goals. Suddenly you have the power (through resources) to adjust and fine-tune your personal wellness plan for maximum benefit. The more you read, the more you will be reminded of your plan and your goals. Cutting-edge awareness is an excellent way to stay focused on your plan and goals. Visit a library or bookstore, find books, materials, or software on the content areas you are interested in developing, and utilize them. Begin now to gather your resources as you create your personal wellness plan.

Despite the ready availability of media resources, many times the most effective support resources are people—people who know you, love you, and believe in you. We often view the term "peer pressure" in a negative light, seeing it as pressure to engage in some type of risky behavior. However, peer pressure can be a positive external source of motivation. Share your goals with a positive support person, someone you see often and with whom you are comfortable. Share with this person your progress toward your goals, as well as the barriers you have encountered. This kind of relationship is built on accountability and is an excellent source of support and motivation.

There is more to a good support resource than just telling a friend or family member your goals. Make sure that the support people you choose know not only your goals, but also how you plan to reach the goals. It is critical to choose people who share your desire to reach those goals. You do not need someone who will say, "Go ahead and skip it just this once; it won't hurt." Be selective and choose only those who will help to keep you accountable. The best support people are involved in your pursuit of wellness on an ongoing basis. They know your difficulties and your triumphs. Some good examples of effective support people are study groups, accountability partners, small group Bible study partners, professional development groups, mentoring relationships, members of your work group, training partners, and instructors. An encouraging note from a mentor or a call from an accountability partner can be a great morale booster. You are much more likely to get out of bed to run if you know someone is waiting for you at the corner. When you have an effective support network around you, progress is no longer totally on your shoulders. Think about who could help you reach your goals. Then talk with those people, explain your plan, and invite them to be a part of your support network.

■ Making the Change

After you have developed a personal wellness plan that addresses benefits, specific action steps, timelines, measurement barriers, and support resources, you are ready for action. Once you implement the plan, you are assured of change. The change likely will be immediate in lifestyle and routine. Other changes will occur on a more gradual basis. As you attain your goals, reevaluate, reassess, and modify your plan to include new challenges and goals. Remember to constantly monitor and adjust your wellness program.

■ A Final Word

The person who successfully addresses each of the components of wholistic wellness is someone who will be better prepared to enjoy life's triumphs and to overcome life's challenges. Each component of wellness is important and related to the other components. If any single area is ignored, it is almost certain that harmony in the other areas will be exceptionally difficult to achieve.

While each wellness component is extremely important for a healthy temporal life, the component of spiritual wellness is important for eternal life. The book of Ecclesiastes tells the story of King Solomon, the wisest man who ever lived. His life was one of endless searching. You name it and King Solomon tried it. You might say that he was in search of wellness. At the end of his story, he reaches a conclusion. King Solomon, the wisest man who ever lived, the man who searched tirelessly for happiness and fulfillment, said this: *"Now all has been heard; here is the conclusion of the matter: Fear God and keep his commandments, for this is the whole duty of man"* (Ecclesiastes 12:13 NIV).

That is pretty clear—straight from the guy who had the resources to try it all. Fear God and keep His commandments. What are God's commandments? When the experts in law asked Jesus which commandment was the greatest, He replied, *"Love the Lord your God with all your heart and with all your soul and with all your mind. This is the first and greatest commandment"* (Matthew 22:37-38 NIV). Jesus Himself has given us the greatest commandment.

So, now we know what the whole duty of man is, according to Solomon and Jesus. What does that have to do with eternal life? What is eternal life? The answer is found in John 17:3: *"Now this is eternal life: that they may know you, the only true God, and Jesus Christ, whom you have sent"* (NIV). Earlier in this text we explained that according to a Christian worldview the only way to spiritual wellness is through a personal relationship with Jesus Christ. *"Now this is eternal life: that they may know you, the only true God, and Jesus Christ."* What is a personal relationship? It is a relationship in which you know someone. According to the Bible, a relationship in which you know Jesus Christ is eternal life. The book of Romans clearly outlines how to begin a relationship with Jesus:

"That if you confess with your mouth, 'Jesus is Lord,' and believe in

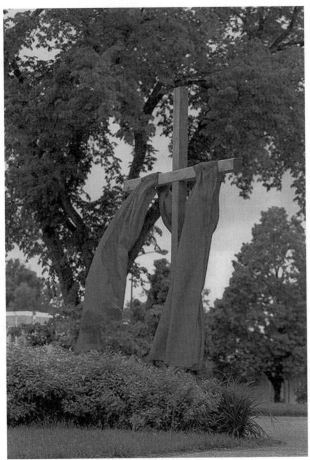

"I tell you, now is the time of God's favor, now is the day of salvation." 2 Corinthians 6:2b NIV

your heart that God raised him from the dead, you will be saved. For it is with your heart that you believe and are justified, and it is with your mouth that you confess and are saved" (Romans 10:9-10 NIV).

The apostle Paul also says, *"I tell you, now is the time of God's favor, now is the day of salvation"* (2 Corinthians 6:2b NIV). Today is the day that you can know Jesus Christ. Today is the day to call upon God and express your need for spiritual wellness. Today is the day. Rest assured that God hears our cries: *"Everyone who calls on the name of the Lord will be saved"* (Romans 10:13 NIV). Today is the day. Call upon God and He will save you from spiritual emptiness.

It is our hope that your life will be enriched by the concepts in this text. If you appropriately address each area of wellness, you should improve the quality of your life and experience fulfillment. Wellness isn't just an empty concept or a pie-in-the-sky theory—it should be the substance of your life. Can you say that about your life at this moment? We trust that you have accepted our challenge to evaluate, diagnose, and effect change that will benefit you and your family for the rest of your lives. Seize the day, seize the opportunity, and reap the benefits!

KEY CONCEPTS

external motivation
internal motivation
long-term goal
short-term goal

Index

H

I

J